Gerontological Social Work in Small Towns and Rural Communities

Sandra S. Butler, PhD
Lenard W. Kaye, DSW
Editors

Gerontological Social Work in Small Towns and Rural Communities has been co-published simultaneously as *Journal of Gerontological Social Work*, Volume 41, Numbers 1/2 and 3/4 2003.

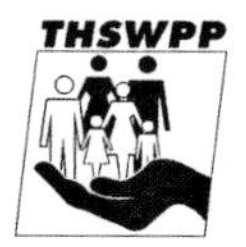

The Haworth Social Work Practice Press
An Imprint of
The Haworth Press, Inc.
New York • London

Published by

The Haworth Social Work Practice Press, 10 Alice Street, Binghamton, NY 13904-1580 USA

The Haworth Social Work Practice Press is an imprint of The Haworth Press, Inc., 10 Alice Street, Binghamton, NY 13904-1580 USA.

Gerontological Social Work in Small Towns and Rural Communities has been co-published simultaneously as *Journal of Gerontological Social Work,* Volume 41, Numbers (1/2) and (3/4) 2003.

© 2003 by The Haworth Press, Inc. All rights reserved. No part of this work may be reproduced or utilized in any form or by any means, electronic or mechanical, including photocopying, microfilm and recording, or by any information storage and retrieval system, without permission in writing from the publisher. Printed in the United States of America.

The development, preparation, and publication of this work has been undertaken with great care. However, the publisher, employees, editors, and agents of The Haworth Press and all imprints of The Haworth Press, Inc., including The Haworth Medical Press® and The Pharmaceutical Products Press®, are not responsible for any errors contained herein or for consequences that may ensue from use of materials or information contained in this work. Opinions expressed by the author(s) are not necessarily those of The Haworth Press, Inc.

Cover design by Jennifer Gaska

Library of Congress Cataloging-in-Publication Data

Gerontological social work in small towns and rural communities / Sandra S. Butler, Lenard W. Kaye, editors.

p. cm.

Has been co-published simultaneously as Journal of gerontological social work, volume 41, numbers 1/2/3/4 2003."

Includes bibliographical references and index.

ISBN 0-7890-1692-3 (alk. paper)–ISBN 0-7890-1693-1 (pbk. : alk. paper)

1. Social work with the aged–United States. 2. Rural aged–United States. 3. Rural aged–Services for–United States. 4. Social service, Rural–United States. 5. Gerontology–United States. I. Butler, Sandra S., 1957- II. Kaye, Lenard W. III. Journal of gerontological social work.

HV1457.G47 2003

362.6′0973′091734–dc22 2003018902

To elders of today and tomorrow who live in small towns and rural communities throughout the United States and world.

Indexing, Abstracting & Website/Internet Coverage

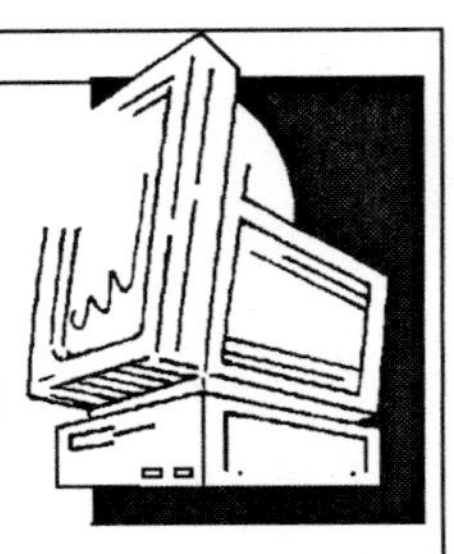

This section provides you with a list of major indexing & abstracting services. That is to say, each service began covering this periodical during the year noted in the right column. Most Websites which are listed below have indicated that they will either post, disseminate, compile, archive, cite or alert their own Website users with research-based content from this work. (This list is as current as the copyright date of this publication.)

Abstracting, Website/Indexing Coverage . . . . Year When Coverage Began

- ***Abstracts in Social Gerontology: Current Literature on Aging*** **1989**
- ***Academic Abstracts/CD-ROM*** **1993**
- ***Academic Search: data base of 2,000 selected academic serials, updated monthly: EBSCO Publishing*** **1995**
- ***Academic Search Elite (EBSCO)*** **1995**
- ***Academic Search Premier (EBSCO)*** **1993**
- ***AgeInfo CD-Rom*** **1995**
- ***AgeLine Database*** **1978**
- ***Alzheimer's Disease Education & Referral Center (ADEAR)*** **1994**
- ***Applied Social Sciences Index & Abstracts (ASSIA) (Online: ASSI via Data-Star) (CDRom: ASSIA Plus) <http://www.csa.com>*** **1987**
- ***Behavioral Medicine Abstracts*** **1992**
- ***Biosciences Information Service of Biological Abstracts (BIOSIS) a centralized source of life science information. <www.biosis.org>*** . . **1993**
- ***caredata CD: the social & community care database <http://www.scie.org.uk>*** **1994**

(continued)

- *CINAHL (Cumulative Index to Nursing & Allied Health Literature), in print, EBSCO, and SilverPlatter, Data-Star, and PaperChase. (Support materials include Subject Heading List, Database Search Guide, and instructional video) <http://www.cinahl.com>* **1994**
- *CNPIEC Reference Guide: Chinese National Directory of Foreign Periodicals* **1995**
- *Criminal Justice Abstracts* **1993**
- *Current Contents/Social & Behavioral Sciences <http://www.isinet.com>* . . . . *
- *e-psyche, LLC <http://www.e-psyche.net>* **2001**
- *Expanded Academic ASAP <http://www.galegroup.com>* **2001**
- *Expanded Academic ASAP–International <http://www.galegroup.com>* . . . **1989**
- *Expanded Academic Index* **1992**
- *Family & Society Studies Worldwide <http://www.nisc.com>* **1996**
- *Family Index Database <http://www.familyscholar.com>* **2001**
- *Family Violence & Sexual Assault Bulletin* **1993**
- *Human Resources Abstracts (HRA)* **1982**
- *IBZ International Bibliography of Periodical Literature <http://www.saur.de>* **1996**
- *Index Guide to College Journals (core list compiled by integrating 48 indexes frequently used to support undergraduate programs in small to medium sized libraries)* **1999**
- *Index to Periodical Articles Related to Law* **1990**
- *InfoTrac Custom <http://www.galegroup.com>* **1996**
- *MasterFILE: updated database from EBSCO Publishing* **1995**
- *National Center for Chronic Disease Prevention & Health Promotion (NCCDPHP)* **1998**
- *National Clearinghouse for Primary Care Information (NCPCI)* . . . **1994**
- *New Literature on Old Age* **1995**
- *OCLC ArticleFirst <http://www.oclc.org/services/databases/>* . . . . *
- *OCLC ContentsFirst <http://www.oclc.org/services/databases/>* . . . . . . *

(continued)

- *OmniFile Full Text: Mega Edition (only available electronically) <http://wwwhwwilson.com>* **1987**
- *Periodical Abstracts, Research II (broad coverage indexing & abstracting data-base from University Microfilms International (UMI))* **1993**
- *Pro Quest 5000. Contents of this publication are indexed and abstracted in the ProQuest 5000 database (includes only abstracts...not full-text), available on ProQuest Information & Learning @www.proquest.co <http://www.proquest.com>* **1993**
- *ProQuest Research Library. Contents of this publication are indexed and abstracted in the ProQuest Research Library database (includes only abstracts...not full-text), available on ProQuest Information & Learning @http://www. proquest.com <http://www.proquest.com>* . . . . *
- *Psychological Abstracts (PsycINFO) <http://www.apa.org>* . . . . *
- *RESEARCH ALERT/ISI Alerting Services <www.isinet.com>* **1985**
- *Periodical Abstracts, Research I (general & basic reference indexing & abstracting data-base from University Microfilms International (UMI))* **1993**
- *Social Sciences Citation Index <www.isinet.com>* **1985**
- *Social Sciences Index (from Volume 1 & continuing) <http://www.hwwilson.com>*. **1999**
- *Social Science Source: coverage of 400 journals in the social sciences area; updated monthly; EBSCO Publishing* **1995**
- *Social Sciences Abstracts <http://www.hwwilson.com>* **1987**
- *Social Sciences Plus Text. Contents of this publication are indexed and abstracted in the Social Sciences PlusText database (includes only abstracts . . . not full-text), available on ProQuest Information & Learning @http://www.proquest.com <http://www.proquest.com>* **1993**
- *Social SciSearch <http://www.isinet.com>* **1985**
- *Social Services Abstracts <http://www.csa.com>* **1989**
- *Social Work Abstracts <http://www.silverplatter.com/catalog/swab.htm>* **1984**
- *SocioAbs <http://www.csa.com>* . . . . *
- *Sociological Abstracts (SA) <http://www.csa.com>* **1989**

***Exact start date to come.**

(continued)

Special Bibliographic Notes related to special journal issues (separates) and indexing/abstracting:

- indexing/abstracting services in this list will also cover material in any "separate" that is co-published simultaneously with Haworth's special thematic journal issue or DocuSerial. Indexing/abstracting usually covers material at the article/chapter level.
- monographic co-editions are intended for either non-subscribers or libraries which intend to purchase a second copy for their circulating collections.
- monographic co-editions are reported to all jobbers/wholesalers/approval plans. The source journal is listed as the "series" to assist the prevention of duplicate purchasing in the same manner utilized for books-in-series.
- to facilitate user/access services all indexing/abstracting services are encouraged to utilize the co-indexing entry note indicated at the bottom of the first page of each article/chapter/contribution.
- this is intended to assist a library user of any reference tool (whether print, electronic, online, or CD-ROM) to locate the monographic version if the library has purchased this version but not a subscription to the source journal.
- individual articles/chapters in any Haworth publication are also available through the Haworth Document Delivery Service (HDDS).

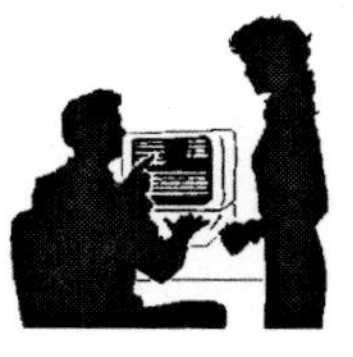

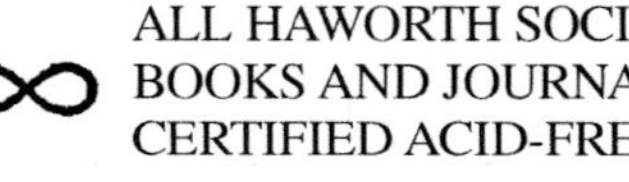

ALL HAWORTH SOCIAL WORK PRACTICE PRESS BOOKS AND JOURNALS ARE PRINTED ON CERTIFIED ACID-FREE PAPER

Gerontological Social Work in Small Towns and Rural Communities

CONTENTS

ABOUT THE EDITORS

Sandra S. Butler, PhD, is Associate Professor in the School of Social Work at the University of Maine. She received her MSW from George Warren Brown School of Social Work at Washington University and her PhD at the University of Washington. From 2001 to 2003, Dr. Butler was a Hartford Geriatric Social Work Faculty Scholar and the Resident Scholar at the UMaine Center on Aging. Her research in aging has included an in-depth study of the impact of the Senior Companion Program in a rural region, a longitudinal study of resident adjustment at a subsidized assisted living facility in a small city, perceptions of rural family caregivers regarding the reliability and adequacy of home care services, rural elder women's conceptions of health and attitudes toward professional and government assistance, and the health care experiences of late middle-aged and elder rural lesbians. In 2002, she was the guest editor of a special issue of the *Geriatric Care Management Journal* on gay, lesbian, bisexual, and transgender elders.

Dr. Butler is the author of one book on middle-aged homeless women, and co-editor of another, soon to be published by SUNY Press, titled *Shut Out: Low Income Mothers and Higher Education in Post-Welfare America*. In 2001, she received the Feminist Scholarship Award from the Commission on Women of the Council on Social Work Education for her research regarding post-secondary education for women on welfare. Dr. Butler sits on the editorial board of the *Journal of Poverty: Innovations on Social, Political, & Economic Inequalities*. She teaches courses in social work practice with older adults, social welfare policy, policy practice, field, and macro practice methods.

Lenard W. Kaye, DSW, is Professor of Social Work at the University of Maine School of Social Work and Director of the UMaine Center on Aging in the College of Business, Public Policy, & Health. Previously, he was Professor of Social Work and Social Research and Director of the PhD Program at the Graduate School of Social Work and Social Research at Bryn Mawr College in Pennsylvania. A prolific writer in the field of social gerontology, he has published approximately 100 journal articles and book chapters and 10 books on specialized topics in aging including older men, home health care, family caregiving, controversial issues in aging, support groups for older women, and congregate housing. A new book, edited by Dr. Kaye, on social work practice with the productive aged will be published in 2003.

Dr. Kaye has been the principal investigator of numerous assessments of innovative community services for older adults. He is currently the co-principal investigator of two U.S. Adminstration on Aging-funded projects: the Maine Primary Partners in Caregiving Program and the Development of a National Osteoporosis Prevention Strategy and Action Plan for Older Post-Menopausal Women.

Dr. Kaye sits on numerous boards including those of the National Advisory Committee on Rural Health and Human Services of the U.S. Department of Health and Human Services, the Senior Health Institute of Jefferson Health System and the Hartford Geriatric Enrichment in Social Work Education Program. He is the immediate past Chair of the National Association of Social Worker's Section on Aging, sits on the editorial boards of *Social Work Today,* the *Journal of Gerontological Social Work,* and *Geriatric Care Management Journal,* and is a Fellow of the Gerontological Society of America.

About the Contributors

Steven Lozano Applewhite, PhD, is Associate Professor, Graduate School of Social Work, University of Houston, Houston, Texas.

Share Bane, PhD, is Assistant Professor, School of Social Work, University of Missouri-Kansas City, Kansas City, Missouri.

Amanda Barusch, PhD, is Professor, College of Social Work, University of Utah, Salt Lake City, Utah.

Cynthia D. Bisman, PhD, is Professor, Graduate School of Social Work and Social Research, Bryn Mawr College, Bryn Mawr, Pennsylvania.

C. Jean Blaser, PhD, is Special Assistant to the Director, Illinois Department on Aging, Springfield, Illinois.

Sandra S. Butler, PhD, is Associate Professor, School of Social Work and Resident Scholar, Center on Aging, University of Maine, Orono, Maine.

The Honorable Josefina Carbonell is Assistant Secretary of Aging, U.S. Department of Health and Human Services, Washington, D.C.

Whitney Cassity-Caywood, MSSW, is a PhD candidate, University of Louisville, and Housing Support Specialist, Bluegrass Regional Mental Health Mental Retardation Board, Lexington, Kentucky.

Elizabeth DePoy, PhD is Professor, School of Social Work, and Interdisciplinary Education Coordinator, Center for Community Inclusion, University of Maine, Orono, Maine.

Lorraine T. Dorfman, PhD, is Professor, School of Social Work and Aging Studies Program, University of Iowa, Iowa City, Iowa.

Stephanie J. FallCreek, DSW, is Executive Director and Chief Executive Officer, Fairhill Center, Cleveland, Ohio.

Stephen French Gilson, PhD, is Associate Professor, School of Social Work, University of Maine, Orono, Maine.

Jane Harris-Bartley, MSW, is Project Director, RSVP Program, Center on Aging and Adjunct Instructor, School of Social Work, University of Maine, Orono, Maine.

Tara C. Healy, PhD, is Associate Professor, Department of Social Work, University of Southern Maine, Portland, Maine.

Ruth Huber, PhD, is Professor and Director of the Doctoral Program, Kent School of Social Work, University of Louisville, Louisville, Kentucky.

Elizabeth Johns, MS, is Senior Program Associate, Center on Aging, University of Maine, Orono, Maine.

Lenard W. Kaye, DSW, is Director, Center on Aging and Professor, School of Social Works, University of Maine, Orono, Maine.

David L. Klemmack, PhD, is Professor of Sociology, New College Program of the College of Arts and Sciences, University of Alabama, Tuscaloosa, Alabama.

Nancy P. Kropf, PhD, is Professor and Director of the Doctoral Program, School of Social Work, University of Georgia, Athens, Georgia.

Hong Li, PhD, is Assistant Professor, School of Social Work, University of Illinois at Urbana-Champaign, Urbana, Illinois.

Kim K. R. McKeage, PhD, is Associate Professor, Maine Business School, University of Maine, Orono, Maine.

Larry Polivka, PhD, is Director, Florida Policy Exchange Center on Aging, Tampa, Florida.

Janice Matthews Rasheed, DSW, is Associate Professor, School of Social Work, Loyola University, Chicago, Illinois.

Mikal N. Rasheed, PhD, is Associate Professor and Director, Social Work Program, Northeastern Illinois University, Chicago, Illinois.

Eloise Rathbone-McCuan, PhD, is Professor, School of Social Work, University of Missouri-Kansas City, Kansas City, Missouri.

Lucinda L. Roff, PhD, is Professor of Social Work and Co-Director of the Center for Mental Health and Aging, University of Alabama, Tuscaloosa, Alabama.

Donald W. Sharland, MSW, is Director of Senior Housing, Maine State Housing Authority, Augusta, Maine.

Christine TenBarge, PhD, is Assistant Professor, College of Social Work, University of Utah, Salt Lake City, Utah.

Cruz Torres, PhD, is Associate Professor and Director of the Hispanic Research Program, Department of Rural Sociology/Agricultural Education, Texas A&M University, College Station, Texas.

Nancy M. Webster, MSW, is Assistant Professor, School of Social Work, and Training Specialist, Center on Aging, University of Maine, Orono, Maine.

Acknowledgments

We would like to thank our colleagues throughout Maine's rural communities, at the University of Maine School of Social Work, and UMaine Center on Aging for sharing their expertise on rural social work and for providing a stimulating context within which to explore the issues examined in this volume. In addition, we would like to acknowledge the John A. Hartford Foundation which provided Sandra Butler with two years (2001-2003) of funding as a Hartford Geriatric Social Work Scholar to concentrate her scholarship in the area of aging. The Foundation has also enabled the School of Social Work to focus especially on developing expanded geriatric curricula opportunities for students and faculty through the Gero-Rich program. This, too, has encouraged thoughtful scholarship by many faculty at the University of Maine in gerontological social work practice.

Preface

We take particular pride in this volume, and urge all of our readers, including those who work with older people in the big cities of our nation, to give it a careful reading. As Butler and Kaye point out in Chapter 1, there have been in the past several decades a number of well written, well researched books about rural and small town elders, but none has had a singular focus on social work practice concerns, principles, and issues. This book fills that void in an admirable way. It combines careful studies of sub-groups of older small town and rural dwellers, with chapters in which attention is directed to specific service networks, and most notably, chapters on intervention models, and the special nature of social work practice in rural communities.

We recommend this volume to you in the certainty that you will find it eminently useful, now and for years to come. We have a number of special volumes in the works, and would welcome suggestions from you for subjects you would like to see receive the focused attention which Butler and Kaye have given in so excellent a fashion to social work practice and rural and small town elderly.

Rose Dobrof, DSW

[Haworth co-indexing entry note]: "Preface." Dobrof, Rose. Co-published simultaneously in *Journal of Gerontological Social Work* (The Haworth Social Work Practice Press, an imprint of The Haworth Press, Inc.) Vol. 41, No. 1/2, 2003, p. xxvii; and: *Gerontological Social Work in Small Towns and Rural Communities* (ed: Sandra S. Butler, and Lenard W. Kaye) The Haworth Social Work Practice Press, an imprint of The Haworth Press, Inc., 2003, p. xxv. Single or multiple copies of this article are available for a fee from The Haworth Document Delivery Service [1-800-HAWORTH, 9:00 a.m. - 5:00 p.m. (EST). E-mail address: docdelivery@haworthpress.com].

http://www.haworthpress.com/web/JGSW
© 2003 by The Haworth Press, Inc. All rights reserved.

PART I

SECTION I
INTRODUCTORY CONCEPTS OF RURALITY AND AGING

Chapter 1

Rurality, Aging and Social Work: Setting the Context

Sandra S. Butler, PhD
Lenard W. Kaye, DSW

SUMMARY. Premised on the argument that the vast majority of literature in gerontological practice continues to emphasize the challenges, problems, crises, and losses experienced by individuals as they age in urbanized settings, this chapter mounts the argument that the unique needs of elders in rural communities and the role of the social work profession in meeting these needs requires more complete examination. Historical context to the discussion of service intervention in rural communities is offered as are alternative definitions of rurality and past and current fed-

[Haworth co-indexing entry note]: "Rurality, Aging and Social Work: Setting the Context." Butler, Sandra S., and Lenard W. Kaye. Co-published simultaneously in *Journal of Gerontological Social Work* (The Haworth Social Work Practice Press, an imprint of The Haworth Press, Inc.) Vol. 41, No. 1/2, 2003, pp. 3-18; and: *Gerontological Social Work in Small Towns and Rural Communities* (ed: Sandra S. Butler, and Lenard W. Kaye) The Haworth Social Work Practice Press, an imprint of The Haworth Press, Inc., 2003, pp. 3-18. Single or multiple copies of this article are available for a fee from The Haworth Document Delivery Service [1-800-HAWORTH, 9:00 a.m. - 5:00 p.m. (EST). E-mail address: docdelivery@ haworth press.com].

http://www.haworthpress.com/web/JGSW
© 2003 by The Haworth Press, Inc. All rights reserved.
Digital Object Identifier: 10.1300/J083v41n01_01

eral stances on the topic. A demographic overview and profile of the major issues facing rural elders and their families is presented and the special set of opportunities and challenges associated with rural gerontological social work practice is underscored, including working with older adults that are less educated, poorer, with fewer retirement benefits, living in inadequate housing, and suffering from more frequent chronic illness. At the same time, rural older adults are likely to value highly their independence while simultaneously having less access to a smaller number of community services. *[Article copies available for a fee from The Haworth Document Delivery Service: 1-800-HAWORTH. E-mail address: <docdelivery@haworthpress.com> Website: <http://www.HaworthPress.com> © 2003 by The Haworth Press, Inc. All rights reserved.]*

KEYWORDS. Rural social work, rural elders, gerontological practice

INTRODUCTION

> While nearly one quarter of our nation's population lives in the rural and outlying communities in this country, almost all our nation's health care and social services continue to be found in the major population centers–sometimes hours away from the people who need them.
>
> –Secretary of Health and Human Services,
> Tommy G. Thompson,
> July 2002 (HRSA, 2002)

In the summer of 2001, Secretary Thompson launched an Initiative on Rural Communities. Having grown up in a town of 1500 in Wisconsin, he perhaps brought a special sensitivity to the needs of rural areas to his Cabinet position in the Bush Administration. He claimed that after talking with people all across the country, he realized: "We had to change the way we thought about rural communities–we could no longer just think of them as 'small cities.' Rural communities have unique challenges that bring with them unique opportunities" (HRSA, 2002). Whether Thompson's Rural Initiative has noticeable impact on the health and social service differential between rural and urban areas is yet to be seen. Nonetheless, the recognition by the federal government of the special circumstances for providing services in rural areas is heartening. Similarly, the motivation for this volume is to draw attention to the particular conditions facing elders and the social workers who work with them in small towns and rural communities and to outline some of the unique practice skills called for by these conditions.

WHY THIS VOLUME?

While a number of edited volumes on rural gerontology have been published over the past two decades (e.g., Bull, 1993; Coward, Bull, Kukulka, & Galliher, 1994; Coward & Lee, 1985; Coward & Krout, 1998; Krout, 1994; Rowles, Beaulieu, & Myers, 1996), no single book or edited volume has looked at the specific practice concerns for social workers assisting older adults in rural areas. The vast majority of research, policy, and practice literature in gerontological practice continues to emphasize the challenges, problems, crises, and losses experienced by individuals as they age in urbanized settings. Concurrently, discussions of social work intervention with older adults center inevitably on strategies for dealing with those problems, crises, and losses based on the resources, programs, technology, and personnel available in metropolitan and suburban regions of the country. Similarly, discussions of productive, vital old age rarely consider the implications that rurality might be expected to have on the quality of the aging experience and the potential functions and roles to be fulfilled by professional social workers.

Likewise, though there has been increasing attention given to rural social work (Ginsberg, 1998; Stoesen, 2002), the unique needs of elders in rural communities and the role of the social work profession in meeting these needs has not been well examined. For twenty years, the journal *Human Services in a Rural Environment* provided one forum for gerontologists working in rural communities in North America to dialogue about innovative programs, policy issues, and practice concerns, but this journal was discontinued in 1996. Currently, the only social work journal devoted specifically to rural concerns is *Rural Social Work* published out of the University of South Australia and not widely distributed in the United States.

The National Association of Social Workers (NASW) has an active Rural Social Work Caucus (*www.uncp.edu/sw/rural/index/html*) whose policy statement appears in the latest version of *Social Work Speaks*. The statement reads:

> The understanding of rural people and cultures is a pressing issue of cultural competence in professional social work . . . Social work practice in rural communities challenges the social worker to embrace and effectively use an impressive range of intervention and community skills . . . NASW must work to develop social work that addresses the needs of clients across all age groups, *particularly the elderly who are the largest growing group in rural communities*. (NASW, in press, italics added)

The chapters in this volume present a range of interventions and community skills aimed precisely at the needs of rural elders, and fill a gap in the existing practice literature.

WHAT DO WE MEAN BY RURAL AND WHO LIVES THERE?

Before the turn of the last century, the United States was predominantly an agrarian, rural society. Rapid changes in agricultural and manufacturing productivity and advances in transportation and communications technology led to the nearly continuous out-migration from rural settlements to emerging urban centers during the 20th century (Longino, 2001). In 1790, when the first U.S. Census was taken, 95% of the population lived in rural areas. One hundred years later–1890–two thirds of the population still lived in rural areas, but by 1990, less than one quarter of the population lived outside of metropolitan areas (Ginsberg, 1998). The growth of the social work profession coincided with these dramatic population shifts and flourished in part due to the social problems accompanying urbanization. It is therefore not surprising that the profession has had an urban bias with its focus on metropolitan problems and issues (Ginsberg, 1998).

Defining what is meant by rural is complex. Bull (1993) states: "The search for a single definition of *rural* has been in progress for so long that many academics and practitioners have almost given up hoping that there will ever be a definition usable to all" (p. xii, italics in the original). The Office of Management and Business (OMB) defines metropolitan and nonmetropolitan differently than does the Census Bureau (Eberhart et al., 2001), while the U.S. Department of Agriculture uses yet another rural-urban continuum (Rogers, 1999). Many authors suggest it is more useful to think of the concept of rural as a continuum rather than a dichotomy, with the large cities on one end and the most sparsely populated areas on the other (Bull, 1993; Coward & Cutler, 1988).

For purposes of comparison across time and among age groups, the U.S. Census Bureau's definitions of rural-urban and metropolitan-nonmetropolitan are useful. Rural areas are defined as those with 2,500 people or fewer, while urban areas have populations greater than 2,500 (Ginsberg, 1998). The designation of Metropolitan Statistical Area (MSA) refers to counties that have either a city with a population of at least 50,000 or an urbanized area of at least 50,000 and a total MSA population of at least 100,000. People living within MSAs are considered in a metropolitan area, and those living outside MSAs are nonmetropolitan (Clifford & Lilley, 1993). In 2000, the total U.S. population was about 281 million and persons 65 and older composed 12.4% of that population. Seventy-nine percent of the entire U.S. population lived in urban areas and, of those, 12.3% were 65 and older. Older adults made up a larger percentage of the rural population (12.8%). The concentration of elders in rural areas appears more dramatic when we look at the metropolitan-nonmetropolitan designation. Four-fifths of the U.S. population lived in metro areas in 2000, of which 11.9% were 65 and older. In the remaining 20% of the U.S. population living in nonmetro areas, 14.7% were over 65–this translates to about 8 million seniors in rural areas (U.S. Census Bureau, 2000).

In general, the nonmetropolitan population has an older age structure than the metropolitan population; the median age for the nonmetro population in 1998 was 36, while it was 34 for the metro population (Rogers, 1999). The greater concentration of elders in rural areas than in urban areas is due, in large part, to older rural adults being less likely to migrate to urban areas than younger adults looking for work and to some degree, to a proportion of more affluent urban seniors moving to rural areas for lifestyle reasons after retirement (Fuguitt & Beale, 1993; Longino, 2001).

WHAT IS THE SITUATION OF RURAL ELDERS?

There are many generalizations we can make about older adults living in rural areas, but it is important to remember there exists tremendous diversity within and between different regions of the country and among the older adults making up the extremely heterogeneous category of people who are "65 years of age and older." For example, a 65-year-old married European-American woman living on a farm in the Midwest has different life experiences and faces different challenges than either a 90-year-old European-American widow living alone in the neighboring town, or a 65-year-old married Latina woman living in southern Texas. In their discussion of long-term care, Rowles, Beaulieu, and Myers (1996) remind us that:

> variation within rural areas is often greater than that between rural and urban areas. Both regional differences in the characteristics and resources of rural areas and differences among rural elderly populations with respect to demography, economic circumstances, life histories and culture, are such that it is unreasonable to expect and inappropriate to seek a universally applicable long-term care system in rural America. (p. 7)

With these caveats in mind, we will outline some of what is known generally about rural elders.

It has been well documented that rural elders face some particular challenges. Compared to their urban counterparts, older adults in rural areas tend to be less educated, to have lower incomes, and to have less adequate housing (Bull, 1993; Glasgow, 1993; Ormond, Wallin, & Goldenson, 2000; Rogers, 1999; Stallman, Deller, & Shields, 2001). The disparity between metro and nonmetro poverty rates increases with age (Stallman et al., 2001); over half of nonmetropolitan persons aged 85 and older were poor or near poor (100% to 149% of poverty level) in 1998 (Rogers, 1999). This is of particular concern given that a higher proportion of rural elders are in this oldest-old category than is true in urban areas. Rural elders have fewer sources of retirement income and are more dependent on transfer payments than are urban elders (Rogers, 1999; Stallman et al., 2001). While older adults in rural areas are more likely to own their homes than is true for urban elders, these homes are often older, and in poorer condition, if not substandard. In addition, older rural elders have fewer options for service-enriched housing (Krout, 2001). Furthermore, while this may change with future cohorts, current rural elders have less formal education than do older adults in urban areas (Bull, 2003; Coward & Dwyer, 1998). On the positive side, rural elders have higher rates of marriage–and thus ready social support–than do urban elders (Coward & Dwyer, 1998), although among the old-old this differential disappears.

While considerable diversity exists among rural older adults–especially between farm and nonfarm elders–there is a greater prevalence of chronic conditions among rural elders than older adults residing in metropolitan areas (Bull, 1993; Coward & Dwyer, 1998). Limitations in activity due to chronic health conditions are more prevalent in nonmetropolitan areas than in metropolitan areas (Eberhart et al., 2001). Moreover, rural elders are less likely to have employer-sponsored supplemental health insurance (Eberhart et al., 2001; Ormond et al., 2000).

Despite these challenges, rural elders do not necessarily see themselves as deprived (Lee & Lassey, 1980). In their exploration of the subjective well-being of rural elders, Lee and Lassey note several factors that may place older adults in small towns at an advantage over their metropolitan counterparts: more involvement in community activities, receipt of more support from local organizations, less fear of crime, and less abrupt retirement. Krout (1988) also submits that rural elders do not see their lives as problematic. He concludes that though rural elders may be "worse off" in many ways, their lives may not be qualitatively inferior–just different. In fact, there is some evidence that life satisfaction for older adults increases as community size decreases (Krout, 1988).

Kivett (1988) reiterates these findings emphasizing that despite negative objective indicators, levels of positive affect among rural older adults generally are found to be equal to or greater than those among urban older adults. Kivett attributes perceived well-being to three factors: values, physical context and relative deprivation. Many people have debated about the nature of "rural values" (Krout, 1988); nonetheless, there appears to be a consensus that differences do exist between the rural and urban elderly in terms of basic values and lifestyle. The values that Kivett lists as being significant to rural elders' perceive well-being include the "high premium placed on usefulness, on the importance of productive time use, on interpersonal relationship and exchanges, and on religious involvement" (p. 126). The second factor in Kivett's list contributing to rural elders' life satisfaction is physical context–"the feeling of open space and the freedom of self it suggests" (p. 126). The third factor explaining higher than expected expressed well-being is relative deprivation–that is, rural elders evaluate their life condition in relation to others they see and know.

It appears that while the nation continues to become ever more metropolitan, with ever great proportions of our population living in urban and suburban environments, we retain a certain nostalgia for our rural past and remaining rural pockets. In a recent *Washington Post* editorial bemoaning the "withering of rural American," Joel Kotkin (2002) states:

> . . . in an intangible way, rural areas project a different notion of America, in their incubation of traditional values regarding community, country, church and the nobility of work. Rural American,

> in sum, represents something different from the larger nation, showing us what we once were and may still want somehow to remain. (p. 22)

Despite this nostalgia, working as a social worker in more remote areas is not all romantic and bucolic–lack of resources and services present many challenges particularly in the field of gerontology.

SERVICES AND RESOURCES FOR ELDERS IN RURAL AREAS

There is substantial evidence that older persons in rural areas have less access to a smaller number and more narrow range of community based services than do elders in urban areas (Glasgow, 1993; Krout, 2001; Ormond et al., 2000; Rogers, 1999). This is particularly true in the area of long-term care, where alternatives to institutionalization are far less available (Coward, Netzer, & Peek, 1996). This dearth of services may lead to premature institutionalization of rural elders (Coward & Dwyer, 1998). Despite the great need due to higher concentrations of older persons and the greater prevalence of chronic conditions in rural areas, there are financial pressures to reduce health services even further by adopting "limited-service" models for rural hospitals (Ormond et al., 2000). In general, rural health services are less accessible in part as they are more costly to deliver (Glasgow, 1993; Rogers, 1999). Sometimes services may be available in the more populated areas of a rural region, but not in the more remote areas, making transportation essential for providing services; not surprisingly, practitioners have repeatedly identified transportation as the key obstacle to providing services to rural elders (Krout, 2001).

While limited transportation services can also be a challenge for elders in metropolitan areas, it is a particular obstacle for rural elders. Burkhardt (2001) notes that in 1990, 45% of rural elderly had no car, and that over a third of the nation's rural residents lived in counties with no public transit. Many communities have no taxi service, and intercity/interstate bus, train and air services are limited and continue to decline. Essentially, in a nation that depends on private automobiles for transportation outside of urban areas, not having a car or being unable to drive is a major barrier to receiving health services and staying connected to society. As Burkhardt states, "[h]igh levels of mobility yield high levels of access, choice, and opportunity, which in turn, help create rich and self-fulfilling lives. Low levels of mobility can lead to isolation and cultural impoverishment" (p. 9).

GERONTOLOGICAL SOCIAL WORK PRACTICE IN RURAL AREAS

In a recent *NASW News* article on rural social work (Stoesen, 2002), the president of the Nevada NASW State Chapter was quoted as saying that generalist practice was "where it's at. The fact is, there is nobody else to help people out here . . . We need to be a lot of different things to a lot of different people" (p. 3). Ginsberg (1998) also emphasizes the need for social work practitioners in less populous areas to be trained as generalists. He submits that those authors who originally developed theories about social work practice in small communities knew that rural areas would have fewer resources–including social workers–than urban areas, and thus social work practitioners would

> [h]ave to know how to do a bit of everything, or at least know how to make a bit of everything available to clients in smaller communities. No matter the setting, the rural social worker would have to provide direct counseling or casework services, community development skills, administrative ability, and research competence. The rural social worker would also have to analyze, develop and implement social policy of all kinds. (p. 9)

Social workers practicing in small towns and rural communities face some particular challenges with regard to privacy, confidentiality and managing dual relationships (Ginsberg, 1998; NASW, in press; Stoesen, 2002). The Rural Social Work Caucus policy statement suggests that:

> Social workers practicing in rural areas must have advanced understanding of ethical responsibilities, not only because dual and multiple relationships are unavoidable, but also because the setting may require that dual or multiple relationships be used and managed as an appropriate method of social work practice. (NASW, in press)

Furthermore, while rural areas may face a shortage of professionals such as gerontological social workers, this does not mean newly arrived practitioners will receive immediate acceptance. Ginsberg (1998) suggests that social workers practicing in nonmetropolitan areas must make a special effort to "fit into the community." Integrating into the community may mean things such as: avoiding offending the leadership of social agencies; being cautious about expressing one's political views; participating in community activities; and being generally conventional in one's person life, dress and associations.

One might wonder why anyone would want to practice social work in rural areas when there are so many challenges: life in the fishbowl, professional isolation, and lack of services for clients. When Stoesen (2002) of *NASW News* asked just that question of social workers practicing in small communities, she heard about the fulfillment practitioners received from their work. For example, one social worker in South Dakota said that

> [r]ural social work is truly the heart of what social work is supposed to be. Helping to decide what they want, when there are so many barriers and obstacles to obtaining it, is truly what social workers are supposed to be doing. (p. 3)

Furthermore, Richard Osborn, the president of the NASW Rural Social Work Caucus, said he believed "rural social work may be 'the last area where a social worker either singly or working with others can make a difference'" (p. 3).

Thus, gerontological social workers simultaneously face the challenges and reap the rewards of practicing in rural regions of this country. The chapters that follow are intended to inform such practitioners who are often working in remote areas with fewer opportunities for continuing education or collegial support and mentoring than are available to their urban counterparts.

STRUCTURE OF THE VOLUME

This volume is divided into five sections. Sections I, II, and III are contained in Part I, while Sections IV and V are included in Part II of the volume. Chapter 2, "The Demographics of Aging in a Rural Perspective" by Lucinda L. Roff and David L. Klemmack, completes *Section I: Introductory Concepts of Rurality and Aging.* Providing further detail regarding the demographic profile of nonmetropolitan elderly which has been introduced in this chapter, Roff and Klemmack describe regional variations, document trends over time, and provide projections regarding future population changes among older persons in nonmetropolitan areas. They conclude with suggestions of ways that rural social workers can use the U.S. Census to improve health and social service delivery.

Section II: Practice Dimensions of Social Work with Rural Elders, is introduced with "Rural Aging: Social Work Practice Models and Intervention Dynamics" (Chapter 3) by Cynthia D. Bisman. Bisman suggests that a biopsychosocial framework–with an emphasis on assessment–should guide social work practice with rural elders and that practice decisions should be based on the social work values of social justice, empowerment, and human dignity. Included in this chapter is a review of theoretical models relevant to rural gerontological social work, such as social support, family systems, group work, and community practice. This broad review chapter is followed by three chapters focusing on particular practice dimensions: advocacy, program planning and marketing.

"Advocacy Techniques with Older Adults in Rural Environments" (Chapter 4), by Sandra S. Butler and Nancy M. Webster, discusses both how advocacy has been defined over the years and how it has been used specifically with older adults. Integrated Case Management is introduced as an advocacy model particularly suited to working with rural elders, and recommendations are offered on incorporating advocacy into rural gerontological social work practice.

The last two chapters of *Section II* address mezzo and macro dimensions of social work practice. In Chapter 5, "Rural Program Planning and Development for Older Adults," Hong Li and C. Jean Blaser discuss program planning and development for older adults in small towns and rural areas. Using Canter's social care systems model, they review rural elders' informal and formal service systems and illuminate the barriers in planning and providing services in rural areas. Strategies for overcoming these barriers are presented and illustrated with case examples from the authors' practice experience.

The final chapter in *Section II*, "A Rural Perspective on Marketing Services to Older Adults," presents a practice dimension that receives scant attention in most compilations on social work practice. Kim K. R. McKeage and Lenard W. Kaye posit that social work practitioners must be familiar with marketing principles if they want to reach those they aim to serve, provide the highest quality service possible and the most needed services for their target populations. These principles are reviewed as they apply particularly to service delivery to older adults in rural areas. Rural gerontological social workers are encouraged to maintain a marketing perspective in their efforts to be responsive and accountable to the clients they serve, the communities in which they are situated, and their funding sources.

The four chapters in *Section III: Special Populations*, describe the circumstances of four subpopulations among rural elders: Native Americans, African Americans, Latinos, and elders with disabilities. Amanda Barusch and Christine TenBarge open this section with Chapter 7, "Indigenous Elders in Rural America," in which they examine the history of forced assimilation and colonization of Native Americans and the impact of that history on rural Indigenous elders. Barusch and TenBarge offer service approaches that can both empower elders and improve their quality of life, suggesting that culturally appropriate interventions should begin with the employment of Indigenous service providers.

The second chapter in *Section III*, "Rural African American Older Adults and the Black Helping Tradition" (Chapter 8) by Mikal N. Rasheed and Janice Matthews Rasheed, begins with a review of the disparities existing between African American and white elders in terms of mental health, service availability, service access, and socioeconomic factors. This is followed by a discussion of the helping tradition in the African American community and the reliance on community-based informal care systems, particularly in the rural context. Rasheed and Rasheed conclude with suggestions regarding how rural gerontological social workers can work with this informal system to meet the needs of rural African American elders.

Chapter 9, "Rural Latino Elders," by Steven Lozano Applewhite and Cruz Torres, offers a discussion of a third racial group among rural elders who face unique and often difficult circumstances. The authors begin by describing the age distribution, economic conditions, living arrangements, language issues, and service utilization among rural Latino elders. They advocate culturally competent practice, which is based on a strong knowledge base, culturally relevant skills, and a value orientation that embraces diversity.

Elizabeth DePoy and Stephen French Gilson are the authors of the final chapter in *Section III*, "Rural Disabled Elder" (Chapter 10). In order to address the complex issue of who fits into the individual categories of disabled, elderly and rural, DePoy and Gilson begin their discussion by defining these terms. Guided by the ideologies of self-determination and legitimacy, they present an approach to social work practice which is informed by a systematic examination and analysis of social problems as they affect individuals and groups. The chapter concludes with suggested principles of practice–which DePoy and Gilson categorize as either positive or negative–for social workers involved with rural, disabled elders.

Section IV: Special Issues and Programs is composed of five chapters covering a range of topics of particular significance for practice with rural elders. Stephanie J. Fallcreek opens this section with Chapter 11, "Older Adult Health Promotion in Rural Settings," in which she demonstrates the similarities between health promotion models and core social work values and competencies. Fallcreek outlines ways in which rural gerontological social workers can incorporate health promotion as part of generalist practice or as a primary practice focus.

The second chapter in *Section IV*, "Older Rural Workers and Retirement Preparation" (Chapter 12) by Lorraine T. Dorfman, examines the impact of the rural environment on work and retirement and the current employment status and income of older rural workers. After discussing job training, job creation, and the retirement needs of rural elders, Dorfman concludes with suggestions for gerontological social work practice in developing employment and retirement services and improving existing services and service delivery.

"Rural Older Adults at Home" (Chapter 13) by Whitney Cassity-Caywood and Ruth Huber is the third chapter in *Section IV*. Utilizing a strengths perspective, the authors encourage readers to consider several alternatives to the deficit-focused mentality that often pervades work with elders. After discussing issues unique to rural areas, Cassity-Caywood and Huber review programs that serve rural seniors at home and offer suggestion for practitioners working with this population.

Chapter 14, "Specialized Housing and Rural Elders" by Sandra S. Butler and Donald W. Sharland, presents the environmental press and empowerment practice models as a framework with which to understand the tension between autonomy and security faced by rural elders and the social workers that assist them. Findings from in-depth interviews with geriatric social workers assisting elders in rural housing settings reveal practice challenges, particular issues related to rurality, and innovative techniques and programs. Drawing from these interviews and the existing literature in this substantive area, the authors conclude with practice and policy guidelines.

Tara C. Healy's "Ethical Practice Issues in Rural Perspective" (Chapter 15) completes this section of the volume. Healy demonstrates how ethical decision making is complicated by the multiple relationships with colleagues, caregiving family members, and elders, which are common in rural areas. She proposes a model for multilevel contextual ethical analysis in order to address the complex situations faced by gerontological social workers practicing in rural areas.

The concluding part of the volume, *Section V: Looking Ahead: Training and Policy Recommendations*, is composed of three chapters. The first of these, Nancy P. Kropf's "Future Training and Education Recommendations for Rural Gerontological Social Workers," discusses curriculum content necessary to prepare students to work with older adults in rural areas; suggested content areas include health care, economics, leadership/decision making and telemedicine interventions. Kropf emphasizes the need to actively seek students who have an interest in working in rural settings and suggests methods for attracting these students.

The second chapter in *Section V*, "Rural Mental Health: A Discussion of Service Capacity Building for Rural Elders" (Chapter 17), by Eloise Rathbone-McCuan and Share Bane, suggests that current mental health services for rural elders are too limited in scope and availability. The authors submit that future mental health services will be dramatically impacted by Medicaid funding decisions. The authors encourage rural gerontological social workers to actively engage in advocacy related to improving the provision of mental health services to old rural citizens.

The final chapter of this section and the volume, Chapter 18, "The Aging Network and the Future of Long-Term Care," is co-authored by Josefina Carbonell and Larry Polivka. Carbonell and Polivka discuss how the United States in general, and the aging network in particular, can become more responsive to the needs and preferences of older people and their families by empowering them to make informed decisions about their life choices and creating more flexible service options from which people can choose. The authors review potential methods for integrating long-term care access and resources; the possibilities for integrated care in rural communities; and the implications of a managed, integrated long-term care system for social workers working with older adults.

An appendix prepared by Elizabeth Johns and Jane Harris-Bartley offers readers a comprehensive set of additional sources to which they can turn for more information on social work with older adults in rural settings.

We invite you to read and learn from this rich compilation of practice wisdom by experts in the field of rural gerontological social work. Taken together, we believe it represents the most complete presentation to date of gerontological social work practice literature directed at the special challenges confronting our colleagues who work in rural America.

REFERENCES

Bull, C.N. (Ed.). (1993). *Aging in rural America.* Newbury Park, CA: Sage.

Burkhardt, J.E. (2001). Transportation for the elderly in rural America. *The Public Policy and Aging Report, 12* (1), 9-13.

Clifford, W.B., & Lilley, S.C. (1993). Rural elderly: Their demographic characteristics. In C.N. Bull (Ed.) *Aging in rural America* (pp. 3-16). Newbury Park, CA: Sage.

Coward, R.T., Bull, C.N., Kukulka, G., & Galliher, J.M. (Eds.). (1994). *Health services for rural elders.* New York: Springer.

Coward, R.T., & Cutler, S.J. (1988). The concept of a continuum of residence: Comparing activities of daily living among the elderly. *Journal of Rural Studies, 4* (2), 159-168.

Coward, R.T., & Dwyer, J.W. (1998). The health and well-being of rural elders. In L.H. Ginsberg (Ed.) *Social work in rural communities,* (3rd ed.) (pp. 213-232). Alexandria, VA: Council on Social Work Education.

Coward, R.T., & Krout, J.A. (Eds.). (1998). *Aging in rural settings: Life circumstances and distinctive features.* New York: Springer.

Coward, R.T., & Lee, G.R. (Eds.). (1985). *The elderly in rural society.* New York: Springer.

Coward, R.T., Netzer, J.K., & Peek, C.W. (1996). Obstacles to creating high-quality long-term care services for rural elders. In G.D. Rowles, J.E. Beaulieu, & W.W. Myers (Eds.) *Long-term care for the rural elderly* (pp. 10-34). New York: Springer.

Eberhart, M.S., Ingram, D.D., Makuc, D.M. et al. (2001). *Urban and rural health chart book: Health, United States, 2001.* Hyattsville, MD: National Center for Health Statistics.

Fuguitt, G.V., & Beale, C.L. (1993). The changing concentration of older nonmetropolitan population, 1960-90. *Journal of Gerontology, 48* (6), S278-S288.

Ginsberg, L.H. (1998). Introduction: An overview of rural social work. In L.H. Ginsberg (Ed.) *Social work in rural communities,* (3rd ed.) (pp. 3-22). Alexandria, VA: Council on Social Work Education.

Glasgow, N. (1993). Poverty among rural elders: Trends, context, and directions for policy. *Journal of Applied Gerontology, 12* (3), 302-319.

Health Resources Services Administration (HRSA). (2002). *Secretary Thompson Remarks–summit on Rural America.* Retrieved January 8, 2003 from *http://ruralhealth.hrsa.gov/RuralAmericanSummit.html.*

Kivett, V.R. (1988). Aging in a rural place: The elusive source of well-being. *Journal of Rural Studies, 4* (2), 125-132.

Kotkin, J. (2002, July 29-August 4). The withering of rural America. *The Washington Post Weekly Edition,* p. 22.

Krout, J.A. (1988). The elderly in rural environments. *Journal of Rural Studies, 4* (2), 103-114.

Krout, J.A. (Ed.). (1994). *Providing community-based services to the rural elderly.* Thousand Oaks, CA: Sage.

Krout, J.A. (2001). Community services and housing for rural elders. *The Public Policy and Aging Report, 12* (1), 6-8.

Lee, G.R., & Lassey, M.L. (1980). Rural-urban differences among the elderly: Economic, social and subjective factors. *Journal of Social Issues, 36* (2), 62-74.

Longino, C.F. (2001). Demographic trends and migration issues for rural communities. *The Public Policy and Aging Report, 12* (1), 20-22.
National Association of Social Workers (NASW). (in press). *Social work speaks.* Washington, DC: NASW Press.
Ormond, B.A., Wallin, S., & Goldenson, S.M. (2000). *Supporting the rural health care safety net.* Part of Urban Institute's Assessing the New Federalism Series. Retrieved May 15, 2000 from *http://www.federalism.urban.org/html.*
Rogers, C.C. (1999). *Changes in the older population and implications for rural areas.* Washington, DC: U.S. Department of Agriculture.
Rowles, G.D., Beaulieu, J.E., & Myers, W.W. (1996). Introduction: Long-term care for rural elderly: The legacy of the twentieth century. In G.D. Rowles, J.E. Beaulieu, & W.W. Myers (Eds.) *Long-term care for the rural elderly* (pp. 1-9). New York: Springer.
Rowles, G.D., Beaulieu, J.E., & Myers, W.W. (Eds.). (1996). *Long-term care for the rural elderly.* New York: Springer.
Stallman, J.I., Deller, S., & Sheilds, M. (2001). Aging and the rural economy. *The Public Policy and Aging Report, 12* (1), 14-19.
Stoesen, L. (2002, October). Rural social workers embrace challenge. *NASW News, 47* (9), 3.
U.S. Census Bureau. (2000). Summary File 1, United States–*Urban/Rural and Inside/Outside Metropolitan Area: Age and Sex.* Retrieved January 11, 2003 from *http://www.census.gov.*

Chapter 2

The Demographics of Aging in Rural Perspective

Lucinda L. Roff, PhD
David L. Klemmack, PhD

SUMMARY. Using data from the Current Population Survey March 2002 Supplement, this article provides a demographic profile of nonmetropolitan elderly in the United States. In addition to providing information on regional variation, the chapter examines nonmetro poverty and health among the elderly in detail. The chapter also reviews changes in the size of the elderly population in nonmetropolitan areas from 1970 through 2000 and in demographic characteristics from 1997 through 2002. This information provides a foundation for projections concerning future population changes among older persons in nonmetropolitan areas. The article concludes by discussing how social workers in local, rural communities can access and use U.S. Census and other data to improve health and social service delivery. *[Article copies available for a fee from The Haworth Document Delivery Service: 1-800-HAWORTH. E-mail address: <docdelivery@haworthpress.com> Website: <http://www.HaworthPress.com> © 2003 by The Haworth Press, Inc. All rights reserved.]*

KEYWORDS. Demographics, rural elder population, census data

[Haworth co-indexing entry note]: "The Demographics of Aging in Rural Perspective." Roff, Lucinda L., and David L. Klemmack. Co-published simultaneously in *Journal of Gerontological Social Work* (The Haworth Social Work Practice Press, an imprint of The Haworth Press, Inc.) Vol. 41, No. 1/2, 2003, pp. 19-35; and: *Gerontological Social Work in Small Towns and Rural Communities* (ed: Sandra S. Butler, and Lenard W. Kaye) The Haworth Social Work Practice Press, an imprint of The Haworth Press, Inc., 2003, pp. 19-35. Single or multiple copies of this article are available for a fee from The Haworth Document Delivery Service [1-800-HAWORTH, 9:00 a.m. - 5:00 p.m. (EST). E-mail address: docdelivery@ haworthpress.com].

http://www.haworthpress.com/web/JGSW
© 2003 by The Haworth Press, Inc. All rights reserved.
Digital Object Identifier: 10.1300/J083v41n01_02

INTRODUCTION

Demographic information about the current population of older adults and how it is likely to change in the years to come is vital to gerontological social workers practicing in small towns and rural communities. In this article we explain our use of the terms rural and urban and metropolitan and nonmetropolitan. We discuss the situation of elders living in nonmetropolitan areas of United States generally, regional variations in their demographic characteristics, demographic issues related to their poverty and health status, and trends and population changes anticipated in the years to come. We conclude with a section on how social workers in rural communities can access and use locally relevant demographic data in their day-to-day practice activities.

WHAT DO WE MEAN BY RURAL?

One would think that defining what we mean by rural would be extraordinarily simple. In one sense, we all know and understand what rural means. As has been noted (Bosak & Perlman, 1982; Hewitt, 1992; Whitaker, 1982), however, there is considerable variation in the use of this term. Thus, to avoid confusion and misunderstanding, it is very important that we be clear in what we mean when using the term "rural" when we discuss information about the demographics of rural aging.

There are two general types of definitions of rural in use today, quantitative definitions and qualitative definitions. Quantitative definitions focus on size, population density, and degree of isolation. Quantitative definitions are frequently used by governmental agencies and others in policy-making and in reporting data and for determining eligibility for grants of various types. Qualitative definitions, on the other hand, focus on culture, human values, and behavior and thus are particularly important in social work practice applications.

The United States Office of Management and Budget (OMB) uses a classification system that divides the country into metropolitan statistical areas (MSA) and nonmetropolitan areas (Office of Budget and Management, 1999) as a basis for collecting statistical data. Several governmental agencies use MSA designations in determining eligibility for program funding. Generally metropolitan areas are defined as one or more central cities with populations greater than 50,000 and the surrounding counties that are linked economically and socially to them.[1] Areas outside of metropolitan areas are classified as nonmetropolitan. In 1993 (the last year for which these determinations were made), there were 837 metropolitan and 2305 nonmetropolitan counties in the U.S. Overall, the nonmetropolitan counties comprise about 80% of the country's land mass and 20% of the population.

The U.S. Bureau of the Census employs the OMB definition of metropolitan/nonmetropolitan as one method of classifying areas but also classifies areas as urban or rural (United States Bureau of the Census, n.d.b). Urban areas include places of 2,500 or more persons incorporated into cities, census designated places of 2,500 or more persons, and other territory included in urbanized areas. Urbanized areas include the central city and densely settled surrounding territory (1,000 persons per square mile) that together have a total population of at least 50,000 persons. Rural areas are defined as all areas that lie outside urban areas.

The OMB definition of metropolitan/nonmetropolitan and the U.S. Bureau of the Census definition of urban/rural are not equivalent. It is possible, for example, to live in a community defined as rural in a county that is classified as metropolitan. For example, the town of Vance, AL (population 464) is located in Tuscaloosa County, a metropolitan county. Similarly there are urban areas in counties classified as nonmetropolitan (e.g., the city of Greensboro, AL, population 2,731, is located in nonmetropolitan Hale County).

Although metropolitan and nonmetropolitan areas both contain rural and urban areas, the metro-nonmetro typology is generally thought to better capture differences in settlement patterns than does the rural-urban typology (Clifford, Heaton, Voss, & Fuguitt, 1985; Clifford & Lilley, 1993). Further, more data and more current data are available using the metro-nonmetro distinction (Clifford & Lilley, 1993). Therefore, most of our discussion in this article uses the metro-nonmetro classification system.

Both the definition of rural-urban developed by the Bureau of the Census and the definition of metropolitan-nonmetropolitan developed by the OMB are dichotomies. The Economic Research Service (n.d.) also provides three different measures of the degree of rurality of an area–rural-urban continuum codes, urban influence codes, and rural-urban commuting area codes. The Economic Research Service further provides two kinds of county typology codes, one where nonmetro counties are divided into six non-overlapping economic types and one where nonmetro counties are divided into five overlapping policy types.

GENERAL UNITED STATES SITUATION

According to the 2000 Census, 12.4% of Americans (35 million people) are 65 years of age or older. Among individuals residing in urban areas, 12.3% (27.4 million) are 65 or older, and among individuals residing in rural areas, 12.8% (7.6 million) are 65 and older. Generally, less densely populated counties have a higher proportion of their population aged 65 or older. Consequently, it is not surprising that, according to the 2000 census, nonmetropolitan areas (which include some less densely populated urban areas) have a higher proportion of their population aged 65 or older (14.7% or 8.1 million) than do metropolitan areas (11.9% or 26.9 million).

The Current Population Survey March 2002 Supplement data file (2002) provides the most current information on non institutionalized persons 65 and older (see Table 1). According to this survey, elderly residents of nonmetropolitan areas are more likely than their metropolitan counterparts to be white, married, male, to be receiving social security benefits, and to have social security as their only pension. Also, a higher proportion of older, nonmetropolitan residents had not completed high school than was the case for metropolitan elders.

What kinds of nonmetropolitan counties are home to high proportions of older persons? The Economic Research Service (n.d.) has divided rural counties into six different categories on the basis of their main economic activity (see Table 2). Rural counties with the highest proportions of older adults are those which are described as farming dependent (Gale, 2002), non-specialized, and services dependent. Those with lower proportions of older persons are government dependent and mining dependent counties.

The nation's rural counties can also be divided into five different, overlapping policy types (Economic Research Service, n.d.). Of these, retirement destination counties (190 counties) have the highest proportion of persons 65 or older, 16.2%. These counties, located in various parts of the nation, have attracted significant numbers of older in-migrants in recent years that have boosted their economic bases (Haas & Serow, 1993; Longino & Smith, 1998; Serow, 2001). Other counties with high proportions of older adults are transfers-dependent counties, where a significant percentage of personal income comes from government transfer payments. Among the nation's rural counties, older residents are least likely to be present in those with a high proportion of Federally-owned land or those described as persistent poverty counties.

Regional Variations

According to the Current Population Survey March 2002 Supplement (2002), nationwide 15.0% of the nonmetro population is 65+,

TABLE 1. Metropolitan by nonmetropolitan differences of those 65 and older by region for age, marital status, education, ethnicity, and receiving social security.

	Total		Northeast		Midwest		South		West	
	Metro %	Nonmetro %	Metro %	Nonmetro %	Metro %	Nonmetro %	Metro %	Nonmetro %	Metro %	Nonmetro %
Age/% 65 +										
65-69	28.8	28.5	27.4	27.6	29.1	26.2	30.4	30.5	27.7	28.5
70-74	24.9	24.6	24.8	24.1	23.4	23.9	25.2	25.6	26.0	23.4
75-79	22.1	21.8	22.3	23.5	22.5	21.5	21.7	20.6	21.9	24.8
80 +	24.2	25.1	25.5	24.8	25.0	28.4	22.7	23.3	24.5	23.3
Percent 65 + of total population	11.3	15.0	13.3	15.3	11.4	15.5	11.3	14.7	9.4	14.8
Gender										
Male	41.9	43.0	41.5	42.4	40.6	43.3	42.1	42.1	43.4	45.7
Female	58.1	57.0	58.5	57.6	59.4	56.7	57.9	57.9	56.6	54.3
Marital Status										
Married	54.9	58.9	51.3	55.9	55.4	60.7	57.2	57.4	55.0	61.7
Widowed	32.4	31.5	34.6	32.3	32.1	30.2	31.9	33.6	30.8	28.0
Divorced/Separated	8.9	6.4	8.2	6.6	3.7	3.0	3.1	2.8	2.6	2.8
Never Married	3.8	3.1	5.9	6.6	3.7	3.0	3.1	2.8	2.6	2.8
Education										
8 years or less	14.1	21.2	14.2	13.1	12.3	18.4	16.3	29.1	12.2	10.5
9-12 years	14.1	15.3	15.9	15.0	14.9	15.3	14.0	15.6	11.1	14.8
High school graduate	35.6	34.4	38.5	38.9	38.4	38.6	34.1	30.2	31.7	34.5
High school +	36.3	29.0	31.4	33.0	34.4	27.6	35.6	25.1	45.0	40.1
Ethnicity										
White	80.6	90.2	84.9	98.0	87.2	97.3	77.6	83.3	73.6	89.4
Black	9.1	5.8	8.0	0.9	9.7	1.3	12.5	12.2	4.1	0.4
Amer Indian/Aleut Eskimo	0.4	1.2	0.2	0.5	0.1	0.7	0.4	1.1	1.2	3.0
Asian/Pacific Islander	3.3	0.4	2.3	0.2	1.3	0.2	1.3	0.1	9.8	2.0
Hispanic	6.6	2.4	4.6	0.3	1.7	0.6	8.1	3.3	11.4	5.2
Social Security										
Receiving	89.0	93.1	89.6	95.6	92.1	94.5	88.9	91.7	86.1	92.5
Only pension	67.2	72.2	67.2	65.4	65.1	71.3	71.3	75.7	69.5	72.0

Note. Source is Current Population Survey March 2002 Supplement (2002)

TABLE 2. Percent of people 65 years of age or older by nonmetropolitan county type.

Definition	Percent 65 or older
Economic Types	
Farming-dependent	16.9%
Mining-dependent	13.6%
Manufacturing-dependent	14.2%
Government-dependent	12.4%
Services-dependent	15.0%
Nonspecialized	15.4%
Policy Types	
Retirement destination	16.2%
Federal lands	13.4%
Commuting	14.0%
Persistent poverty	13.8%
Transfers-dependent	15.3%

Note. Population data from county population dataset produced by U.S. Bureau of the Census and online at: http://eire.census.gov/popest/data/counties.php and 1989 county type definitions from http://www.ers.usda.gov/Briefing/Rurality/Typology/Data/typology89.xls.

compared with 11.3% of the metro population. The higher proportion of elders in nonmetro areas holds in every region of the country, with the largest differences in the West and the Midwest and smallest in the Northeast (see Table 1). Nonmetropolitan elders are more likely to be married than metropolitan elders in all regions, with the highest proportions of married persons in the Midwest (60.76%) and the West (61.7%). With the exception of the South, metropolitan older persons are more likely to be widowed than their nonmetropolitan counterparts (see Table 1).

The proportion of older persons with an eighth grade education or less is substantially higher in nonmetropolitan areas than in metropolitan areas (see Table 1). However, this is not characteristic of all regions. In both the Northeast and the West, the proportion of nonmetropolitan residents with an eighth grade education or less is lower than for metropolitan residents. In all but the Northeast, the proportion of elders who had completed more than a high school education is higher in the metro areas than in the nonmetro areas.

Nonmetro elderly persons are more likely to be White than are those living in metro areas (see Table 1). This is particularly the case in the Northeast, where 98.0% of nonmetro elders are White, and the Midwest, where 97.3% of nonmetro older persons are White. In every region, the proportion of older Blacks, Asian/Pacific Islanders, and Hispanics is higher in the metro than the nonmetro areas, and the proportion of American Indians/Aleut Eskimos is higher in the nonmetro than in the metropolitan areas. However, the proportion of nonmetro elderly Blacks is quite similar to the proportion of metro elderly Blacks in the South (12.2% nonmetro vs. 12.5% metro).

Poverty Status

The economic well-being of older adults has improved dramatically in recent decades, with the percentage living below the poverty level declining from 35% in 1959 (Federal Interagency Forum on Aging-Related Statistics, 2000) to 9.9% in 2000 (U.S. Bureau of the Census, n.d.a). In nonmetro areas, however, the percentages of older adults living in poverty and in near-poverty exceed those in metro areas in the U.S. overall and in nearly every geographic region of the nation (see Table 3). Over 12% of nonmetro elders live in poverty nationwide, compared with 9.5% of metro elders, and 16.5% of nonmetro elders live below 150% of the poverty line, compared with 13.4% of metro elders. Among America's nonmetro elders, nearly 29% live below 150% of the poverty line, an issue of major concern for social workers in rural communities.

Regional comparisons indicate that Southern nonmetro elders are more likely to have low incomes than those in any other area of the nation, while nonmetro elders in the Midwest are least likely to be poor or near poor. In the Northeast region, metro older persons are more likely to live below the poverty line than their nonmetro counterparts.

Poverty rates increase with advancing age, both for metro and nonmetro elders, with poverty rates higher in every age category for nonmetro elders. In all age categories, the poverty rate for nonmetro elders exceeds the 65+ national average of 9.9%, with the rate for nonmetro elders who are 80+ being 14.5%. The percentage of poor and near-poor nonmetro elders in the 80+ category exceeds 35%.

Nonmetro elderly women are particularly at risk of poverty (14.4%) or near-poverty (18.9%). These rates of low-income status for women are particularly striking when compared with the poverty rate for males living in metro areas (6.3%). Older males in non metro areas are more likely to live in poverty (9.4% vs. 6.3%) and in near-poverty (13.3% vs. 10.2%) than their metro counterparts.

TABLE 3. Metropolitan by nonmetropolitan differences in poverty and near poverty rates for persons 65 and older by region, age, gender, marital status, education, ethnicity, and health status.

	Below		100% - 149% Above	
	Metro%	Nonmetro %	Metro %	Nonmetro %
Total U.S.	9.5	12.2	13.4	16.5
Region				
Northeast	10.5	9.1	13.4	15.4
Midwest	7.1	9.7	12.2	15.0
South	11.0	16.1	14.3	17.9
West	8.2	9.1	13.0	16.5
Age				
65-69	8.9	10.5	8.8	15.3
70-74	8.4	11.0	12.7	14.6
75-79	9.6	13.4	15.3	15.4
80 +	11.2	14.5	17.7	20.6
Gender				
Male	6.3	9.4	10.2	13.3
Female	11.8	14.4	15.7	18.9
Marital Status				
Married	4.4	5.8	7.9	11.5
Widowed	13.9	20.1	20.7	24.4
Divorced/Separated	20.9	22.9	17.5	24.8
Never Married	18.4	33.7	20.3	13.9
Education				
8 years or less	20.6	26.5	21.1	25.1
9-12 years	14.2	14.8	19.3	24.6
High school graduate	7.7	8.5	13.3	14.7
High school +	5.1	4.9	8.1	8.0
Ethnicity				
White (non-Hispanic)	7.3	10.4	12.4	15.6
Black (non-Hispanic)	19.7	33.3	18.2	25.2
American Indian/Aleut Eskimo	6.5	28.6	16.7	25.7
Asian/Pacific Islander	10.3	5.9	10.9	6.7
Hispanic	21.8	22.1	19.6	26.8
Health				
Fair/poor	13.4	18.5	17.1	21.4
Good or better	7.4	8.3	11.4	13.4

Note: Source is Current Population Survey March 2002 Supplement (2002).

Married persons are considerably less likely than unmarried persons to live below the poverty line, regardless of whether they live in metro or nonmetro areas. Married persons in metro areas are the least likely (4.4%) and never-married persons in nonmetro areas are the most likely (33.7%) to live below the poverty line. Over 20% of all widowed and divorced/separated nonmetro elders live below the poverty line, and more than an additional 24% live in the near-poverty category. Thus unmarried, nonmetro elders who tend to be predominately female are those at greatest risk for low-income status.

Level of educational attainment is directly related to poverty and near-poverty status. For both metro and nonmetro elders, the percentages in poverty and near-poverty categories decline with increased education. Nonmetro elders most at risk of living in poverty are those with an 8th grade education or less (26.5%), while those with more than a high school education are least likely to live below the poverty line (4.9%).

Poverty status comparisons by ethnicity reveal considerable variability across groups and by metro/nonmetro status. In most cases, nonmetro elders are more economically disadvantaged than are their metro counterparts. Among nonmetro elders, those least likely to be in poverty status are Asian/Pacific Islanders (5.9%), and those most likely to be in poverty status are Black non-Hispanics (33.3%). Nonmetro elders in other ethnic groups exceed the national poverty level average of 9.9%, including American Indians/Aleut Eskimos (28.5%), Hispanics (22.1%), and White non-Hispanics (10.4%).

In 2002, approximately 8.8 million metro and 3.0 million nonmetro older Americans reported being in fair or poor health (Current Population Survey March 2002 Supplement, 2002). Among those living in nonmetro areas, 18.5% were also living below the poverty level and an additional 21.4% were elders living in near poverty. Thus, nearly 40% of nonmetro older Americans who assessed their health as fair or poor (or 1.2 million people) had incomes below 150% of the poverty level.

Glasgow (1993) advances a dynamic life course perspective to explain why poverty and near poverty rates are higher for older adults in nonmetro areas. Her model takes into account the lifetime experiences of nonmetro older persons whose work histories were characterized by low-wage, part-time, and seasonal employment with limited pension coverage in comparison to their metropolitan counterparts. Women in nonmetro areas historically participated in the labor force at lower rates than did metro women (Bokemeier, Sachs, & Keith, 1983). Widowed or divorced women are particularly at risk if, as is often the case, their survivors' pensions are inadequate. The result for nonmetro elders' economic status in later life is reduced lifetime earnings, pension accumulation, and opportunities to save for old age. These problems are compounded by their tendency to be in poorer health (Glasgow & Beale, 1985), a situation which has further implications for depleting financial resources. Social workers' efforts in direct practice, advocacy, and social policy development activities must take into account higher rates of poverty among nonmetro elders, particularly among the oldest old, women, unmarried persons, ethnic minorities of color, and people who are poorly educated.

Health

One important indicator of overall well being is whether people describe their health as "excellent," "very good," "good," "fair," or "poor" (Rogers, 2002). Most older Americans report their health as excellent, very good, or good. Because social workers are particularly concerned with persons at greatest risk, we focus here on the approximately one-third of the 65+ population who rate their health status as fair or poor (see Table 4).

Nationwide, nonmetropolitan elders are more likely to report being in fair or poor health (38.7%) than were metropolitan elders (34.1%). There is considerable variability by region of the country, with the highest proportion of nonmetro elders reporting fair or poor health in the South (49.2%) and the lowest proportion in the Northeast (27.7%). In the Northeast and West elders in fair and poor health are more likely to reside in metro areas. In the Midwest there is no difference (33.2%) between metro and nonmetro older adults in their assessment of fair and poor health, while in the South nonmetro elders gave considerably more negative health assessments. Despite these regional variations, nonmetro older adults in all age, marital status, education, ethnicity and poverty status categories, however, consistently report poorer health than their metro counterparts.

In both metro and nonmetro areas older Americans positive health evaluations decline with age. Nearly half (47.3%) of persons 80+ in nonmetro areas report being in fair or poor health. Non-metro residents who are widowed, divorced/separated, or never married are at greatest risk, with more than 45% of nonmetro elders among the least healthy.

Health status is related to educational level for both nonmetro and metro elders, with those least well educated most likely to report fair or poor health. Among nonmetro elders, 56.1% of persons with eight or fewer years of education are in the least healthy category, compared

TABLE 4. Metropolitan by nonmetropolitan differences in percent in fair or poor health for persons 65 and older by region, age, gender, marital status, education, ethnicity, and poverty status.

	Metro %	Nonmetro %
Total U.S.	34.1	38.7
Region		
Northeast	32.3	27.7
Midwest	33.2	33.2
South	37.3	49.2
West	31.8	28.6
Age		
65-69	27.2	34.0
70-74	30.3	34.7
75-79	37.5	39.7
80 +	43.0	47.3
Gender		
Male	32.2	38.0
Female	35.4	39.3
Marital Status		
Married	31.1	34.4
Widowed	38.6	45.2
Divorced/Separated	34.7	44.6
Never Married	37.6	43.1
Education		
8 years or less	53.7	56.1
9-12 years	43.4	46.6
High school graduate	32.7	33.6
High school +	24.2	28.1
Ethnicity		
White (non-Hispanic)	31.7	36.6
Black (non-Hispanic)	47.1	64.4
American Indian/Aleut Eskimo	45.6	46.5
Asian/Pacific Islander	33.4	38.4
Hispanic	45.1	53.8
Poverty status		
Below poverty level	48.2	58.5
100%-149% poverty level	43.6	50.3

Note: Source is Current Population Survey March 2002 Supplement (2002).

with 28.1% of those who reported education beyond the high school level.

Nonmetro older adults in all ethnic categories assess their health less favorably than metro residents. The disparity is greatest for Black Americans, with 64.4% of nonmetro elders in poorer health compared with 47.1% of metropolitan Blacks. Nonmetropolitan Blacks are most likely to rate their health unfavorably followed by Hispanics (53.8%) and American Indians/Aleut Eskimos (46.5%). Nonmetro Blacks are more than twice as likely to rate their health as fair or poor than metro Whites.

Over half of nonmetro elders below the poverty line and in the near-poverty category rate their health as fair or poor. Below poverty-level nonmetro elders (58.5%) are considerably more likely than their urban counterparts (48.2%) to rate their health unfavorably, and near-poor nonmetro elders (50.3%) also rate their health more unfavorably than near-poor metro elders (43.6%).

Elders in nonmetro areas are at greater risk for self-assessed poor health than are those in more metropolitan areas, with those most at risk being nonmetro elders of color and those living below or near the poverty level. As Rogers (2002) has noted, problems of poor health in nonmetro communities are exacerbated by structural barriers to accessing health care services, including physicians, hospitals and other health facilities that tend to be concentrated in urbanized areas. Gerontological social workers in rural places are often challenged to help nonmetro elders find affordable and accessible transportation to needed health services and to advocate for continuation or expansion of needed services in areas of low population density.

TRENDS

The rate of growth in the elderly population in nonmetropolitan areas has slowed over the past 30 years (Fuguitt, Beale, & Tordella, 2002), both because of declines in the natural increase in the numbers of elderly persons and because of declines in the net migration rates to nonmetro areas. Two factors contributed to the decline in the natural increase of older persons in nonmetro areas. First, large numbers of men and women left farming during the 1940s and 1950s, decreasing the base of nonmetro persons available to age in place (Gale, 2002). Second, the nation experienced lowered birth rates during the post depression years, further reducing the available base population overall

(Fuguitt et al., 2002). Net migration rates to nonmetropolitan counties also declined, particularly in counties located away from metro areas, counties with low population density, and counties with few natural amenities (McGranahan & Beale, 2002).

There was substantial regional variation in growth patterns of the nonmetro elderly population. The Southwest and Mountain West experienced high growth both because of natural increase and net migration. The growth in the size of the elderly population in nonmetro, Great Plains counties was substantially lower than in other areas and actually showed a small loss (1.4%) from 1990 to 2000. Finally, the nonmetro, elderly population growth rates were highest in recreation counties and, to a lesser extent, in manufacturing counties (Fuguitt et al., 2002).

Over the past five years, the growth rate in the nonmetro elderly population (8.6%) exceeded the 5.8% rate for the metro elderly population (Current Population Survey March 2002 Supplement, 2002; Current Population Survey March 1997 Supplement, 1997). The growth rate among nonmetro elderly in the West region was 24.6% (compared with a metro growth rate of 0.7%), and in the Northeast region was 18.5% (compared with a metro growth rate of 5.8%). The nonmetro growth rate among those age 80 or older was 22.0% (compared with a metro growth rate of 13.9%) and among those age 75-79 was 16.9% (compared with a metro growth rate of 8.1%). However, the growth rate for those age 70-74 was negative for both nonmetro and metro areas and was only two percent for those age 65-69. Finally, the nonmetro elderly growth rates were higher than the metro elderly growth rates for Hispanics, Black non-Hispanics, and White non-Hispanics, but lower for Asian/Pacific Islanders and American Indians/Aleut Eskimos.

By 2020, persons born in the post World War II baby boom will reach age 65, resulting in substantial increases in the numbers of elderly nonmetropolitan and metropolitan residents. Boomers are forward looking (Keegan, Gross, Fisher, & Remez, 2002) individuals who are better educated than the current generation of older persons. The health care technology available to them is superior to that which was available to today's elders when they were in their 40s and 50s. Consequently we should expect an increase in the numbers of frail elderly surviving into their 80s and 90s, stressing the social service and health delivery systems of rural communities.

Since those in their 40s and 50s have higher levels of educational attainment than current elders, the educational attainment among the elderly in 2020 will be higher in all regions. However, nonmetro-metro disparities will remain in the South.

The movement of middle aged and younger Blacks and Hispanics into nonmetropolitan areas suggests that the nonmetropolitan elderly in 2020 will be more diverse ethnically than today's nonmetro elderly are. More specifically, there should be substantial numbers of elderly Blacks and Hispanics residing in the nonmetro South and West regions.

Finally, McGranahan and Beale (2002) suggest that nonmetropolitan population loss occurs primarily in counties remote from metropolitan areas (and thus far from specialized services) that are thinly settled (small labor market) and lack compensating natural amenities. There is every reason to believe that this trend will continue, making it even more difficult to provide services for older adults residing in such areas.

DEMOGRAPHIC INFORMATION FOR DEVELOPMENT AND PLANNING FOR RURAL COMMUNITIES

This article provides demographic information about older adults in rural America and discusses variations by geographic regions or kinds of communities and expectations about changes that will occur in the future. The typical rural social worker, however, is concerned about the very particular community, county, or set of counties where he or she works. The worker needs current information about what the demographic conditions in that specific area are and what the trends for the future might be.

Specific county or community level data are often necessary to understand the full range and distinctiveness of the older population to be served, to anticipate trends and future needs and issues, and to plan new programs that will be responsive to the aging population. These data can also be used to support clinical impressions and anecdotal evidence in writing grant applications, to answer specific questions that members of one's agency board may have about community needs, and to advocate for better services for the elders in the community.

One approach to gathering information about the characteristics of elders in a local area is to conduct a survey or series of focus groups. This is, however, a time-consuming and expensive task. In fact, it may not be necessary. A number of U.S. government agencies routinely collect information at the community or county level. In some states, state level planners summarize these data at the county or community level and make them available to local users (CARES, 1990). Some state agencies on aging provide this service. Where this does not occur, or where the available data do not address the specific questions that a local worker needs to answer, the worker with Internet access can go directly to the data sources and gain a wealth of information.

Data from the U.S. Bureau of the Census are available through *www.census.gov/main/www/cen2000.html.* By using the American Fact Finder feature of this website, the worker can quickly find information about a county, place, or (in some cases) a census tract that includes numbers of persons 65+ by race and gender, veteran status, poverty status and mobility or self care limitations. Considerably more information is readily available that enables one to compare the status of the elders in the population with younger residents and/or with elders statewide or in adjacent counties. Further, general contextual information about the economic base of the community, general educational level, housing characteristics, percent native and foreign born, and sources of income of residents, is also available.

U.S. Department of Agriculture, through its Economic Research Service, provides another rich data source specifically on rural areas at *www.ers.usda.gov/data/RuralMapMachine/.* This source provides information about median county income, percentage of various ethnic/racial groupings, county typology code, unemployment rates, and metropolitan status, among other types of information. Useful county-level information pertaining to the older population is also collected by the department of public heath in each state, and the information may be available on-line or through contacts with state health departments' offices for health statistics.

CONCLUSION

This article presents an overview of the U.S. population in rural perspective. Most older adults live in metropolitan areas, but some 7.8 million or 23.3% of the nation's elders live in counties classified as nonmetropolitan. Older persons comprise a substantially larger proportion of nonmetro counties' populations than they do in metro counties (15.0% v 11.3%). Because of this, their needs and concerns may be of special concern to social workers in small towns and rural communities. Counties with the highest proportion of older adults can also be described as farming dependent, non-specialized, services-dependent, retirement destination and transfer-dependent counties.

The profiles of nonmetro elders vary by region, as do the ways in which they differ from their metropolitan counterparts. Overall, nonmetro elders are more likely to be White, married, less well educated, to be receiving social security, and to have social security as their only pension. On the key indicators of poverty and self-assessed health status, Southern nonmetro elders are particularly at risk. Social work must be particularly sensitive to nonmetro elders who are 80+, female, unmarried, of low educational attainment and minorities of color, because these persons are most likely to live below or near the poverty level. Similarly older adults who are unmarried, poorly educated, minorities of color, living near or below the poverty line, and 80 years old or older are at greatest risk for poor health.

As we consider the situation of older adults in nonmetropolitan areas over the next 20 years, they are less likely to be poor and poorly educated than today's generation of nonmetro older adults. Moreover, although living in areas classified as nonmetropolitan, they will not be as isolated from health and social services as today's nonmetro elders are.

Neither national nor regional data can provide an adequate substitute for local demographic information when a social worker is planning a specific program or policy advocacy activity. Now that U.S. Census Bureau data for every community in the nation have become readily accessible to Internet users, local social workers can use up-to-date information in understanding and planning for the older population in the areas that they serve.

NOTE

1. OMB has just completed new standards for defining metropolitan and micropolitan statistical areas. The new standards are accessible through the Bureau of the Census's home page, *http://www.census.gov*, and will be used in analyses beginning in 2003.

REFERENCES

Bokemeier, J.L., Sachs, C., & Keith, V. (1983). Labor force participation of metropolitan, nonmetropolitan and farm women: A comparative study. *Rural Sociology, 48*, 515-539.

Bosak, J., & Perlman, B. (1982). A review of the definition of rural. *Journal of Rural Community Psychology, 3*, 3-33.

CARES (Center for Aging Research and Educational Services), North Carolina Comes of Age, prepared by the Center for Aging Research and Educational Services, School of Social Work, University of North Carolina for the North Carolina Division of Social Work, University of North Carolina for the North Carolina Division of Aging, CARES, Chapel Hill, North Carolina, 1990.

Clifford, W.B., Heaton, T.B., Voss, P.R., & Fuguitt, G.V. (1985). The rural elderly in demographic perspective. (pp. 22-55). In R.T. Coward & G.R. Lee (Eds.) *The elderly in rural society: Every fourth elder.* New York: Springer.

Clifford, W.B., & Lilley, S.C. (1993). Rural elderly: Their demographic characteristics. (pp. 3-16). In C. N. Bull (Ed.) *Aging in rural America*. Newbury Park, CA: Sage.

Current Population Survey March 2002 Supplement. (2002). [Data file]. Available from *http://ferret.bls.census.gov/cgi-bin/ferret*.

Current Population Survey March 1997 Supplement. (1997). [Data file]. Available from *http://ferret.bls.census.gov/cgi-bin/ferret*.

Economic Research Service. (n.d.). Measuring rurality. Retrieved March 26, 2003, from U.S. Department of Agriculture Web Site: *http://www.ers.usda.gov/Briefing/ Rurality*.

Federal Interagency Forum on Aging-Related Statistics. (2000). Older Americans 2000: Key indicators of well-being. Washington, DC: U.S. Government Printing Office.

Fuguitt, G.V., Beale, C.L., & Tordella, S.J. (2002). Recent trends in older population change and migration for nonmetro areas, 1970-2000. *Rural America, 17*, 11-19.

Gale, F. (2002). The graying farm sector: Legacy of off-farm migration. *Rural America, 17*, 28-31.

Glasgow, N. (1993). Poverty among rural elders: Trends, context, and directions for policy. *The Journal of Applied Gerontology, 12*, 302-319.

Glasgow, N., & Beale, C. (1985). Rural elderly in demographic perspective. *Rural Development Perspectives, 2*, 22-26.

Haas, W.H., & Serow, W.J. (1993). Amenity retirement migration process: A model and preliminary evidence. *The Gerontologist, 33*, 212-220.

Hewitt, M. (1992). Defining "rural" areas: Impact on health care policy and research. (pp. 25-54) In W.M. Gesler & T.C. Ricketts (Eds.), *Health in Rural North America*. New Brunswick: Rutgers University Press.

Keegan, C., Gross, S., Fisher, L., & Remez, S. (2002). Boomers at midlife: *The AARP Life stage study executive summary*. Washington, DC: AARP.

Longino, C.F., & Smith, M.H. (1998). Theoretical and methodological approaches to migration research on rural aging populations. (pp. 67-96). In W.M. Gesler, D.J. Rabiner, & G.H. DeFriese, *Rural health and aging research: Theory, methods and practical applications*. Amityville, NY: Baywood, 67.

McGranahan, D.A., & Beale, C.L. (2002). Understanding rural population loss. *Rural America, 17*, 2-11.

Office of Budget and Management. (1999). OMB Bulletin 99-04. Retrieved March 26, 2003, from *http://www.whitehouse.gov/omb/inforeg/msa-bull99-04.html*.

Rogers, C.C. (1997). Growth of the oldest old population and future implications for rural areas. *Rural Development Perspectives, 14*, 22-26.

Rogers, C.C. (2002). Rural health issues for the older population. *Rural America, 17*, 30-36.

Serow, W.J. (2002). Retirement migration counties in the southeastern United States: Geographic, demographic and economic correlates. *The Gerontologist, 41*, 220-228.

United States Bureau of the Census. (n.d.a). Table GCT-P14 Income and Poverty in 1999: 2000. Retrieved March 25, 2003, from United States Bureau of the Census Web Site: *http://www.census.gov/main/www/cen2000.html*.

United States Bureau of the Census Bureau (n.d.b). *Census 2000 Urban and Rural Classification*. Retrieved March 26, 2003b, from United State Census Bureau Web Site: *http://www.census.gov/geo/www/ua/ua_2k.html*.

Whitaker, W.H. (1982, July 26). The many faces of Ephraim: In search of a functional typology of rural areas. Paper presented at the meeting of the Seventh Annual National Institute on Social Work in Rural Areas. Dubuque, Iowa.

SECTION II PRACTICE DIMENSIONS OF SOCIAL WORK WITH RURAL ELDERS

Chapter 3

Rural Aging: Social Work Practice Models and Intervention Dynamics

Cynthia D. Bisman, PhD

SUMMARY. This chapter presents a biopsychosocial framework, with an emphasis on assessment, to guide social work practice with the rural elderly. Social work values of social justice and human dignity, its mission of human well-being and its special commitment to empower vulnerable populations are reviewed as the basis for practice decisions. Discussion focuses on theoretical models relevant to practice with this population including social support, family systems, group work, and

[Haworth co-indexing entry note]: "Rural Aging: Social Work Practice Models and Intervention Dynamics." Bisman, Cynthia D. Co-published simultaneously in *Journal of Gerontological Social Work* (The Haworth Social Work Practice Press, an imprint of The Haworth Press, Inc.) Vol. 41, No. 1/2, 2003, pp. 37-58; and: *Gerontological Social Work in Small Towns and Rural Communities* (ed: Sandra S. Butler, and Lenard W. Kaye) The Haworth Social Work Practice Press, an imprint of The Haworth Press, Inc., 2003, pp. 37-58. Single or multiple copies of this article are available for a fee from The Haworth Document Delivery Service [1-800-HAWORTH, 9:00 a.m. - 5:00 p.m. (EST). E-mail address: docdelivery@haworth press.com].

http://www.haworthpress.com/web/JGSW
© 2003 by The Haworth Press, Inc. All rights reserved.
Digital Object Identifier: 10.1300/J083v41n01_03

case management and community practice. Conceptual material is directly linked with intervention approaches that target the multiple areas of the social work domain. *[Article copies available for a fee from The Haworth Document Delivery Service: 1-800-HAWORTH. E-mail address: <docdelivery@haworthpress.com> Website: <http://www.HaworthPress.com>*
© 2003 by The Haworth Press, Inc. All rights reserved.]

KEYWORDS. Practice models with elders, gerontological practice, interventions with elders

INTRODUCTION

The domain of inquiry in this chapter, models of social work practice for the rural elderly, contains complex phenomena in varying stages of change. Categories used in the past may no longer capture the nuances and multiple realities for thinking about the population of the rural aging. At the same time, the models of practice are broader than a particular set of persons or problems. Current seismic shifts in the nature and delivery of social work services including privatization and the blurring of professional boundaries only add to the importance of recognizing the many layers of diversity we confront as social workers practicing with the elderly who reside in rural areas.

Moreover, advances in technology, especially television and the Internet, have permanently changed communication and altered the traditional association of rural with isolation. Small family farms are losing out to large corporate-owned agri-businesses turning farmers into workers. Sensitive to these challenges this chapter presents a practice framework followed by concepts and intervention approaches specifically relevant for social work practice with the rural elderly. First we consider the social work profession's unique commitment and expertise to provide services to the elderly in rural areas.

SOCIAL WORK'S EXPERTISE

It is the nature and continuing challenge of professional occupations to be relevant to the contemporary social context while remaining attentive to the profession's historical traditions, especially its values, code of ethics and mission. The mission to enhance human well-being, which necessarily encompasses both individual and social well-being, strongly roots the profession of social work in the perspective of person *and* environment. Individual change and social reform go hand-in-hand in effective social work practice. Those who engage in direct practice with individuals, families and small groups must also attend to needed environmental changes including legislation and service delivery. Similarly, social workers whose primary responsibilities focus on policies and programs must also address the individuals and families in need of help.

Such a mixture of macro and micro, the person and the environment, individual change and social reform, meshes beautifully with serving the needs of the rural elderly. Social work's breadth of domain can meet the diverse needs of this population for advocacy and direct practice, attention to the family and to community resources, interventions that include therapy and financial help.

Social work's values and code of ethics provide strong support for practice that simultaneously targets multiple levels of intervention. The mission of human well-being is rooted in the profession's core values of service, social justice, dignity and worth of each individual, and the primacy of human relationships. Emerging from the values and mission, the ethical standards in the Code of Ethics guide such practice. The following standards are especially relevant: engagement in social and political action (6.04, p. 27); promotion of the general welfare (6.01, p. 26); promote the wellbeing of individual clients (1.01, p. 7); respect client self-determination (1.02, p. 7); provide informed consent (1.03, p. 7); and respect social diversity (1.05, p. 9) (NASW, 1999). Farley, Griffiths, Skidmore, and Thackeray (1982) stress that the small size of rural communities makes it even more important that in recording notes and reports, social workers respect clients' privacy and confidentiality.

Related to its mission, values and ethical code, the social work profession has particular concerns to empower vulnerable populations including those who are oppressed and poor. While all elderly are not financially vulnerable, they are all potentially vulnerable socially. Ginsberg (2001) asserts that the biggest and most vulnerable social work client populations are the elderly and children. The elderly benefit from several social welfare programs such as Medicare and Social Security, and receive a range of social work related services including adult protective services, day care, nutrition assistance, hospital care.

Browne (1995) broadens Solomon's 1976 seminal approach to empowerment to include interdependence and societal good in addition to independence and individual good. This contemporary re-conceptualization which emphasizes community and connection further supports social work's person and environment perspective. For Browne, the following can enhance empowerment for the elderly: friendships, community connections, mutual aid and support groups, family support, education, and peer counseling. I discuss these in the later section on theoretical models and interventions. Next I present the components of a framework for practice with the rural elderly.

A PRACTICE FRAMEWORK

There are components that are central to social work whether practicing with an individual, a family, or the community. These include assessment, the biopsychosocial perspective and practitioner observation or self-awareness/use of self (see Bisman, 1994, for full development). These components are supported by much of the practice literature (see Greene, 2000; Compton and Galaway, 1998, among others). We consider each of these in turn.

Assessment and Case Theory

Richards (2000) warns about tensions between agency and user-centered practice. For her, assessment is not merely an administrative task that requires fitting the elderly into predetermined categories, but is rather a process of gathering and providing information that is meaningful to the elderly and responsive to their problems. Nieto, Coward, and Horsley point out that assessment is an "incremental process that augments, on a continuing basis, what is known about the client" (1989, p. 16), and that it should focus on all persons significant in the client's support system. Holosko and Holosko (1996) agree that assessment is best handled over several sessions so that it goes beyond pathology and problem solving. The use of significant others will enrich the data gathering and increase the assessment's relevance. Assessment is as well a mutual process; the client's autonomy must be respected. Ryan, Merdeith, and MacLean (1995) comment on the value of careful attention to narrative to determine how the elderly clients themselves make sense of their situation.

Barker (1987) emphasizes the importance of a thorough assessment. In addition to mental and physical variables, practitioners should consider values, economic factors, religious orientation, support systems, sociocultural history and data from family members. Territo, Nathanson, and Langer (1996) add the need for an extensive medical history and the inclusion of functional capacities and support systems. They also suggest consideration of the assessment data in comparison to the client's peers. Other basic variables should include appearance, affect, intellect, memory, judgment, orientation, level of independence, and physical limitations.

All the pieces of practice should be driven by the assessment since it is where the social worker makes sense of the data and formulates a case theory that provides an explanation unique to this client and situation. Kivnick and Murray (2001) urge social workers to go beyond the basic data to find the uniqueness of each elderly human. Keller and Bromley admonish that "viewing all elderly as alike is a common mistake that disregards their variability of experiences, situations, and expectations" (1989, p. 30). Moreover, they stress the importance of context in understanding the needs of older persons; their problems are not solely products of aging.

It is the case theory that links together the range of relevant data collected and organizes it into a coherent whole to understand a specific client and to intervene. The idiographic (applies only to a specific case) nature of case theory distinguishes it from the nomothetic (applies to groups of persons) social and behavioral theories (see Bisman, 1999, for fuller discussion). The assessment and case theory grounds the social worker's decision-making in choosing from the range of social and behavioral theories discussed later in the section on theoretical models. In fact, it is likely that in practice with the rural elderly the social worker might well draw from all of them including social support, family systems, group work, and case management and community practice.

Biopsychosocial. It is critically important that social work assessments with the elderly are truly biopsychosocial in scope. Greene (2000) points to the need for a functional assessment that takes into account the social work perspective inclusive of the biological, psychological and social. She explains that the biological addresses health related issues, medications and drug effects, disorders and brain functioning. The psychological includes history of affective and emotional functioning, and thoughts about one's own aging. Sociocultural for Greene refers to role and status, and the meaning of work and retirement.

Kivnick and Murray (2001) also support exploration of the physiological and psychosocial and suggest using, but not limiting oneself to, agency mandated assessment tools such as the Resident Assessment Instrument (RAI) in nursing homes or the Minimum Data Set (MDS) that had been available from the Health Care Financing Administration. McQuellon and Reifler (1989), as well, stress the importance of a comprehensive assessment that presents the what and the why. For them it must be biopsychosocial in breadth and family centered, presenting symptoms, the problem situation and the worker's judgments. Many agencies and funding sources require completion of specific intake forms, inventories or scales, and social workers must be familiar with them. Yet, as important as these forms are, they cannot substitute for the case theory which integrates the range of information collected with the relevant theoretical models into the social worker's biopsychosocial theory of this particular case. Social work's mission requires this breadth and practice with the rural elderly demands that social workers address the physical, psychological and social problems that can benefit from intervention (Keller and Bromley, 1989). Morse (1989) adds that for 'good' old age one needs "good health, good feelings of self-worth and a good sense of economic security" (1989, p. 133), pointing again to the bio, psycho and social aspects of aging and the need to include these in assessments of the elderly.

Family assessments should address intergenerational and historical issues and include such factors as caregiving, role shifts, family life cycle, education and income level, financial health, access to resources, and level of family support.

Practitioner Observation. Distinction between the professional and personal selves was recognized early by social work (Reynolds, 1970, 1942; Hamilton, 1946). Practitioner observation is central to social workers' ability to be aware of and monitor their personal reactions and biases so that they can maintain focus on what is happening and on what is best for the client.

Mercer (1992) encourages those who practice with the elderly to acknowledge and articulate their own feelings about aging and death and cautions that frailty does not need to equate with loss of autonomy or independence. Those who are elderly are still expert on their own lives and have the right to be self-determining. Marino (1996) concurs, emphasizing the multitude of losses the elderly face including death and dying, functioning (physical and mental), finances, life style, relationships, privacy and independence (the latter two are often especially important to the rural elderly). Social workers may become overly emotional or involved with these compelling changes unless they become aware of their own attitudes about aging, loss, dependency, and family responsibility.

Richards (2000) advises that practitioners attend to their own assumptions such as that the elderly are passive or unable to state their needs. Silverstone (1996) cautions about prejudices against the elderly and rural areas as well as sexism and classism and discusses the importance of overcoming these biases. Silverstone and Burack-Weiss (1983) further encourage practitioners to confront their own vulnerability, and that warmth and caring should not become patronizing.

Ginsberg reminds us that "there is probably a greater range in the capacities and socioeconomic characteristics of older adults than of any other population group . . . " (2001, p. 139). Differences may include ethnicity, culture, income, education, gender, life experience, health history, personality, and, moreover, aging is uneven. It is critical that social workers not treat the elderly as one homogeneous group.

THEORETICAL MODELS AND INTERVENTIONS

In this section I consider four theoretical models, including interventions, that are relevant for practice with the rural elderly. These models are social support, family systems, group work, and case management and community practice. For effective practice, social workers need concepts and theories that relate to the problems experienced by the rural elderly. Yet, social workers must also appreciate the distinction between concepts and theories and understand their relationship to interventions.

Theories are broad explanations to make sense of a range of phenomena in the world while concepts are the mental constructions, represented by a label, that help comprise the theory (see Bisman and Hardcastle, 1999, for further development). For example, in the sections below I consider family systems theory along with its concepts of boundaries, homeostasis and feedback. Interventions are the activities and behaviors specifically planned and implemented to change the elderly person's situation. Included are short- and long-term goals, contracts, environmental outcomes, measurement and evaluation. For treatment integrity and practitioner accountability, social workers must be able to measure the treatment's implementation, control intervention drift (unintentional change) and shift interventions when necessary.

The cultural and social features of rural areas are factors to consider in choosing a theoretical model and intervention approach. Of the many models relevant to practice with this population, social support and family systems seem especially germane, and we begin with social support. There are many other models that are also pertinent which I discuss or have cited earlier, including problem-solving, psycho-social, brief treatment, ecological and psychoanalytic.

Social Support

Concepts. In his seminal article, Specht (1986) seeks to clarify some of the definitional problems with social support and its related concepts.

While *social support* is broad and refers to social interaction, Specht explains that *social network* is more specific and unique for each person referring to a "specific set of interrelated persons" (p. 220) including memberships and relationships. Social exchange involves the power of individuals in their network; increases in the number of exchanges correspondingly increases the power. *Density* concerns the proportion of actual exchanges to the potential number. *Collaterals* are the others who constitute the networks, those who exchange the resources. He points to the need for further research to study the relationship between social support and better health or well-being as it may be that well-being increases social supports (instead of the commonly accepted opposite). In the same vein, he points out the confusions with this concept. Although in the literature, social support generally means social interaction, it is often not distinguished from the subjective sense felt by someone and the actual supportive behaviors.

Haber's (1999) definition of social support refers to this subjectivity, the "perceived caring, esteem, and assistance people receive from others. Support can come from spouses, family members, friends, neighbors, colleagues, health professionals, or pets" (p. 212). Haber identifies three types of support (1) *emotional*–sense of love, belonging, reassurance, (2) *instrumental*–tangible aid and services), (3) *informational*–advice, feedback. Cohen and Syme (1985) share some of Specht's concerns, pointing to the difficulty in differentiating effects of social support from other psychological and social factors. They also discuss the functions that the structures serve, including the provision of affection and feelings of belonging. These authors believe that individuals' perceptions of their functional levels may be able to provide psychological representations of support systems while objective measures of the structural supports could help to determine the resources that affect health and behavior.

Over these past two decades empirical data to clarify the meaning, functions and effects of social support remain elusive. Although the concept endures in the literature, the research findings are not conclusive. Pearlin, Aneshensel, Mullan, and Whitlatch (1996) comment on the necessity of social supports for the well-being of the elderly, and Monohan and Hooker (1997) state that "*perceived support* is an essential dimension of social support in caregiving relationships" (p. 289). They argue that spouse caregivers of Alzheimer's need more attention from providers than caregivers of Parkinson's. Their claim is supported by Tebb and Jivanjee's (2000) assertions that caregivers of Alzheimer's are often isolated. As the "hidden patient," the caregivers' social contacts have decreased, and as well they experience a loss of a sense of wholeness. This becomes cumulative covering biophysical, psychoemotional, social and economic. The authors assume that supportive interventions early in the process will reduce caregiver isolation.

On the other hand, Heenan (2000) finds in her study of farming families that farm wives experience the caregiving as rewarding and positive. While resisting formal social services, these rural women are able to place the caring within the context of a complex ongoing relationship. And, although Israel and Schurman (1990) assert that *social isolation* has as strong an effect on mortality as smoking or high cholesterol, they do admit that while there has been support in the literature for this claim, rigorous studies are lacking. These authors also acknowledge that there seems to be a greater correlation of negative relationships (mistrust and troubles) with poor mental health than that of social support with good mental health. Antonucci and Jackson offer an additional perspective "that social support operates by transferring the beliefs of the supportive other in the ability of the target person to perform a task, thereby increasing the target person's self-efficacy" (1987, p. 301). Perhaps, social support is a necessary but not sufficient condition for overall health, but more research is needed.

Minkler (1985) cautions about assuming homogeneity of the elderly, believing that the relationships among social supports, networks and health for the elderly may be similar to the rest of the population (although acknowledging that those who are isolated or institutionalized may be disadvantaged). For her, the elderly often confront a contracting of their social world because of deaths and geographic moves, but they still possess the basic ingredients for social supports.

Interventions. The rural elderly may face a particular set of social support issues due to geographic distances, limitations of mobility, and the contracting to which Minkler refers. In a follow-up study of families initially interviewed in the 1950s, Phillips, Bernard, Phillipson, and Ogg (2000) found differences in the extent to which the elderly rely on family supportive relationships. Traditionally, family has been viewed as the linchpin of a support network with the spouse, daughter, son–in that order–most crucial. But the authors found the number of family intimates shrinking, to about nine and for some, five or less. The questions the authors raise in the 2000 study are not whether family provides support but how is the support given and what are its limits.

> Social work with older people must address issues about where people live, and the pressures they experience in these environments. A more holistic assessment of people's needs is therefore

> called for, spanning their wider housing and environmental needs and not being confined to health and social issues. (p. 851)

These authors admonish that practitioners not assume that all family members are equally involved and that they should look beyond family to close friends. Practitioners must know and understand the clients' informal and formal networks of social supports, actual and potential primary supports (family, kin), and possible secondary supports (neighbors, friends, community). In this study, interestingly, it was the middle income families that made greater use of tertiary supports (formal support agencies such as welfare services).

It is necessary to note that when this study was first conducted, forty years ago, the British communities studied were close and geographically distinct. Changes in American rural communities, as in Britain, will continue to impact on the social supports available from family members and close friends. Finally, practitioners will need community assessment skills in order to capture the different patterns of service in each community.

Antonucci and Jackson (1987) believe there is a relationship between social support and psychological and physical health. They suggest targeting both the older person and the support providers for efficacy enhancing (sensitize them to the difficulty of certain tasks, etc.) with a focus on specific health behaviors. They further propose a reciprocity perspective with use of accumulated credits in a 'support bank.' Antonucci (1988) later considers a variable reciprocity wherein the elderly may receive more from their children but still engage in reciprocal relationships with friends and neighbors. She encourages health care advocacy and interventions to develop peer and group services. Goals of practice should seek to improve interactions between the elderly and social institutions.

Territo, Nathanson, and Langer (1996) also discuss the importance of improving connections between the elderly and community systems. These include the community gatekeepers (non-traditional neighborhood personnel such as pharmacists, postal deliverers, meter readers) and informal social supports (enduring, non-professional relationships). Carstensen (1987) believes there is no consensus about the importance of social activity for the elderly and that the best indicator of the optimal level of activity is the individual's prior level of contacts. If these differ significantly, the social worker should examine the physical and social barriers, using both phone contact and visitation. She further posits that loneliness is related to loss of confidantes, not necessarily to a low rate of activity. Carstensen encourages maintenance of previous contacts because "humans are social animals . . . <we> live most of our lives in highly complex interdependent social systems that provide us with a sense of purpose and identity" (p. 234).

Despite the lack of research consensus on the meaning of social support, there is agreement on the relevance of the social world for the rural elderly. The task for social workers is to make sense of the research and to gain familiarity with the range of theories, concepts and interventions. This is especially important in practice with the rural elderly where distances may make frequent visitation difficult (for the social worker as well as for the family members). Territo, Nathanson, and Langer stress that an emphasis on social functioning in practice with the elderly is to help them "achieve fulfillment and function as productive and contributing members of society" (1996, p. 116). Social interactions, be they by and/or with organizations, communities, friends, individuals, or families are the thrust of social work interventions. We next consider family systems as a conceptual framework for interventions with the rural elderly.

Family Systems

Concepts. Systems theory has remained the foundation for most of the major schools of family therapy since the late 1960s. The following concepts (italicized) are central to understanding the family as a system. The extent to which the family is *open or closed* refers to the capacity of the family to engage in exchanges with its environment. A system that is open can receive input, ideas and energy while a closed system tends to entropy through its lack of adaptability. *Boundaries* establish the invisible lines that separate what is inside the family from the external world and as well the different family subsystems from each other (members belong to more than one subsystem such as mother and child, mother and father, etc.). These boundary lines may be expressed by family rules and the roles of family members. The flexibility of the boundaries helps to determine the system's openness and its ability to receive *feedback*, without which the family cannot adjust its future by changing its behavior based on received information. *Homeostasis* refers to the family's push to maintain stability.

These concepts are intricately linked with each other, and a finely tuned balance of each of these attributes can result in a high-functioning family. The elderly have been members of a family for a long time and have likely had experiences of open and closed systems, balance and chaos, adaptability and rigidity. Yet, for many elderly, their family life is undergoing major alteration. Individuals' perceptions of family are highly emotional and primitive. It is through family, after all, that each person shapes a sense of identity and belonging at home and in the wider world. Family changes in the later years challenge these basic assumptions.

Interventions. Greene (1989) explains that increases in life expectancy have resulted in the need for greater attention to parent-child relationships. She points to the reciprocal interactions among generations and links based on indebtedness, loyalty and reciprocity. For Greene, the family system is adaptive. Family therapy looks at the impact of members' behavior on each other and should seek to alleviate problems by modifying structure and patterns of communication and mobilizing the family as a resource for itself and its members.

Silverman, Kahn, and Anderson remind us that "aging is not a sudden, drastic event, it is a continuous process, the evolution of patterns established earlier in life. . . . It is a mistake to consider them as one group or treat them as isolated beings" (1986, p. 171). They emphasize that the life styles of elderly persons are rooted in family subsystems, requiring practitioners to consider the elder's place in the family dynamics and to use the whole family as a resource. These authors suggest including the younger generations in treatment of the elderly to increase their knowledge about the aging process and awareness of their responses to the parents' aging. This approach can utilize group problem-solving, produce wider access to community supports and improve the support system in the family.

Nieto, Coward and Horsley (1989) offer principles to guide interactions with later-life families. They emphasize that practitioners use their professional authority, cast the net widely to increase levels of participation and collaboration by all members of the family, employ the least disruptive intervention, and seek to clarify perceptions, expectations, rules and roles. Bonjean (1989) favors combining individual therapy for the primary caregiver with family therapy. She begins with the patient as the problem, then shifts to the family and its adjustment. Emphasizing a strengths perspective, Bonjean believes it important to convey belief in the capacities of the family while helping to diffuse old battles. She assesses the physical and psychological and addresses feelings, day care decisions, and community resources. Morse (1989) advises practitioners to consider the role of money in the family, and underscores the need to help with financial planning, wills and funeral plans.

Perspectives differ on the use of psychotherapy with elderly families. Tepper (1996) states that problems for these families are often in daily living, suggesting there is no need for long-term focus on personality change, but rather a need to problem-solve and to use empathy. He encourages practitioners to facilitate (1) setting of realistic goals, (2) sharing by family members, (3) defining the problem, (4) full participation of family, (5) discussion of anger, and (6) a mobilization of energy.

While Keller and Bromley (1989) believe that physical, social and psychological changes can accrue for families from a psychotherapeutic approach, they do caution practitioners to assure that the family has adequate support systems for income, diet, health and health care resources, housing, and transportation. These authors suggest a focus on family patterns via the following techniques: (1) emotional connections review, (2) family meeting, (3) probing for strengths, (4) counter-pointing realities (unfold multiple realities), (5) structured reminiscence. Christopherson (1989) supports insight-oriented therapy but acknowledges that it can be a mixed blessing. For him, acceptance of responsibility must accompany increased awareness and understanding of dynamics.

Issues of loss are of concern for some authors. Osgood (1989) comments on the high rate of suicide among the elderly, relating this phenomenon to cultural issues (modernization and urbanization), social change, reduction of status and psychological problems (loss, depression, alcoholism). She encourages practitioners to assess suicidal risk, and if necessary, provide family therapy for suicide prevention. Williams distinguishes grief "complex painful effects and the emotional response to loss" from mourning "the process that one goes through in bereavement, including the many and varied rituals associated with loss" (1989, p. 226). He believes that in order to be able to talk directly about death practitioners need to attend to their own history of loss (discussed earlier in the section on practitioner observation) as well as to provide help with concrete needs, comfort, support and consolation, and the acceptance of loss.

Several authors support use of reminiscence with aging families. Hughston and Cooledge (1989) encourage reviewing the family's history through the use of tapes, journals or direct narrative. The reminiscence can include life span successes and problems as well as recognition of conflicting recollections. Confronting the past may help deal with the present and generate new interests, while the reminiscence may offer meaning, assist mourning and stimulate cognition. This process can provide validation and support self-esteem. Territo, Nathanson, and Langer (1996) recommend use of reminiscence in psychotherapy on a case by case basis. Coleman (1986) considers reminiscence a potentially productive therapeutic approach as part of an assessment that seeks to understand the client's view by learning about life history and circumstances. For him, positive memories are strengths to draw from. While this process seems to come naturally to older people, they may need prompting by the social worker.

Reminiscence seems a particularly useful technique for practice with rural families. Although this population may not be especially receptive to formal programs (Filinson, 1986), the opportunity to review the past via telling stories, especially 'passing down' the family's history to the younger folks, is likely to seem appealing and even enjoyable.

Group Work

Concepts. Reid (1997) explains that the purpose of the social work method of group work is to help members cope and reach a higher level of social functioning. Groups become vehicles for their members to create positive change outside the group setting. This process relies on the following concepts. *Self-observation* refers to the capacity for self-awareness that may include some introspection and insight about one's thoughts, feelings, perceptions and communications. *Empowerment* is at its core "self-action and self-definition, with individuals acting singly or collectively to achieve greater control over their loves and destinies" (p. 16). An emphasis on s*trengths* involves a focus on the client's assets, capacities, coping strategies and desire to change. Those who have managed to reach the state of being elderly have much strength to emphasize, praise and draw from in this new phase of their lives. For some elderly, there are shifts from reliance on family to a greater connection to group memberships.

Interventions. In rural areas it is likely that group members will know each other and that the group leader is the primary unknown. Such situations require the social worker to gain the trust of the participants and engage them through the development of group rules, contracts and expectations. Farley, Griffiths, Skidmore, and Thackeray (1982) identify ways for social workers to prepare for an effective group work process. They discuss such specifics as identification of criteria for membership, whether the group is open or closed, using a co-leader (especially important if one does not reside in the community), frequency and length of meeting times. Social or recreational groups can be inter-generational. Planning and activity groups can engage the rural elderly in advocacy for community resources and development. Religious groups may also offer possibilities to engage this population.

Filinson (1986) indicates that the rural elderly tend not to seek formal help, partly due to resource limitation and partly out of their wish to remain independent. Self-help (mutual help and peer support) is flexible, less costly and likely more amenable to this population. Furthermore, it can provide a compensatory social support network, a forum for sharing experiences. Self-help groups can target caregivers, focus on behavior modification or problem-solving, and build self esteem. Cohen and Syme (1985) suggest use of social support groups to alter behaviors and emotions such as substance abuse and depression. Barker (1987) discusses a range of group approaches including life review, peer counseling, reality therapy. Cautioning to respect participants' fears, in his view, groups provide a viable milieu to cover such personal areas as the needs for touch, intimacy, and sex.

Israel and Schurman (1990) believe that neighbors, churches and community groups can provide lay support by complementing professional helpers, creating an exciting synergy. Professionals can aid these peer supports by providing training in facilitation skills, offering knowledge, and arranging for referrals to existing groups. Coleman (1986) recommends the use of group reminiscence therapy with the use of visual aids to help elders share experiences and stimulate memories. He cautions that practitioners should use this tool to stimulate and preserve mental functioning, rather than to brood on the past.

The rural elderly may not be as willing to join support groups but may rather participate in task or activity groups such as wood-working, gardening, quilt-making, sewing, knitting (Farley, Griffiths, Skidmore, and Thackeray, 1982). Pets are increasingly a resource with the elderly and those with disabilities, and are often used in nursing homes for companionship and bonding. There are creative ways to connect those rural elderly who can no longer care for their own pets (but who may have extensive prior experience) with animals on farms or in shelters.

Case Management and Community Practice

Concepts. Hardcastle, Wenocur, and Powers (1997) frame case management as community and inter-organizational practice. Similar to family practice, they draw from systems theorists for conceptual grounding. Although they see "communities as systems composed of subsystems such as mental health systems, community support systems, social service systems" (p. 399), they are concerned that social workers make sure that these systems are functional for clients. For them, case management "entails direct practice, community organization, and management . . . " (p. 390) and is distinguished by its emphasis on the social component and context of the client's condition and on the achievement of goals and objectives. This requires an orientation to management as well as to community practice. For them *community practice* "is the application of practice skills to alter the behavioral patterns of community groups, organizations, and institutions or people's relationships and interactions with these entities" (p. 1). *Management* refers to the social worker's responsibility to "integrate the array of services and social supports into a social system so that the client can achieve the objectives" (p. 391).

Interventions. Losses of family ties may increase the needs for case managers to organize the various elements necessary for healthy functioning. Yet, Ginsberg (1993) explains that rural areas often lack the necessary numbers of professionals and resources. Furthermore, while professional resources are scarce, they are not necessarily accepted. Often, rural populations rely on services where they know the providers. Social workers, therefore, need to know the community and have others know them, perhaps through providing some services informally, such as breakfast or coffee in a local place.

York, Denton, and Moran (1983) acknowledge some of the difficulties in defining rurality, but urge identification of the sociocultural factors of a community that will be important in shaping practice including geography, social problems, values, and types of service providers. Martinez-Brawley (1993) emphasizes that good community practice is egalitarian and non-bureaucratic. Mermelstein and Sundet (1993) encourage the targeting of community norms for change such as views about substance abuse, depression and dependency. They stress the importance of the role of case manager as a social broker and advocate. Silverstone and Burack-Weiss (1983) discuss case management in terms of providing an auxiliary function, filling in for losses and providing temporary strength for families while building community resources.

Austin (1996) discusses the outreach function of the case manager including the following tasks: (1) screening, (2) assessment, (3) care planning, (4) service arrangements, (5) monitoring and re-assessments. She expects case managers to not only publicize agency services but to identify those who qualify and to assure the delivery of appropriate services. To function as both advocate and agency employee social workers must be able to manage potential role conflict. Austin sees case management as the bridge between the institution and the community and anticipates that it "will continue to be a central function and service in the provision of community-based, long-term care services" (p. 173). Cicerelli and Browne (1986) explain that day care services for elderly people can serve to maintain, restore and rehabilitate individuals and also promote socialization and respite for caretakers. As case managers, social workers may need to assist rural areas to develop day care programs including related services such as congregate meal sites.

Jeffrey (1986) argues for direct involvement by therapists in services to elderly, stating that "it may well be no more cost-effective to work indirectly through care staff and carers than it is to work directly with a few people" (p. 125). Yet he also stresses the necessity of systemic change, "in order successfully to implement meaningful cost-effective therapy, it is necessary to pay attention to the factors of social organization . . . and the nature of the relationship between the therapist/innovator and the care staff who will implement the therapy" (p. 126). The organization is as much the client as are the individuals needing help and the communities in which they reside. Additionally, Jeffrey identifies the following approaches to strengthen residential care for the elderly: (1) gain support of senior management, (2) choose responsive homes, (3) facilitate development of managers, (4) improve communication between managers and staff, (5) remain sensitive to the change process, (6) encourage and participate in team meetings, (7) utilize a systems perspective for problem solving and decision making.

Tobin (1997) emphasizes the importance of community services such as senior centers, congregate dining, and counseling and as well as those that are home-based including transporting clients, arranging for home repair, and regular phone contact. McIntosh, Pearson, and Lebowitz (1997) believe that the elderly may be good candidates for individual, family and group therapies and psychotropic medications but may need to be identified and to receive help in reaching services. They suggest (1) a buddy system to identify new clients, (2) reaching out to community locations, (3) providing transportation services, and (4) delivery of mental health services in community locations outside of traditional clinics.

Successful case management in rural areas involves collaboration with other professionals and with the range of agencies providing service to the elderly. Farley, Griffiths, Skidmore, and Thackeray (1982) comment on the need for social workers to have the ability to practice with institutions of all sizes and to engage in interdisciplinary collaboration and cooperation. This is necessary to engage in prevention activities. They explain primary prevention as increasing the capacities of individuals and communities for general health and well-being. Activities might include stress management, activity groups and senior centers. For them, secondary prevention is through institutions including adult protective services and regular health checks. Tertiary prevention focuses on chronic illnesses by helping the elderly use resources to reduce pain and suffering.

Bassuk and Lessem (2001) emphasize the importance of outreach in rural areas and suggest the building of linkages with physicians and attorneys. Giannetti (1996) concurs, cautioning social workers to refer for medical intervention and, as well, to advocate, educate, monitor, and coordinate. He suggests working with the elderly client in creative ways such as teaching a client to use generic, color-coded charts that match the required pills. Territo, Nathanson, and Langer (1996) discuss the value of multidisciplinary teams to which each profession contributes its distinctive orientation; this mix of differing perspectives can be valuable in analyzing and solving problems. For them, collaborative practice allows for a holistic and integrated service delivery.

CONCLUSION

Social workers who practice with the rural elderly must embrace the person and environment perspective and target the biological, psychological and social domains. This means addressing intrapsychic and interactional problems as well as difficulties with health, and access to financial and other resources in both assessments and interventions. Additionally, this work requires an engagement with multiple levels of practice including individuals, families, groups, organizations and communities. Roles are also varied, incorporating at different times or simultaneously administrator, organizer, planner, consultant, case manager, and therapist. The social worker should be able to collaborate with others and integrate services, yet be able to work independently.

Changes in rural areas are rapid and complex. To practice effectively, social workers can draw guidance from their professional mission to enhance human well-being (which incorporates individual and social well-being) and their ethics including social justice and the dignity and worth of each individual. Theoretical models including, among others, social support, family systems, group work, and case management and community practice must inform and guide interventions.

The diversity and rapid change in this population challenges social workers and makes very real Hassbrook's cautions about the need in rural areas to create opportunities and build better communities (2002). As with all good professional interventions, there is demand not only for wide-ranging knowledge, but also for the capacity to make decisions about the particular theoretical models that are relevant to client problems. Provision of effective practice with the rural elderly requires social work assessments and case theories that reflect sound, knowledgeable, yet creative decision-making.

REFERENCES

Antonucci, T., & Jackson, J. (1987). Social support, interpersonal efficacy and health: A life course perspective. In L. Carstensen & B. Edelstein (Eds.), *Handbook of clinical gerontology* (pp. 291-311). New York: Pergamon.

Antonucci, T. (1988). Reciprocal and nonreciprocal social support: Contrasting sides of intimate relationships. *Journal of Gerontology, 43* (3), 565-73.

Austin, C. (1996). Case management practice with the elderly. Medication utilization problems among the elderly: Implications for social work practice. In M. Holosko, & M. Feit (Eds.), *Social work practice with the elderly* (pp. 151-175). Toronto, Ontario: Canadian Scholars' Press.

Barker, R. (1987). Fears and Phobias. In L. Carstensen, & B. Edelstein (Eds.), *Handbook of clinical gerontology* (pp. 271-303). New York: Pergamon.

Bassuk, K., & Lessem, J. (2001). Collaboration of social workers and attorneys in geriatric community based organizations. *Journal of Gerontological Social Work, 34* (3), 93-108.

Bisman, C., & Hardcastle, D. (1999). *Integrating research into practice: A model for effective social work.* Pacific Grove, CA: Brooks/Cole.

Bisman, C. (1999). Social work assessment: Case theory construction. *Families in Society, 80* (3), 240-246.

Bisman, C. (1994). *Social work practice: Cases and principles.* Pacific Grove, CA: Brooks/Cole.

Bonjean. (1989). Solution focused psychotherapy with families caring for an Alzheimer's patient. In G. Hughston, V. Christopherson, & M. Bonjean (Eds.), *Aging and family therapy: Practitioner perspectives on Golden Pond* (pp. 197-210). New York: The Haworth Press, Inc.

Browne, C. (1995). Empowerment in social work practice with older women. *Social Work, 40*, 358-364.

Carstensen, L. (1987). Age-related changes in social activity. In L. Carstensen & B. Edelstein (Eds.), *Handbook of clinical gerontology* (pp. 222-237). New York: Pergamon.

Christopherson, V. (1989). The burden of insight: A basis for constructive response. In Hughston, G., Christopherson, V., & Bonjean, M. (Eds.), *Aging and family therapy:*

Practitioner perspectives on Golden Pond (pp. 185-196). New York: The Haworth Press, Inc.

Cicerelli, V., & Browne, E. (1986). Psychological considerations in the day care of elderly people. In I. Hanley, & M. Gilhooly (Eds.), *Psychological therapies for the elderly* (pp. 80-100). New York: NYU Press.

Cohen, S., & Syme, L. (Eds.). (1985). *Social support and health.* Orlando, FL: Academic Press.

Coleman, P. (1986). Issues in the therapeutic use of reminiscence with elderly people. In I. Hanley, & M. Gilhooly (Eds.), *Psychological therapies for the elderly* (pp. 41-64). New York: NYU Press.

Compton, B. R., & Galaway, B. (1998). *Social work processes.* Pacific Grove, CA: Brooks/Cole.

Farley, O., Griffiths, K., Skidmore, R., & Thackeray, M. (1982). *Rural social work practice.* New York: Free Press.

Filinson, R. (1986). Self help and family support groups. In I. Hanley. & M. Gilhooly (Eds.), *Psychological therapies for the elderly* (pp. 101-123). New York: NYU Press.

Giannetti, V. (1996). Medication utilization problems among the elderly: Implications for social work practice. In M. Holosko, & M. Feit (Eds.), *Social work practice with the elderly* (pp. 87-101). Toronto, Ontario: Canadian Scholars' Press.

Ginsberg, L. (2001). *Careers in social work.* Needham Heights, MA.

Ginsberg, L. (Ed.). (1993). *Social work in rural communities* (2nd ed.). Alexandria, VA: CSWE.

Greene, R. (2000). Serving the aged and their families in the 21st century using a revised practice model. *Journal of Gerontological Social Work, 34* (1), 43-62.

Greene, R. (1989). A life systems approach to understanding parent-child relationships in aging families. In G. Hughston, V. Christopherson, & M. Bonjean (Eds.), *Aging and family therapy: Practitioner perspectives on Golden Pond* (pp. 57-69). New York: The Haworth Press, Inc.

Haber, D. (1999). *Health promotion and aging* (2nd ed.). New York: Springer.

Hamilton, G. (1946). *Social casework.* New York: Columbia University Press.

Hassbrook, C. (2002, April 14). Will rural America have a future. *The New York Times*, pp. WIR, 13.

Hardcastle, D., Wenocur, S., & Powers, P. (1997). *Community practice: Theories and skills for social workers.* Pacific Grove, CA: Brooks/Cole.

Heenan, D. (2000, December). Informal care in farming families in Northern Ireland: Some considerations for social work. *The British Journal of Social Work, 30* (6), 855-866.

Holosko, M., & Holosko, A. (1996). What's unique about social work practice with the elderly, In M. Holosko, & M. Feit (Eds.), *Social work practice with the elderly* (pp. 21-35). Toronto, Ontario: Canadian Scholars' Press.

Hughston, G., & Cooledge, N. (1989). The life review: An underutilized strategy for systemic family intervention. In G. Hughston, V. Christopherson, & M. Bonjean (Eds.), *Aging and family therapy: Practitioner perspectives on Golden Pond* (pp. 47-55). New York: The Haworth Press, Inc.

Israel, B., & Schurman, S. (1990). Social support, control and the stress process. In K. Glanz (Ed.), *Health behavior and health education: Theory, research and practice* (pp. 196-201). Pacific Grove, CA: Jossey Bass.

Jeffrey, D. (1986). The systems approach to changing practice in residential care. In I. Hanley, & M. Gilhooly (Eds.), *Psychological therapies for the elderly* (pp. 124-150). New York: NYU Press.

Keller, J., & Bromley, M. (1989). Psychotherapy with the elderly: A systemic model. In G. Hughston, V. Christopherson, & M. Bonjean (Eds.), *Aging and family therapy: Practitioner perspectives on Golden Pond* (pp. 29-46). New York: The Haworth Press, Inc.

Kivnick, H., & Murray, S. (2001). Life strengths interview guide: Assessing elder clients' strengths. *Journal of Gerontological Social Work, 34* (4), 7-31.

Marino, S. (1996). Selected problems in counselling the elderly. In M. Holosko, & M. Feit (Eds.), *Social work practice with the elderly* (pp. 54-85). Toronto, Ontario: Canadian Scholars' Press.

Martinez-Brawley, E. (1993). Community-oriented rural practice. In Ginsberg, L. (Ed.). *Social work in rural communities* (2nd ed., pp. 67-81). Alexandria, VA: CSWE.

McIntosh, J., Pearson, J., & Lebowitz, B. (1997). Mental disorders of elderly men. In J. Kosberg, & L. Kaye (Eds.), *Elderly men: Special problems and professional challenges* (pp. 193-215). New York: Springer.

McQuellon, R., & Reifler, B. (1989). Caring for the depressed elderly and their families. In G. Hughston, V. Christopherson, & M. Bonjean (Eds.), *Aging and family therapy: Practitioner perspectives on Golden Pond* (pp. 97-116). NY: The Haworth Press, Inc.

Mercer, S. (1992). Suicide and the elderly, In F. Turner (Ed.), *Mental health and the elderly: A social work perspective* (pp. 425-453). New York: Free Press.

Mermelstein, J., & Sundet, P. (1993). Social work practice in rural mental health. In L. Ginsberg (Ed.). *Social work in rural communities* (2nd ed., pp. 82-98). Alexandria, VA: CSWE.

Minkler, M. (1985). Social support and the elderly. In Cohen, S., & Syme, L. (Eds.), *Social support and health* (pp. 199-216.) Orlando, FL: Academic Press.

Monohan, D., & Hooker, K. (1997). Caregiving and social support in two illness groups. *Social Work, 42*, 278-287.

Morse, R. (1989). Roles of the psychotherapist in family financial counseling: A systems approach to prolongation of independence. In G. Hughston, V. Christopherson, & M. Bonjean (Eds.), *Aging and family therapy: Practitioner perspectives on Golden Pond* (pp. 133-147). New York: The Haworth Press, Inc.

NASW. (1999). *Code of Ethics*. Washington, DC: NASW.

Nieto, D., Coward, R., & Horsley, D. (1989). Principles of therapeutic intervention with elders and their families. In G. Hughston, V. Christopherson, & M. Bonjean (Eds.), *Aging and family therapy: Practitioner perspectives on Golden Pond* (pp. 13-27. New York: The Haworth Press, Inc.

Osgood, N. (1989). A systems approach to suicide prevention. In G. Hughston, V. Christopherson, & M. Bonjean (Eds.), *Aging and family therapy: Practitioner perspectives on Golden Pond* (pp. 117-131). New York: The Haworth Press, Inc.

Pearlin, L.I., Aneshensel, C.S., Mullan, J.T., & Whitlatch, C.J. (1996). Caregiving and its social support. In R.H. Binstock, & L. George (Eds.), *Handbook of aging and the social sciences* (pp. 283-302). San Diego: Academic Press.

Phillips, J., Bernard, M., Phillipson, C., & Ogg, J. (2000, December).Social support in later life: A study of three areas. *The British Journal of Social Work, 30* (6), 837-859.

Reynolds, B. (1970, 1942). *Learning and teaching in the practice of social work.* New York: Russell and Russell.

Reid, K. (1997). *Social work practice with groups: A clinical perspective.* Pacific Grove, CA: Brooks/Cole.

Richards, S. (2000). Bridging the divide: Elders and the assessment process. *British Journal of Social Work, 30*, 37-49.

Ryan, E., Merdeith, S., & MacLean, M. (1995). Changing the way we talk with elders: Promoting health using the communication enhancement model. *International Journal of Aging and Human Development, 41* (2), 89-107.

Silverman, A., Kahn, B., & Anderson, G. (1986). A model for working with multigenerational families. In Meyer, C. (Ed.), *Social work with the aging* (pp. 171-175). Silver Spring, MD: NASW.

Silverstone, B., & Burack-Weiss, A. (1983). *Social work practice with the frail elderly and their families: The auxiliary function model.* Springfield, IL: Charles C. Thomas.

Silverstone, B. (1996). Practice with older persons: Challenges and opportunities. In I. Gutheil (Ed.), *Work with older people: Challenges and opportunities*, (pp. 9-28). New York: Fordham University Press.

Specht, H. (1986). Social support, social networks, social exchange, and social work practice. *Social Service Review, 60*, 218-240.

Solomon, B. (1976). *Black empowerment: Social work in oppressed communities.* New York: Columbia University Press.

Tebb, S., & Jivanjee, P. (2000). Caregiving isolation: An ecological model. *Journal of Gerontological Social Work, 34* (2), 51-72.

Tepper, L. (1996). Family relationships in later life. In I. Gutheil (Ed.), *Work with older people: Challenges and opportunities* (pp. 42-62). New York: Fordham University Press.

Territo, T., Nathanson, I., & Langer, N. (1996). *Elder practice: A multidisciplinary approach to working with older adults in the community.* Columbia, SC: University of South Carolina Press.

Tobin, S. (1997). Community programs and services. In J. Kosberg, & L. Kaye (Eds.), *Elderly men: Special problems and professional challenges* (pp. 250-261). New York: Springer.

Williams, F. (1989). Bereavement and the elderly: The role of the psychotherapist. In G. Hughston, V. Christopherson, & M. Bonjean (Eds.), *Aging and family therapy: Practitioner perspectives on Golden Pond* (pp. 225-241). New York: The Haworth Press, Inc.

York, R., Denton, R., & Moran, J. (1993). Rural and urban social work practice: Is there a difference. In L. Ginsberg (Ed.), *Social work in rural communities* (2nd ed., pp. 53-66). Alexandria, VA: CSWE.

Chapter 4

Advocacy Techniques with Older Adults in Rural Environments

Sandra S. Butler, PhD
Nancy M. Webster, MSW

SUMMARY. This chapter examines the essential social work practice role of advocacy and its implementation for gerontological social work practice in rural areas. We begin by reviewing some of the many ways social work advocacy has been defined over the years and specifically how advocacy can be used in social work practice with older adults. Particular attention is given to an advocacy model currently utilized in rural Maine–the Integrated Case Management model–and how it is precisely well-suited to the needs of rural elders. We conclude with recommendations regarding the incorporation of advocacy into rural gerontological social work practice. *[Article copies available for a fee from The Haworth Document Delivery Service: 1-800-HAWORTH. E-mail address: <docdelivery@haworthpress.com> Website: <http://www.HaworthPress.com> © 2003 by The Haworth Press, Inc. All rights reserved.]*

KEYWORDS. Advocacy, rural social work, rural elders

[Haworth co-indexing entry note]: "Advocacy Techniques with Older Adults in Rural Environments." Butler, Sandra, S., and Nancy M. Webster. Co-published simultaneously in *Journal of Gerontological Social Work* (The Haworth Social Work Practice Press, an imprint of The Haworth Press, Inc.) Vol. 41, No. 1/2, 2003, pp. 59-74; and: *Gerontological Social Work in Small Towns and Rural Communities* (ed: Sandra S. Butler, and Lenard W. Kaye) The Haworth Social Work Practice Press, an imprint of The Haworth Press, Inc., 2003, pp. 59-74. Single or multiple copies of this article are available for a fee from The Haworth Document Delivery Service [1-800-HAWORTH, 9:00 a.m. - 5:00 p.m. (EST). E-mail address: docdelivery@haworthpress.com].

http://www.haworthpress.com/web/JGSW
© 2003 by The Haworth Press, Inc. All rights reserved.
Digital Object Identifier: 10.1300/J083v41n01_04

INTRODUCTION

The practice role of advocacy is firmly situated in the social work profession's *Code of Ethics*. The ethical obligation of social workers to advocate for individual and societal well-being is reiterated throughout the document (NASW, 1996). For example, under Section 3, "Social Workers' Ethical Responsibility in Practice Settings," practitioners are told to "advocate within and outside their agencies for adequate resources to meet clients' needs" (NASW, Sec. 3.07a, p. 20) and to "advocate for resource allocation procedures that are open and fair" (NASW, Sec. 3.07b, p. 21). Under Section 6, "Social Workers' Ethical Responsibilities to the Broader Society," we learn that we should "advocate for living conditions conducive to the fulfillment of basic human needs and should promote social, economic, political and cultural values and institutions that are compatible with the realization of social justice" (NASW, Sec. 6.04a, p. 27).

In this chapter, we will examine this essential social work practice role of advocacy and its implementation for gerontological social work practice in rural areas. After reviewing some of the many ways that social work advocacy has been defined over the years, we will compare and contrast advocacy to other practice roles and look specifically at how advocacy can be used in social work practice with older adults. The challenges and opportunities for advocacy work with elders in rural areas will be explored and illustrated with a case example from the literature of an outreach program in the Southeast, and one from our practice experience in rural Maine. This latter example will describe an innovative rural advocacy program, currently assisting families with children, but which will soon be expanded to include elder services. We will conclude with recommendations regarding doing advocacy with older adults in rural areas and small communities.

DEFINING ADVOCACY

Advocacy is one of those practice roles which distinguishes social workers from other helping professions (Sosin & Caulum, 1983). Almost all social workers do some sort of advocacy in their work whether at the individual or institutional level. Nonetheless, we do not all have the same idea of what advocacy means. Defining advocacy can be a slippery endeavor. In reviewing the literature on advocacy twenty years ago, Sosin and Caulum (1983) lamented that "[t]he role of the advocate

. . . seems to be practically synonymous with almost all social work roles" (p.12). One area of confusion regarding advocacy in social work practice is that it is frequently thought of on two levels: case advocacy and cause advocacy. Case advocacy, on the one hand, operates at the micro-level and involves helping clients who are unable to make successful connections to necessary resources. "Advocacy means that social workers collaborate with clients to influence the way other systems respond to a client's attempts to gather resources" (Miley, O'Malia, & DuBois, 2001, p. 319). Cause advocacy, on the other hand, operates at the macro-level, involving the partnership of vulnerable or disenfranchised groups of clients with social workers, who recognize the public issues inherent in personal problems (Miley et al.).

Sosin and Caulum (1983) attempted to bridge these dichotomous meanings of advocacy in order to provide a framework that might be more useful to the social work practitioner. They proposed the following definition:

> An attempt, having greater than zero probability of success, by an individual or group to influence another individual or group to make a decision that would not have been made otherwise and that concerns the welfare or interests of a third party who is in a less powerful status than the decision maker. (p. 13)

According to this definition, advocacy can take place at the individual, administrative or policy level, and chosen strategies will depend on one's relationship to the decision maker and decision making structure.

Nearly 20 years later, Schneider and Lester (2001) return to this problem of describing what has been referred to by some students of the topic as a "conceptual disaster" (p. 58). Schneider and Lester have also attempted to distill a definition of advocacy which is both clear and comprehensive. They suggest that "social work advocacy is the exclusive and mutual representation of a client(s) or a cause in a forum, attempting to systematically influence decision making in an unjust or unresponsive system" (p. 65). Writing at about the same time, Ezell (2001) emphasizes the need for the definition of advocacy to focus on activities rather than roles. He defines advocacy as "those purposive efforts to change specific existing or proposed policies or practices on behalf of or with a specific client or group of clients" (p. 23). The emphasis of this definition is on purposive change of policies and practices as they relate to clients.

To better understand what advocacy is, it is instructive to look at how it differs from other social work activities with which it is closely associated and sometimes confused. For example, how does advocacy differ from brokering, social reform, and social action? While brokering may help an elder get needed services, it is advocacy which comes into play when the brokering is ineffective (Schneider & Lester, 2001). The difference between advocacy and social reform lies mostly in scale: "while the reformer's vision is primarily a large vision about correcting a societal ill, the advocate's perspective will be highly focused on clients' identifiable needs" (Schneider & Lester, p. 70). Sosin and Caulum (1983) further delimit advocacy by stipulating that advocacy occurs within an existing power structure, thereby distinguishing it from social movement or social reform work. Of the various practice roles, advocacy may be most closely related to social action. In fact, advocacy can be viewed as one form of social action, but a form that needs to be directly related to the needs of a particular client or clients (Schneider & Lester, 2001).

ADVOCACY WITH OLDER ADULTS

Hanna (1981), in his exploration of advocacy and the elderly, was also concerned with the multiple definitions of the term advocacy. Nonetheless, he too has settled on a broad definition not unlike those discussed above: An advocate either causes something to happen that will aid in correcting an injustice or prevents something from happening that would create or intensify an injustice. His illustrations of the various ways aging advocacy can be implemented are useful in understanding the scope of this practice role for gerontological social workers:

> [Aging advocacy] can be an *individual* challenging the tactics of a hearing aid salesman, or a *coalition* of national organizations seeking comprehensive health care legislation. It can be an organized *lobby* seeking a more effective legislative policy on aging. It can seek to change individual and societal stereotypes and attitudes through *consciousness-raising* activities. It can be case advocacy, working to assure the rights and benefits of an individual older person; or it can be *class advocacy* representing the rights and benefits of all or large numbers of older persons. It can be *reactive* responding to the actions of others which have a positive or negative affect [sic] on the elderly; or it can be *proactive*, taking

> the initiative in proposing its own new directions and solutions. (Hanna, 1981, p. 299 [italics in the original])

Hyduk and Moxley (2000; 1997) have further defined advocacy with older adults by emphasizing the need to incorporate an empowerment perspective that promotes client control over their daily lives and over the resources they need to live with dignity. These authors label this "personal advocacy" and distinguish it from a more case management approach in that "personal advocacy works to identify user-defined issues and to establish an effort to attack and resolve these issues using the satisfaction of the user as the principal outcome" (1997, p. 89)–a sort of consumer-driven case management (Hyduk & Moxley, 2000). The connection of empowerment practice with advocacy activities is particularly important with populations who are at risk of reduced autonomy and self-determination, as is the case for many of our elderly clients. Advocacy, within the empowerment perspective, enables people without power to articulate and advance their needs, and aims to help vulnerable individuals gain more control over their lives (Hyduk & Moxley, 2000).

One important aspect of social work advocacy with the aged is the training of elders to advocate for themselves (Epstein, West, & Riegel, 2000). Seniors advocating for themselves, with and without the support of social workers, is no longer just social worker advocacy, but rather aging activism. For a fuller discussion of activism among older adults and the benefits of activism for healthy aging, see Butler (in press). For the purposes of this chapter, we will confine our discussion to advocacy by social workers who incorporate an empowerment approach in their work with clients.

ADVOCACY WITH OLDER ADULTS IN RURAL AREAS

One might ask if advocating for older clients takes a different form for social workers practicing in rural areas. Interestingly, a study comparing urban and rural social work practice in North Carolina found few differences between the two groups of respondents with regards to emphasis on the various practice roles, including advocacy (York, Denton, & Moran, 1998). Nonetheless, it is likely that the issues for which rural geriatric social workers must advocate are affected by the special conditions found in non-metropolitan areas (Ritchie, Wieland, Tully, Rowe, Sims, & Bodner, 2002). Rural aging research over the past decades has revealed that services are neither sufficiently available nor accessible to meet the needs of rural elders. For example, rural elders generally have access to a smaller number of community-based services than do urban elders; gaps exist in the continuum of care in rural communities; and service delivery models are rarely designed specifically for rural areas (Krout, 2001). Moreover, there is a higher rate of poverty among rural elders than among their urban counterparts (Stallman, Deller, & Shields, 2001), and some researchers have found rural elders to have more functional health limitations and a greater number of medical conditions than do non-rural elders (Dorfman, 2002). Lack of transportation is one key issue faced by rural practitioners working with older adults. According to the 1990 census, 45% of the rural elderly and 57% of the rural poor had no car (Burkhardt, 2001). Many rural areas have no public transportation whatsoever, making trips to the grocery store and medical appointments difficult, not to mention outings for social interaction.

RURAL ADVOCACY IN GERIATRIC MENTAL HEALTH

Snustad and her colleagues (1993) discuss the particular psychosocial challenges faced by rural elders and an innovative outreach intervention to meet the needs of this population in the rural Southeast. While nearly 25% of the nation's rural elderly population is reported to manifest psychiatric problems, there exists a paucity of local mental health services in rural areas and few psychiatric beds in community hospitals (Snustad, Thompson-Heisterman, Neese, & Abrahm, 1993). Geriatric services, when they do exist, tend to be too narrow in scope to meet the needs of elders and their families, and the absence of formal geriatric mental health services results in higher utilization of local emergency services (Snustad et al.) Mental health care is also inaccessible to rural elders due to fewer trained health professionals in geriatric mental health and the closure of physician practices and community hospitals. As described by Snustad et al.:

> Other barriers to delivering mental health services relate to general lack of knowledge among rural families about mental health and available services, geographic and social isolation, lack of transportation, large catchment areas (encompassing up to 60,000 square miles), concerns about confidentiality, a dearth of suitable service models, and ageism, or relative negative attitudes toward the elderly on the part of health care professionals. (p. 97)

The Jefferson Area Rural Elder Health Outreach Program (REOP) was created in Charlottesville, Virginia to increase equity and accessibility of mental health services to rural elders (Snustad et al., 1993). Advocacy is one of the primary goals of the multidisciplinary teams–including social workers–conducting outreach services for REOP. In addition to its goals of providing assessment and intervention; integrating community services and assuring access; offering counseling and caregiver support; completing psychiatric evaluation and treatment; and carrying out crisis intervention, REOP outreach teams place considerable emphasis on their task of advocacy. Their approach to advocacy exemplifies two of the definitions of advocacy discussed above: advocacy within an empowerment model emphasizing client control (Hyduk & Moxley, 2000; 1997) and the mutual and exclusive representation of clients or causes to systematically influence an unresponsive system (Schneider & Lester, 2001). Snustad et al. describe how REOP integrates advocacy for rural elders into their outreach work:

> Individual advocacy is aimed at empowering clients in their use of the health or social care system, and to enhance patients' and families' self-reliance for self-care. At the community level, bringing the groups caring for the rural elderly together into a coalition has strengthened the power, visibility, and planning abilities of these organizations. Through work with various community groups and participation in public hearings on the health care needs of rural elderly, public attention has been focused on the plight of this population and the issues surrounding rural mental health delivery. Advocacy at the national level has included the preparation of briefing papers for congressional personnel, and presentations to national meetings and conferences. (1993, p. 108)

Social work advocates in rural areas are less likely to have the established advocacy networks existing in metropolitan areas, due to the difficulties associated with building and sustaining these networks in smaller communities (Rathbone-McCuan, 2002). Therefore, rural geriatric social workers must be creative in their advocacy, looking to clients' existing networks to assist in problem solving (Martinez-Brawley, 1998). Moreover, local leadership must feel ownership of programs and services and be involved in generating community solutions for community problems. In other words, social work advocates in rural areas must be political (Martinez-Brawley). Recently, we asked the director of an Area Agency on Aging in rural northeastern Maine if she thought advocacy for elders in rural areas was different from advocacy in non-rural areas. After a moment of thought, she said she thought it was distinct in two ways: On the negative side, there are fewer resources and services for which to advocate, but on the positive side, it is probably easier to get the attention of local and statewide decision makers in trying to bring about change (personal communication with Roberta Downey, January 11, 2002).

We will turn now to describing in detail one model of rural advocacy which has worked extremely well for families with children needing mental health and social services in the State of Maine. We discuss the potential for replicating this model in order to better meet the needs of rural elders.

CASE STUDY OF RURAL ADVOCACY: THE INTENSIVE CASE MANAGEMENT MODEL

Partnering. Bringing advocacy to the rural service arena, whether case or cause, needs to be strengths-based, consumer driven, adherent to natural neighborhood systems and utilize community networks. Bruner (1994) submits that professional expertise is only one form of knowledge. The experience of the consumer and community must also be recognized and valued. Bruner further recommends the concept of "partnering"–utilizing community expertise in conjunction with client insights of day-to-day coping and social worker experience of institutional systems. There is a need to utilize the indigenous capacity of those in the rural communities to construct natural helping networks, an imperative when there is a minimum of services.

In rural areas the issues of the elderly as they relate to case and cause advocacy are myriad, complicated and very frequently merge. For example, transportation issues compound the problems of serving the rural aging population. Additionally, there is less access to social workers that can "partner" with the elderly, less service penetration, and because of this, potentially more need. Moreover, services to rural areas are often fragmented, rule bound and paternalistic. The most useful rural programs are those that focus on helping aging individuals gain control over their lives by managing day-to-day stress, overcoming social isolation, establishing goals and taking steps to meet them. Such programs must be persistent and creative in their outreach to the socially and geographically isolated individual. From a micro practice perspective, helping individuals or families through the morass of services and service providers, understanding and being able to articulate availability of services, and determining what services are needed, can be challenging for the gerontological social worker.

Cause advocacy, as previously described in this chapter, while operating at the macro level, utilizes the concept of "partnering" vulnerable or disenfranchised groups of clients with social workers. Indeed, locating local or regional service providers and designing a plan of integrated services to meet the needs of the rural individual or family is a complex endeavor both for the families and the service providers. Recently, in the State of Maine, a group of concerned individuals used cause advocacy to gain support for a novel approach to meeting the needs of rural children and families and complementing the components of service provision; the new approach was the Integrated Case Management (ICM) model. After describing this model, which is now fully systemized and operational for children and families in the state of Maine, we will apply the concepts of ICM to the elderly rural population–a group the State plans to serve with this model in the near future.

The ICM Model. Integrated Case Management was initially developed by the Maine Department of Human Services for use with children and families. Integrated Case Management was conceptualized in response to a question posed by Maine Governor Angus King in 1997, and as a response to the frustration of families and individuals navigating the demands and requirements of multiple systems and social service organizations. Governor King's question was simply, "How do we know that families being served by more than one department are receiving coordinated, effective and efficient services?" (Maine Children's Cabinet, 2000, p. 3). This question emerged as individuals and family members receiving support from state and local agencies were wrestling with the complex requirements and were apparently being either over-served or underserved. Additionally, few social work "partners" existed in the numerous agencies serving this population–agencies which were neither designed to simplify the issues nor provide integrated service.

The ICM vision was to provide Maine families and children with access to services that were well planned, carefully managed and delivered in a holistic, inclusive and thoughtful manner. Partnering families with social workers in community agencies was paramount and allowed for shared leadership and control, a shared vision, a team approach and continuous assessment (Maine Children's Cabinet, 2000). In order to achieve the vision, several steps were identified and undertaken, including the establishment of Regional ICM Steering Committees; identifying families to participate at two pilot sites; identifying resources needed to make this succeed; and developing training committees to design and conduct training. In spite of the challenges, there was a strong consensus and commitment that actually "doing the work" was the best vehicle for sorting out the strengths and weaknesses of ICM. At both the case and cause advocacy level, the piloting of ICM would determine whether the model was "workable" (Becky Hayes Boober, ICM Steering Committee Member, personal communication, Feb. 12, 2002).

The State of Maine appears a logical testing ground for the concept of Integrated Case Management Services. The state is highly rural with few pockets of urban cluster. Within the state, large geographic distances create transportation challenges. Weather and geography can induce significant isolation. Rural community services are scarce and the state lacks a well-developed network of regional services. Further, while individuals and families were connected to their communities, community resource were fragmented and disconnected. After a comprehensive and in depth study of families receiving multiple services (Maine Children's Cabinet, 2000) and the establishment of two regional pilot projects in the State of Maine, the Integrated Case Management program for children and families became fully systemized in 2000. Currently, plans have begun to extend the ICM program to encompass the elder population in Maine.

How ICM Works. The concept of Integrated Case Management utilizes the social service delivery systems to bring together social workers and the client to determine what services are needed, what services are available, what services are requested, and what services the client believes he or she needs to function optimally. Generally, with the ICM program, service delivery is shared between agencies, dramatically reducing the number of service providers in a family's life and allowing the remaining service providers to more effectively do their job. The family is given a voice, and provided with the support of an individual in the form of a Lead Case Manager (LCM). There is a reduction in the amount of outside intervention in clients' lives and improved utilization of those service providers remaining in their lives.

A recent example of ICM in a family social work intervention began with the realization by social workers that a particular family, consisting of a mother and three children, was utilizing 27 service providers due to their myriad, complex, and interagency needs. The mother was overwhelmed with the amount of social service individuals and support staff moving through her life. She struggled to meet all appointments, which was clearly impossible, and then, when she failed to get to an appointment, she was held accountable and seen as non-compliant. The system that proposed to serve this woman and her children had turned on her by over-serving. This family was recommended to participate in the ICM project at one of the regional sites; meetings were held with all service providers including school personnel. Services were evaluated with an ear to both the objective and "felt" needs of the family. Service providers were able to share particular services through inter-agency agreements; school personnel were kept informed by the Lead Case Manager; transportation issues were addressed, though not fully resolved; housing needs were improved; and the total number of service providers were reduced to seven, including the Lead Case Manager. The family reported feeling heard, understood, relieved, and more able to function autonomously as a family unit without being overwhelmed by the provision of services. Integrated Case Management clearly represented a persistent and creative form of outreach to a socially isolated family. This same approach appears to be well suited to rural elders who also are often either over-served or underserved.

Our current society produces multiple, interwoven, and complex stresses and issues. These components tend to fold in on themselves in rural areas due to geography; poverty; the limited availability of services; the often independent nature of rural individuals; and frequently, a lack of knowledge of how to ask for and utilize services. The result is often an underserved individual or an individual who is overwhelmed with services and service providers. When serving and advocating for rural elders, the spoken and felt need of the individual may be quite simple, but the systems that serve the individual are complex, and unfortunately, service providers may well believe they know what the individual "needs" without truly listening. Because of the complexity of the advocacy response to individual needs in rural areas, including the geographical dispersion of individuals served and the tendency to centralize social service agencies in large communities, ICM services appear to be as ideally suited for social work advocacy with rural elderly recipients of social services as it has been for children and families in Maine.

The ICM model is unique in that it is a collaborative model of service provision, based on what the individual or family knows that they need. It is a strengths-based model that considers: a safety and crisis plan, economic stability, mental health, physical health, spiritual and community natural supports, recreation and social development, and housing and living situations (B. Boober, personal communication, Feb. 12, 2002); of primary importance is that individual and family are major advocates for their own needs. As mentioned earlier, ICM pulls service providers together, allowing all providers to be in the same room with the family, to work for short and long term change, and perhaps most importantly, to work from a strengths based position in providing comprehensive services.

Simply described, the ICM model of advocacy utilizes wraparound case management services, but leaves the family in charge. Lead Case Managers (LCM) are independent facilitators, trained in the local community, and therefore fully aware of community resources. Under the current ICM model, LCMs, in collaboration with the client, convene the ICM team. The ICM team is comprised of social service providers in the region, providers currently serving the family, the child and any family members. The LCM functions in an advocacy role with the client to determine what services are needed, what services are being provided, whether there is duplication of services, and the client's felt or objective needs. There is also assistance and support for the client in developing a comprehensive service plan. The LCM stays involved with the individual or family and can reconvene the ICM team to further assist the family in realizing and honing the plan.

The Potential of ICM for Rural Elders. For elders, the LCM would remain available to the individual for consultation, for discontinuing or for enhancing services. The LCM would also be a resource for the individual and would mitigate the need to state a single request repeatedly to different agency staff, and different service providers. In addition to providing assistance and support the LCM, as a locally trained individual, would be aware of community resources and might be able to assist the individual in developing natural networks with community resources.

Natural support systems are a vital link in supporting aging individuals in all areas but are particularly important in supporting and advocating for individuals in rural areas. Distance and transportation are enormous obstacles in obtaining coherent and holistic services in rural areas. Providing an arena for all individuals serving, and individuals served, to be in one room at one time, not only resolves the challenges for service, but also is a "solution fed" problem solving collaboration for services. The potential compromises of providing services to an individual are illustrated, solutions brainstormed, plans formulated and services implemented. Because the LCM is a local individual and locally trained, he or she is much more likely to have a knowledge base, particularly of natural support systems, than individuals in regionalized offices some distance from the service recipient. As community individuals, LCMs would also be aware of the barriers and impediments to developing a comprehensive, coherent and workable plan for the elderly client and potentially for the client's family.

For success to be achieved in the ICM process, we must consider the provider of services as respectfully as the elderly recipient of service. Successful service delivery will necessitate a "buy in" from community agencies providing services to the rural elderly. The "buy in" includes shared leadership and control; considering the community and the agencies as partners; a willingness to alter policy, procedures, and practices; a shared vision; a team approach; and continuous assessment. This "buy-in" was the focus of the cause advocacy that allowed the ICM program for children and families to succeed in Maine. The "buy in" calls for us to challenge our assumptions about service provision in rural areas from an agency model to a model of collaboration, and to stretch our thinking to include "access to services that are planned for, managed, and delivered in a holistic and integrated manner in order to improve the family's self-sufficiency, safety, economic stability, health and quality of life" (Maine Children's Cabinet, 2000, p. 7). However, the "buy in" also challenges us, as social workers, in compelling ways. The "buy in" demands we step down from our position of authority and assume a "partnering" role. Integrated Case Management utilizes client involvement in all phases of implementation; this requires both a realization that how we structure the process itself often creates barriers to client involvement, and a commitment to reducing those barriers. Using cause advocacy to solicit such a "buy in" from social workers and agencies serving elders is the first step toward establishing an ICM program for rural seniors.

In summary, the ICM program exemplifies a practice model that would allow rural elderly clients to exercise considerable autonomy, independence and decision-making in choosing the level and nature of intervention. The ICM model advocates a holistic approach to providing case management and advocacy and seeks to provide services in as normal and flexible an environment as possible. This model considers not only the individual, but also the individual within natural support systems, the individual as a spiritual being and the individual as someone who recreates. Further, the use of a locally trained LCM, allows for local and regional knowledge of services and lack of services, and allows for an understanding of barriers to implementation of services. Ultimately, with ICM, the elderly client would be the manager of his or her own "case"; in other words, ICM exemplifies consumer-driven case management or "personal advocacy" as described by Hyduk and Moxley (2000; 1997).

CONCLUSIONS AND RECOMMENDATIONS FOR PRACTICE

Clearly advocacy is an essential social work role for practitioners working in all geographic areas. We are obligated as social workers to advocate for our clients at both the individual and societal levels. Drawing from the advocacy literature, the case example of REOP in the Southeast, and our practice experience with ICM in Maine, we offer the following recommendations to gerontological social workers practicing in rural areas:

- Be creative in your advocacy and draw on the client's existing networks to assist in problem solving.
- Involve local leadership in generating community solutions for community problems so that the leadership feels ownership for, and "buy-in" to, the resulting programs and services.
- Bring a client's multiple service providers together with the client to make sure the client's voice is heard, to creatively problem-solve, and to avoid over-serving and underserving.
- Consult local experts who are aware of both formal and informal community resources.
- Respect the client's need for autonomy and independence, and assure that he or she remains in control of advocacy efforts on his or her behalf.
- Be cognizant of transportation concerns in all client interventions and make ameliorating transportation problems for isolated elders a primary advocacy goal.
- Look for opportunities to "partner" community expertise with client insights in all advocacy efforts, whether at the case or cause level.

Social worker practitioners working with elders in small towns and rural areas are faced daily with situations that warrant their advocacy efforts. By allowing their clients to remain in control, respecting culture and expertise of local communities, and working to reduce geographic obstacles, social workers will be more successful in their advocacy interventions. The examples and recommendations presented in this chapter should serve as guidelines to gerontological social workers in non-metropolitan areas as they work toward the National Association of Social Work Code of Ethics' goal (NASW, Sec. 6.04a, p. 27) of advocating "for living conditions conducive to the fulfillment of basic human needs" and promoting "social, economic, political and cultural values and institutions that are compatible with realization of social justice."

REFERENCES

Bruner, C. (1994). Toward improved outcomes for children and families–A framework for measuring the potential of comprehensive service strategies, *Occasional Paper #8*, CFPC Publications. (August, 1994). Retrieved May 29, 2002 from *http://www.cfpciowa.org/publicationscfpc8PUB.shtml.*

Burkhardt, J.E. (2001). Transportation for the elderly in rural America. *The Public Policy and Aging Report, 12* (1), 9-13.

Butler, S.S. (in press). "We are the most free to take the risks required": Activism among elders. In L.W. Kaye (ed.) *Productive aging and social work practice.* Washington DC: NASW Press.

Dorfman, L. (2002). Family relations and networks among rural elders: Implications for geriatric care management. *Geriatric Care Management Journal, 12* (1), 16-21.

Epstein, D., West, A.J., & Riegel, D.G. (2000). The Institute for Senior Action: Training senior leaders for advocacy. *Journal of Gerontological Social Work, 33* (4), 91-99.

Ezell, M. (2001). *Advocacy in the human services.* Belmont, CA: Brooks/Cole Thomas Learning Center.

Hanna, W.J. (1981). Advocacy and the elderly. In R.H. Davis (ed.) *Aging: Prospects and issues* (pp. 297-316). Los Angeles, CA: The University of Southern California Press.

Hyduk, C.A., & Moxley, D. (2000). Challenges to the implementation of personal advocacy for older adults. *Families in Society, 81* (5), 455-466.

Hyduk, C.A., & Moxley, D. (1997). A personal advocacy model for serving older adults. *Journal of Gerontological Social Work, 28* (4), 75-90.

Krout, J.A. (2001). Community services and housing for rural elders. *The Public Policy and Aging Report, 12* (1), 6-8.

Maine Children's Cabinet. (2000). *Integrated case management initiative assessment report.* Augusta, ME: Edmund S. Muskie School of Public Service.

Martinez-Brawley, E.E. (1998). Community-oriented practice in rural social work. In L.H. Ginsberg (Ed.) *Social work in rural communities* (3rd ed.) (pp. 99-113). Alexandria, VA: Council on Social Work Education.

Miley, K.K., O'Malia, M., & DuBois, B. (2001). *Generalist social work practice: An empowerment approach* (3rd ed.). Boston: Allyn & Bacon.

National Association of Social Workers (NASW). (1996). *Code of Ethics.* Washington DC: Author.

Rathbone-McCuan, E. (2002). Perspectives on rural mental health services: Limited options for older persons. *Geriatric Care Management Journal, 12* (1), 4-6.

Ritchie, C., Wieland, D., Tully, C., Rowe, J., Sims, R., & Bodner, E. (2002). Coordination and advocacy for rural elders (CARE): A model of rural case management with veterans. *The Gerontologist, 42* (3), 399-405.

Schneider, R.L., & Lester, L. (2001). *Social work advocacy.* Belmont, CA: Brooks/Cole Thomson Learning Center.

Snustad, D.G., Thompson-Heisterman, A.A., Neese, J.B., & Abrahm, I.L. (1993). Mental health outreach to rural elderly: Service delivery to a forgotten risk group. *Clinical Gerontologist, 14* (1), 95-111.

Sosin, M., & Caulum, S. (1983). Advocacy: A conceptualization for social work practice. *Social Work, 28,* 12-17.

Stallman, J.I., Deller, S., & Shields, M. (2001). Aging and the rural economy. *The Public Policy and Aging Report, 12* (1), 14-19.

York, R.O., Denton, R.T., & Moran, J.R. (1998). Rural and urban social work practice: Is there a difference? In L.H. Ginsberg (Ed.) *Social work in rural communities* (3rd ed.) (pp. 83-97). Alexandria, VA: Council on Social Work Education.

Chapter 5

Rural Program Planning and Development for Older Adults

Hong Li, PhD
C. Jean Blaser, PhD

SUMMARY. Building on Canter's social care systems model, this chapter reviews rural elders' informal and formal service systems, summarizes the barriers in planning and providing services in rural areas, and suggests strategies that social workers can adopt to overcome these barriers to meet the needs of rural elders and their families. Strategies considered include: integrating formal services with informal care; knowing the culture or tradition of local communities and residents; identifying and involving community leaders in the development and planning process; building into the community and contributing to the community; and encouraging implementation flexibility, creativity and innovation. *[Article copies available for a fee from The Haworth Document Delivery Service: 1-800-HAWORTH. E-mail address: <docdelivery@haworthpress.com> Website: <http://www.HaworthPress.com> © 2003 by The Haworth Press, Inc. All rights reserved.]*

KEYWORDS. Program planning, service systems, rural service delivery

[Haworth co-indexing entry note]: "Rural Program Planning and Development for Older Adults." Li, Hong, and C. Jean Blaser. Co-published simultaneously in *Journal of Gerontological Social Work* (The Haworth Social Work Practice Press, an imprint of The Haworth Press, Inc.) Vol. 41, No. 1/2, 2003, pp. 75-89; and: *Gerontological Social Work in Small Towns and Rural Communities* (ed: Sandra S. Butler, and Lenard W. Kaye) The Haworth Social Work Practice Press, an imprint of The Haworth Press, Inc., 2003, pp. 75-89. Single or multiple copies of this article are available for a fee from The Haworth Document Delivery Service [1-800-HAWORTH, 9:00 a.m. - 5:00 p.m. (EST). E-mail address: docdelivery@ haworthpress.com].

http://www.haworthpress.com/web/JGSW
© 2003 by The Haworth Press, Inc. All rights reserved.
Digital Object Identifier: 10.1300/J083v41n01_05

INTRODUCTION

Planning and developing programs for elders living in rural communities are challenging. More than two decades of inquiry have clearly demonstrated that rural elders are in less optimal health and living with lower incomes than their urban counterparts (Rogers, 1999), and rural elders present, if not more, at least similar types of needs for services (Krout & Coward, 1998). Although substantial efforts have been made to improve the services for rural elders, barriers such as long-distance traveling, narrow range of services, lack of financial resources, and strong preference for family caregiving have limited rural elders' access to and use of formal services (Krout & Coward, 1998).

Based on Canter's social care systems model, we will review rural elders' informal and formal service systems, summarize the barriers in planning and providing services in rural areas, and suggest strategies that social workers can adopt to overcome these barriers to meet the needs of rural elders and their families.

SOCIAL CARE SYSTEMS MODEL

From an ecological perspective, Canter (1991) conceptualized social care systems for supporting older adults. In the system, older adults are the center of a series of subsystems ranging hierarchically from their informal networks, such as family caregivers, friends, and neighbors; to community organizations, such as religious organizations and racial cultural groups; and finally to formal service organizations, such as home health care agencies, and adult day care centers. At the time of needing services, older adults often prefer to turn to their informal support networks first and then maybe to formal organizations when the informal support networks are not available or are inadequate. The ultimate outcome of the social care system is to maintain and improve older adults' independence and quality of life. This outcome is achieved through the support from subsystems and the interaction between and/or among the subsystems. Although the empirical evidence has not been consistent on the interaction of subsystems, the layout of the social care system is clearly supported.

The patterns of social care systems conceptualized by Cantor (1991) have been found in rural communities. In an ethnographic study, Magilvy and colleagues (1994) used "circle of care" to depict the elder care systems in rural communities and found the circle of care fits well with rural culture and traditions. Similar to the subsystems in Canter's model, the circle of care includes service providers, community leaders, family, friends, and neighbors. They conclude that these circles lay the foundation of rural service planning and development, and that cooperation and networking between and among the people in each circle is the key to the success of rural programs and services (Magilvy, Congdon, & Martinez, 1994). Using national survey data, Coward, Cutler, and Mullens (1990) showed that 82 percent of impaired elders in rural areas used informal support, 7.7 percent used both informal and formal support, and 9.8 percent only used formal support. The social care systems model lays a solid foundation for social service planners and program developers to understand the elder care system in rural environments and develop acceptable, appropriate services. It is advantageous over other models because it is flexible, maps out the context of elder care systems, and emphasizes the interaction between different care systems.

SOCIAL CARE SYSTEMS FOR RURAL ELDERS

Informal Care Networks

A majority of rural elders are healthy and living independently. Like elders of other residential areas, as they age, rural elders are likely to experience a decline in health and functional status. A recent population report on rural older adults showed that 37 percent of rural elders at age 65 to 70 reported fair or poor health, but by age 85 and older, 56 percent reported fair or poor health (Rogers, 1999). The self-reported health status is often related to chronic conditions and functional limitations that elders have developed. Although researchers may still debate about whether rural elders are better or worse off than urban elders, given rural elders' poorer economic conditions, lower education attainment, and limited access to health care services, the general consensus is that many rural elders are in great need of social services (Krout, 1994; Rogers, 1999).

Informal support networks are the main source of elder care in rural areas (Coward & Cutler, 1989). Data from a national representative sample showed that 82 percent of rural elders reported using informal caregivers, and elders with more severe impairments used both more informal and formal services (Coward, Cutler, & Mullens, 1990). Informal support networks for rural elders often include their spouses, adult children, siblings, other relatives, friends, and neighbors. Using 1982 National Long-Term Care Survey Data, Dwyer and Miller (1990) found that about 50 percent of the primary caregivers for rural elders were spouses, 28 percent were adult children, and 22 percent were other relatives, friends, or neighbors. Departing from one of the rural myths, they also found only minor differences in rural and urban elders' informal support networks. For example, rural elders received more frequent visits from relatives than urban elders, but there were no significant differences in size of informal support networks (Dwyer & Miller, 1990). Members of informal support networks provided intensive assistance to rural elderly persons. Informal caregivers helped elders with activities of daily living (ADL) and instrumental activities of daily living (IADL). On average, they provided 4.4 hours of care daily for an average of 6.5 years (Dwyer & Miller, 1990).

However, informal support networks are not an unlimited resource for elder care. Out-migration of younger generations has weakened the informal support networks for rural elders (Coward, Lee, & Dwyer, 1993). Although rural elders have more adult children, the children often live far away from the impaired elders (Lee, Dwyer, & Coward, 1990). Geographic proximity was found to be one of the important factors affecting levels of care provided to rural elders (Powers & Kivett, 1992). Meanwhile, rural primary caregivers are more likely to live on limited incomes than urban caregivers. The low-income status may further limit rural caregivers' ability to provide elder care because low-income caregivers may have fewer resources as well as longer work hours (Stoller & Lee, 1994). When the elder care demands exceed the capacity of caregivers, either the quality of elder care or the elder and/or caregivers' well-being may be compromised. Many rural informal caregivers have experienced caregiving stress, which has been found to be higher than their urban counterparts have experienced (Dwyer & Miller, 1990).

Formal Care Services

To enhance the informal support network and assist impaired elders, a wide range of formal programs and services have been developed and delivered in many diverse rural areas. These programs include information and assistance, case management, adult day care, respite care, home health care, homemaker services, nutrition programs, transportation and escort services, senior centers, home delivered and congregated meals, and many other types of programs. The majority of these programs and services are supported by Medicare, Medicaid, or the Older Americans Act with states and local areas contributing as well. Data from the 1984 supplement on aging to the National Health Interview Survey showed that about 17.5 percent of rural elders used formal services (Coward, Cutler, & Mullens, 1990). Netzer and colleagues (1997) examined four frequently used formal services in rural areas and found that 18 percent of the rural elders used senior centers, 9.3 percent used homemaker services, 6.7 percent used special transportation, and 8.6 percent used home health services. Kenney and Dubay (1992) found that Medicare beneficiaries in rural areas were 17 percent less likely to use home health benefits than were those in urban areas. Cautions need to be taken in interpreting the above findings as they are confounded by rural diversity and service availability.

The difficulties that rural service planners and providers face are clear, and include geographic distance, financial ability to purchase services, knowledge of services, eligibility constraints, and willingness to utilize existing services (Krout, 1994; Krout & Coward, 1998). The consequences of the above difficulties have been reported. Rural formal services are provided in a narrower range and are limited in meeting the needs of elders with more severe conditions (Nelson, 1994). The lack of community-based services may push rural elders to nursing home care prematurely (Kenney & Dubay, 1992).

In sum, many elders in rural communities are impaired and need informal and formal assistance. Although the tradition of informal caregiving is still strong in rural areas, informal support networks are vulnerable especially when the caregiving demands exceed the capability of informal caregivers. Formal services in rural areas reach a proportion of rural elders in need; however, many of these services face the challenges of great geographic distances and funding limitations. At the same time, rural elders' reliance on informal caregiving networks and lack of information or knowledge of formal services further complicate the process of planning and developing rural services. In this rural environment, are we able to overcome the difficulties and plan and develop social services that meet elders' and their families' needs?

USEFUL STRATEGIES FOR RURAL SERVICE AND PROGRAM DEVELOPMENT: IMPLICATIONS OF THE SOCIAL CARE SYSTEMS MODEL

As suggested in the social care systems model, successful social services must be rooted in local communities, and interact with elders' informal networks and other local organizations and existing services and programs. Because of the considerable differences in rural areas, rural social workers need to be creative and innovative in exploring what works and what does not work. There are some general strategies that rural social workers can use in developing and providing services in diverse rural communities. They are: integrate formal services with informal care; know the culture or tradition of local communities and residents; identify and involve community leaders into the development and planning process; build into the community and contribute to the community; and be flexible, creative and innovative. In the following sections we are going to highlight the services in rural New Mexico and Southern Illinois to illustrate these strategies. This area of Illinois is very rural, with over 17 percent of the population over 65 years of age, and 15 percent with incomes below the federal poverty level. The population density is a little more than 31 persons per square mile (Illinois Institute for Rural Affairs, 1999).

Integrate Formal Services into Informal Care

As discussed in the earlier section, rural elders are typically cared for by a social care system that includes informal support networks and formal service organizations. One way to strengthen the function of the rural elders' social care systems is through integrating formal services with existing informal care.

For example, in Illinois, case managers under contract with the Department on Aging have taken several steps to understand and integrate the formal and informal care systems to meet the needs of older persons. The case manager develops and implements a care plan which integrates the formal and informal systems of care and targets additional services to meet the unmet needs of the older person. Eligibility criteria for home and community-based services focus on two groups, those with relatively moderate impairment but no or limited informal supports, and those with considerable impairment but a great deal of informal support. For the latter clients, formal services provide respite for the informal support system.

Case managers use a standard assessment instrument, the Determination of Need, to identify the functional abilities of the older persons and the availability of resources to meet these needs (Paveza, Cohen, Blaser, Hagopian, Prohaska, & Brauner, 1990). Older persons are evaluated on their ability to perform each of sixteen activities of daily living and instrumental activities of daily living. For each task with which the older person experiences difficulty, the case manager inquires if the individual has someone, or something, to help him with that task. The completion of the assessment provides a clear picture of what the individual needs and what the informal system is able and willing to do, along with what formal services already are being provided.

The assessment takes place in the home of the older person, in order to observe first hand the accessibility and condition of the home. Informal caregivers may participate in the assessment, providing information about the needs of the older persons, and the informal support system. With the implementation of the National Family Caregiver Support Program, the case manager is able to offer support for the informal system of caregivers, as well.

An earlier evaluation of this system showed that those with a great deal of family support were more impaired when they requested home and community services, compared to those with little or no family support. It would appear that the family provided needed care at first, and sought formal assistance only when the burden became considerable (Armstrong, 1989).

Armstrong (1989) also found that when the formal services were provided, family caregivers noted they no longer did the tasks performed by the formal services, but adjusted their activities to supplement and complement the formal services. She found the family caregivers did not reduce the hours spent caregiving, but rather continued to provide emotional support, special transportation, special meals, and emergency services.

These findings are consistent with the conceptualization that describes the link between informal and formal services. In the literature, several approaches have been suggested to assist in integrating informal and formal services. In the social care system model, Canter (1991) suggested formal services should target the areas that informal caregivers are not able to provide. In the task-specific model, Litwak (1985) suggested that formal services can be used to handle the tasks that are specialized and technical, and informal services can be used to handle the tasks that are unpredictable and nontechnical. Contrasting with this finding, Edelmen and Hughes (1990) found that many elders used formal services to supplement informal services and formal service providers and informal caregivers shared the caregiving tasks. However, further research is needed regarding the most effective way to integrate informal and formal services.

KNOW THE CULTURE OR TRADITION OF LOCAL COMMUNITY AND RESIDENTS

The program and service planners need to know the culture of the people living in the area. Years ago, the second author of this chapter was funded by the U.S. Administration on Aging to conduct a needs assessment of the Pueblo Indians of New Mexico (Rogers & Gallion, 1978). We learned it was not enough to ask if the older person had a telephone, since many feared to use a phone, and instead learned to ask if the person would use a phone. We also learned to differentiate among homes when we asked about the conveniences in the home, because some Pueblos, e.g., Taos Pueblo, maintained at least three homes, the federally-funded home on the outskirts of the pueblo, the traditional home in the pueblo, and the more spiritual home of their ancestors, which they visited and resided in for a few weeks each year for ceremonies. And, we learned the more usual type of home energy assistance was of little value to an older person who was gathering sticks to heat her home.

In Northern New Mexico, some rural Hispanics practice beliefs that date back centuries. In one training session for homemakers employed under the state's Title XX (of the Social Security Act) program, the trainer (the second author of this chapter) was asked how to break spells. An elderly gentleman was convinced a spell had been cast upon him by a neighbor, so that the man's wife had died, his cow had gone dry (was not giving milk), and he had no money. The homemakers were told how to break a spell by a graduate student who had grown up in the area and knew the culture. Once the spell was broken, the homemakers were advised to help the gentleman sign up for benefits for which he was eligible, including SSI (Supplemental Security Income). This combination of the old and new ways, building upon the culture of the area, is also exemplified by a practice at the medical school at the University of New Mexico, where Native American medicine men and Hispanic curanderos are invited to work with the medical doctors to heal patients.

While other rural areas may not display such dramatic differences from the more urban mainstream cultures, subtle differences may exist that are not as readily noticed. Numerous authors have suggested people in rural areas may be more reluctant to accept services, branding the services as "welfare," which is to be avoided (Coward & Cutler, 1989; Nelson, 1994). While this is true in some areas and for some people, others may decline services, fearing that to accept services is to admit to a family deficiency, since it is the family duty to provide services. On the other hand, some elders will accept services to avoid "bothering" their children.

Identify and Involve Community Leaders in Planning and Development

In each rural community, there are people who are viewed as leaders, who have a track record of getting things done and who know the community. These are the people who will know the local culture and the history of service delivery in the area, what worked and what did not, and who can bring along the larger community to endorse and develop an idea. People living in small rural communities know most of the people residing there, as well as their histories, so selecting the wrong person, known to be lazy or a thief or a procrastinator (or descended from a family with these characteristics) will doom a project before it gets off the ground. Community leaders may be elected officials, leaders in local churches, educators, doctors, or associations/organizations, such as the local health care center, the senior center, or the Kiwanis. Most importantly, they have a track record of acceptability in the community and of successfully building a program or initiative.

A successful example of involving the community is the State of Illinois' Gatekeeper Program. In this program, the staff from the Department on Aging and Area Agencies on Aging train meter readers, utility workers, librarians and direct service personnel to recognize signs indicating an older person may need help. These "Gatekeepers" have made approximately 6,000 referrals to the Aging Network since 1987. As a result, older people in need have received such services as in-home care, financial assistance, home-delivered meals and elder abuse intervention assistance. Over the past seven years, the Department on Aging has expanded the program to a "Youth Gatekeeper Program," that involves Illinois newspapers and their local paper carriers. In a similar reliance on local, community-based agencies, the Service PLESE effort (Service Program for the Limited English Speaking Elderly) relies on ethnic agencies who represent their respective cultures and languages to perform outreach, interpretation, and services to their communities.

Affordable housing undergirds efforts to assist older persons to remain in the community. Clearly, home services can not be provided unless there is a home. Rural areas are known to have more persons who are home owners, compared to renters, and the housing stock is known to be older and more in need of repairs and renovation (Prosper & Clark, 1994). In addition to the problems with the physical condition of the homes, they are often a great distance from services. In rural Southern Illinois, where assisted living housing has been practically non-existent, elderly are forced to relocate to more urban areas to gain access to health and social services. They are often unnecessarily institutionalized in nursing homes because they and their families cannot find either services closer to home or other affordable supportive housing options.

After identifying a significant need in the region for both personal care services and affordable housing, the River to River Corporation teamed with local providers, the Illinois Department on Aging, and the NCB Development Services to develop low-income, assisted living facilities in Southern Illinois as part of the Coming Home project funded by the Robert Wood Johnson Foundation. The River to River Corporation has made a conscious effort to involve the community leaders and experts, forming a board composed of representatives from each of the major community-based health care providers in the 13 county region. A publication on Cache Valley Services, the first of now three assisted living facilities, notes "the challenge in trying to create this type of project is to bring together the right group of people who offer local credibility and technical expertise" (NCB Development Corporation, 1999, p. 11). The providers have a long history of service in the area and know the rural culture and how it varies in different sections of Southern Illinois. The advisory council represents "a who's who" in the area, including city officials, housing representatives, health and senior service providers, and social workers. Without the involvement of these individuals, it is doubtful the project could have succeeded.

Build Social Services Which Contribute to Local Communities

In each community, even though it may be economically depressed, there are some resources that can be used for service development and planning. The resource may be a church, and a new adult day care may be located there. Or, the old fire hall could be renovated for senior services, and local contractors would be hired to do the renovation. Staff should be hired from the community, and every effort should be made to purchase goods and services from the local businesses. In these ways, the new program becomes part of the economic fabric of the community, increasing the possibility of acceptance by the community as more and more members of the community have a stake in the success of the project.

Gunter (1985) describes an innovative approach to delivering adult day services in Southern Illinois. To overcome the barriers of low population density, the high cost of transportation, and extensive client travel time, a model of satellite sites was developed whereby the staff, rather than the clients, were transported. Each day for four days of the week, professional staff traveled to a different community, delivering adult day services to small community units. In one community, the services were delivered in a fire station. The other sites included a converted school house, an old jail, and a store front facility. Participants received transportation, hot meals, medication administration, health monitoring, and socialization. At the time of the report, a total of 110 individuals received services at the four sites. Additionally, the communities were involved in the provision of equipment, including chairs, a sofa, refrigerator, and supplies. At the end of the three year development period, when all four sites were up and operating, they were transferred to a local agency for continuation. Since that time, several rural areas around the country have sought information about the project and the U.S. Administration on Aging has funded a similar project in Georgia.

In addition to maximizing the community resources, social service programs and services also can bring opportunities to the residents in local communities and help local economies. For example, an assisted living program can be very helpful in providing services to rural elders by locating the older people in a congregate setting where the services, including meals, health and medication monitoring, homemaker and laundry services, and social activities can be accessed. However, assisted living facilities are rarely built in poor, rural areas. As noted, an exception is Cache Valley Apartments, an assisted living facility in Ullin, Illinois. Ullin is exceptionally rural, with a population of only 500 and is characterized by a high percentage of elders and high rates of unemployment and poverty. In the area, 77 percent of elders had incomes below $15,000 a year. The Cache Valley Apartments have not only become a focal point for delivering social services, they also support the economy of the town, with staff hired locally, along with the use of local contractors, pharmacies, and grocery stores. At the grand opening of the apartments, the newest building project in the community in 100 years, the popular saying was that the population of the town doubled on that day as people from all over Southern Illinois attended the event. In 1998, Cache Valley Apartments received a "Best of Home Award" by the Assisted Living Federation of America.

Be Flexible, Creative and Innovative

Two components of generally accepted definitions of rural are density, number of persons per square mile, and distance to services. The urban model of older persons coming to the service does not work well in rural areas. Unlike the urban dweller, most rural older persons have very limited access to public transportation. If transportation is provided by a service agency, the cost of going to the client's home to get the client, bringing the client to the service, returning the client to his or her home, and returning to the central dispatch point means the individual client has spent a considerable time on the bus and the bus has made two trips without a customer. Some agencies may not be able to provide services due to expenses involved in long-distance traveling and inadequate funding, while others have developed innovative solutions to the time and distance problems.

Shawnee Alliance for Seniors is a case management agency serving the 13 southernmost counties of Illinois and over 2700 older persons. The agency has contracts with the local Area Agency on Aging and two state agencies to provide nursing home preadmission screening for all persons entering nursing facilities in the area and to determine eligibility for home- and community-based services for persons 60 years of age and older. The agency also provides protective services to prevent elder abuse and serves as the ombudsman for nursing home residents in the area. To respond to barriers of low density and great distance, Shawnee Alliance for Seniors decentralized the case managers to six regional offices, so that the case managers could reach their clients from these regional offices. Furthermore, this agency analyzed and divided the tasks of the case managers into tasks requiring professional skills such as nursing home preadmission screening, elder abuse assessments, and eligibility determinations and redeterminations for home and community-based services, and tasks requiring administrative skills such as completion of paper work and billing forms.

To best utilize the time of case managers, the agencies assigned those professional tasks to case managers and left the other tasks to administrative staff at the central office. In addition, the agency developed software that schedules clients for an assessment or reassessment based on geographic area. For example, if a client requests that a case manager assess a change in needs, the program will generate a list of other clients in the vicinity who are due for assessments in the next few weeks. Since the agency is reimbursed for specific tasks, there is a great effort to reduce the time the case manager spends in non-reimbursed time traveling from home to home. As a further economy, the case managers are "generalists," able to assess individuals for a variety of programs, so that more than one case manager does not have to travel to the home.

Another response to the time and distance problems in rural areas is to deliver the service to the client, e.g., home delivered meals, or visiting nurse services. Here the total miles traveled are reduced, but the cost of "down time" while the provider is traveling from one home to another must be factored in. The more the service provider costs in terms of salary, the less likely it is that this approach will prove to be cost effective. For example, the cost differential between having a volunteer deliver a meal versus having a physician make a house call is substantial.

Whether one should bring the client to the service or the service to the client depends upon the results of an analysis of reimbursements and costs, both to the service agency and the client. One agency which provides homemaker service in Illinois determined that transporting one person living in Community A to dialysis in Community B cost far more than the reimbursement which would be received from the funding source. However, the agency was very resourceful and developed a work plan for the homemaker that involved picking up a client in Community A, where the homemaker resided, traveling to Community C (which was on the way) to pick up a second client needing dialysis, and taking both to the scheduled dialysis in Community B. During the time the two clients were undergoing dialysis, the homemaker visited and served another client in his home in community B. Then the homemaker retraced the route, picking up the two dialysis clients and returning them to their respective communities. The agency was reimbursed for the time spent transporting each client and serving the third, covering the cost of the worker and her mileage (Illinois Department on Aging, 2000).

CONCLUSION

Planning and developing rural services for elders are challenging. There are no quick and easy ways to meet the challenges. However, the social care systems model is a useful theoretical framework that can be used to understand rural elders' care systems, cultures, traditions, and rural environments. Its emphasis on the interaction between informal care and formal services provides insight on how to use limited formal services to support informal caregiving, and its emphasis on coordination among different formal agencies and local resources sheds light on how to enhance the often fragmented rural aging network. The successful programs presented in this chapter highlighted these strategies. As we discussed in the chapter, rurality is characterized with diversity and variations. We know "scaled down" urban service models may not work in rural areas. We also know a successful rural program from one area may not be generalizable to another rural area. Given rural diversity and limited financial resources, rural social workers need to be creative and innovative to explore and develop programs that meet the needs of local rural elders.

REFERENCES

Armstrong, C.J. (1989). *The reciprocal impact of the community care program upon family caregivers in Southern Illinois.* Unpublished Doctoral Dissertation, Southern Illinois University, Carbondale, IL.

Cantor, M. (1991). Family and community: Changing roles in an aging society. *The Gerontologist, 31*(3), 337-346.

Coward, R., Lee, G., & Dwyer, J. (1993). The family relations of rural elders. In N. Bull (Eds.) *Aging in rural America* (pp. 216-231). Thousand Oaks, CA: Sage.

Coward, R., & Cutler, S. (1989). Informal and formal health care systems for the rural elderly. *Health Services Research, 23*(6), 785-806.

Coward, R., Cutler, S., & Mullens, R. (1990). Residential differences in the composition of the helping networks of impaired elders. *Family Relations, 39*(1), 44-50.

Dwyer, J., & Miller, M. (1990). Difference in characteristics of the caregiving network by areas of residence: Implications for primary caregiver stress and burden. *Family Relations, 39*, 27-37.

Edelman, P., & Hughes, S. (1990). The impact of community care on provision of informal care to homebound elderly persons. *Journal of Gerontology: Social Science, 45*(2), S74-84.

Gunter, P.L. (1985) Four rural centers use non-traditional delivery. *Perspectives on Aging, 14*(6), 8-9, 18.

Illinois Department on Aging. (2000). *Internal program reports.* Springfield, IL: Author.

Illinois Institute for Rural Affairs. (1999). *Building a brighter future for rural Illinois.* Springfield, IL: Author.

Kenney, G., & Dubay, L. (1992). Explaining area variation in the use of Medicare home health services. *Medical Care, 30*(1), 43-57.

Krout, J.A., & Coward, R.T. (1998). Aging in Rural Environments. In R. Coward, & J. Krout (Eds.) *Aging in rural settings: Life circumstances and distinctive features* (pp. 3-14). New York, NY: Springer.

Krout, J. (Ed.). (1994). *Providing community-based services to the rural elderly.* Thousand Oaks, CA: Sage.

Lee, G., Dwyer, J., & Coward, R. (1990). Residential location and proximity to children among impaired elderly parents. *Rural Sociology, 55*, 579-589.

Litwak, E. (1985). *Helping the elderly.* New York: Guilford.

Magilvy, J., Congdon, J., & Martinez, R. (1994). Circles of care: Home care and community support for rural older adults. *Advanced Nursing Science, 16*(3), 22-33.

NCB Development Corporation. (1999). *The coming home program.* Oakland, CA: Author.

Netzer, J., Coward, R., Peek, C., Henretta, J., Duncan, R., & Dougherty, M. (1997). Race and residence differences in the use of formal services by older adults. *Research on Aging, 19*(3), 300-322.

Nelson, G. (1994). In-home services for rural elders. In R. Coward, N. Bull, G. Kukulka, & J. Galliher (Eds.), *Health services for rural elders*, (pp. 65-83). New York, NY: Springer.

Paveza, G.J., Cohen, D., Blaser, C.J., Hagopian, M., Prohaska, T., & Brauner, D. (1990). A brief assessment tool for determining eligibility and need for community-based long-term care services, *Behavior, Health, and Aging*, *1*(2), 121-132.

Powers, E., & Kivett, V. (1992). Kin expectations and kin support among older rural adults. *Rural Sociology*, *57*, 194-215.

Prosper, V., & Clark, S. (1994). Housing America's Rural Elderly. In Krout, J. (Ed.) *Providing community-based services to the rural elderly* (pp. 133-155). Thousand Oaks, CA: Sage.

Rogers, C. (1993). Health status and use of health care services by the older population. Washington, DC: U.S. Department of Agriculture.

Rogers, C. (1999). *Changes in the older population and implications for rural areas.* Washington, DC: U.S. Department of Agriculture.

Rogers, C.J., & Gallion, T.E. (1978). Characteristics of elderly Pueblo Indians in New Mexico. *The Gerontologist*, *18*(5), 482-487.

Stoller, E., & Lee, G. (1994). Informal care of rural elders. In R. Coward, N. Bull, G. Kukulka, & J. Galliher (Eds.), *Health services for rural elders* (pp. 33-64). New York, NY: Springer.

Chapter 6

A Rural Perspective on Marketing Services to Older Adults

Kim K. R. McKeage, PhD
Lenard W. Kaye, DSW

SUMMARY. In the scarce resource environment of rural communities, social workers have a special obligation to both embrace and contribute to the human service agency's marketing campaign. This chapter begins by clarifying the differences between goods and services and then develops a profile of the older adult as health and social service consumer. The unique features of rural older consumers are considered and approaches to segmenting a rural agency's target population are reviewed. Such concepts as outshopping, segmentation, destination marketing, and virtual servicescapes are considered as are the "Four P's" and the "Four I's" of marketing services. An organization-wide marketing philosophy is strongly encouraged in rural human service organizations. *[Article copies available for a fee from The Haworth Document Delivery Service: 1-800-HAWORTH. E-mail address: <docdelivery@haworthpress.com> Website: <http://www.HaworthPress.com> © 2003 by The Haworth Press, Inc. All rights reserved.]*

KEYWORDS. Marketing, older consumers, rural human service administration

[Haworth co-indexing entry note]: "A Rural Perspective on Marketing Services to Older Adults." McKeage, Kim K. R., and Lenard W. Kaye. Co-published simultaneously in *Journal of Gerontological Social Work* (The Haworth Social Work Practice Press, an imprint of The Haworth Press, Inc.) Vol. 41, No. 1/2, 2003, pp. 91-120; and: *Gerontological Social Work in Small Towns and Rural Communities* (ed: Sandra S. Butler, and Lenard W. Kaye) The Haworth Social Work Practice Press, an imprint of The Haworth Press, Inc., 2003, pp. 91-120. Single or multiple copies of this article are available for a fee from The Haworth Document Delivery Service [1-800-HAWORTH, 9:00 a.m. - 5:00 p.m. (EST). E-mail address: docdelivery@haworthpress.com].

http://www.haworthpress.com/web/JGSW
© 2003 by The Haworth Press, Inc. All rights reserved.
Digital Object Identifier: 10.1300/J083v41n01_06

INTRODUCTION

The greatest disservice that could be done to both marketing and to rural older adults would be to promote the familiar perspective of the "snake oil salesman" whereby marketing is seen as a powerful tool in the exploitation and manipulation of this consumer population. This is the perspective that sees marketing as solely the selling or advertising function of customer communication (Cooper, 1995), and can bring about a number of undesired consequences, such as creating desires not previously considered by the consumer, promotion of age segregation, and neglecting low-income elders (Kaye, 1996, p. 29). Rather, let it be clear that marketing takes as its fundamental premise the assertion that understanding consumers is the key to success in any endeavor and that the failure to market health and human services for older adults can result in the highest quality and most needed of such services being discontinued because potential consumers of those services don't know they exist. Put simply, "when done properly, better marketing insures that an agency's services will be used [effectively]" (Kaye, 1995b, p. 134). Therefore, we will try to elucidate an approach that will serve those who wish to reach any segment of the rural older adult population–affluent or poor, old or very old, home based or institutionalized, etc. As Cutter (2001) notes:

> Elders work and are retired; they go to school; they are grandparents and raise children; they fall in love, divorce, remarry, and become widows or widowers. They pay taxes and collect entitlements. (p. 15)

In other words, all consumers have a variety of needs that must be met, and the task of the program planner is to determine which ones he or she can meet, and how that will be done.

This chapter is also premised on the belief that social workers and other health and human service professionals who work with rural elders have an obligation to both embrace and in many cases contribute to various aspects of an agency's marketing campaign. Indeed, in rural settings, it is argued that scarce resources obligate social workers and others, regardless of their primary responsibilities to assume a more broad range of an organization's planning and administrative functions (such as marketing), than would otherwise have been expected.

In the area of health care in particular, a true marketing orientation is finally gaining institutional recognition. The Joint Commission on Accreditation of Healthcare Organizations revised its standards to include public expectations of hospitals and the needs of patients and other customers (LaFleur, Taylor, and Sumrall, 1997). Cooper (1995) proposes that health care marketing is moving toward this more inclusive orientation, and proposes that resources can fruitfully be reallocated toward:

1. Market research on specific consumer groups
2. Developing new products, processes and services
3. Placing services in more convenient locations
4. Timing the availability of services to match the needs of the market (pp. 57-58).

Note that while Cooper was discussing health care, his prescriptions are good ones for marketers of any service including rural gerontological social service programs.

While institutions need to adopt a marketing orientation, it is not enough for the executives to do so. The marketing orientation requires that everyone in the organization must be, at some level, a marketer (Yasin and Green, 1995). An organization-wide marketing orientation speaks to the importance of engaging all levels of the rural social service agency in various marketing functions including direct service workers, support staff, and consumers of the services offered (Kaye, 1995b). Obviously not everyone will partake of formal marketing training, though. Thus, there is a growing need for marketers to work with interdisciplinary teams that include marketers, executives, service providers, and even service consumers. Everyone involved must be flexible and able to see his or her role as part of meeting the consumer's needs.

DIFFERENCES BETWEEN MARKETING GOODS AND SERVICES

Anybody who has worked in the field of social services no doubt has an intuitive understanding that services are different from tangible products. However, the ways in which services differ from "goods" (as the tangibles are called) must be understood in order to, in turn, understand the care which must be taken in providing services.

In marketing, the differences between goods and services are generally categorized into four concepts. These can be thought of as the "Four I's" of services. They are Intangibility, Inseparability, Inventory, and Inconsistency. We will discuss each of these in turn.

Intangibility

The fundamental characteristic of services, whether provided in urban or rural settings, is that they are Intangible. That is, "service" occurs in the mind of the customer. Until a consumer feels that he or she has "been served" there is no service episode to consider. Because service is intangible, it is not amenable to technical descriptions of quality or characteristics. Consider a service such as entertainment. Two viewers can watch the same movie, comedy show, or play and have very different reactions. One viewer can be quite entertained, another not at all. With services, it is very difficult to appeal to objective sensory perspectives in describing the service.

Services display varying degrees of Intangibility. At one extreme are services such as mental health treatment. The service can be described as providing "mental health," which is extremely intangible. At the other end of a continuum could be the provision of durable medical equipment. The equipment itself is quite tangible, and the intangible part is making these goods available and facilitating access and installation. Services that are the most intangible must be given special consideration in adapting product marketing principles.

Inseparability

Another characteristic of social services is that they are Inseparable from the consumer and the service provider. Because of the intangible nature of these services, the consumer's perceptions are key in determining what service was actually delivered. Because the social work service provider is often an integral part of the service episode, the consumer also cannot disentangle his or her perceptions of the service from those of the service provider. An excellent example of this is mental health care. A rural elder who was recently widowed seeks advice from a mental health professional. The care provider diagnoses the client's problem to the best of his or her ability, and prescribes a solution such as counseling to address the client's sense of loss and loneliness. If the prescription fails, however, it is difficult to determine where the service breakdown occurred. It could be that the client did not adequately describe the symptoms. It could be that the care provider did not conduct an adequate assessment, did not get the correct diagnosis based on the information at hand, or did not prescribe an adequate treatment intervention. Finally, it could be that the client did not follow the care provider's interventive recommendations that included becoming involved in the programs of the local senior center and a self-help support group for recently widowed older adults. The problematic part of this is that the client will most likely be dissatisfied with the service no matter who is responsible.

Inventory

Inventory is the storage of goods or capacity as a buffer against variation in demand. Goods manufacturers know that production and demand may be difficult to align completely. Therefore, many manufacturers will carry excess inventory in case demand rises above their current ability to supply. This system has worked well in the production of goods for a long time.

Services, on the other hand, cannot be inventoried. If a rural geriatric care manager is ready and waiting to give service, and no elders or family members appear, then that capacity is wasted. This is true whether the service provider is mechanical or human. If an ATM machine sits idle, or the social workers in the local Area Agency on Aging do, in either case service capacity is wasted. Not only is it wasted, it is lost forever. Because services are consumed in a time space, they cannot be retrieved from the past. Once the opportunity to provide service is gone, it is gone forever.

Inconsistency

Inconsistency is a double-edged sword. On the negative side, it is considered a problem of service provision and something that must be controlled. On the positive side, it is called customization, and it is something that many older adults seek.

Inconsistency simply means that service varies from provider to provider, even within the same social service agency. With human service providers this is easy to see, as humans all have different capabilities, moods, needs, tolerances, etc. Even with mechanical service provision, though, there can be temporary breakdowns or conditions that cause service inconsistency. And finally, no matter how they are provided, elder services are ultimately assessed in the mind of the service consumer whether it be the older adult him- or herself or a relative, and each consumer will have his or her own perceptual biases that cause inconsistent service evaluations.

Managing the Four I's

Service marketers have developed many ways of dealing with the Four I's. These will be discussed and illustrated in the sections to follow. It is important, though, to keep these characteristics in mind when applying any marketing techniques, especially those that have been developed in the realm of tangible goods marketing. This framework will provide the insight needed to adapt marketing techniques with special attention to their application by social work and allied human service professionals in rural communities.

UNDERSTANDING YOUR CLIENTS

One of the first tenets of marketing is the importance of understanding your consumers. Marketing is the art and science of effectively meeting clients' unmet needs in a way that gives the service provider a competitive advantage over alternate service providers. In order to do that, you must understand your clients.

It is dangerous to over generalize about rural older consumers just as it is any other large group. And this group is large–approximately one out of every four older adults in the United States lives in rural America (Coward and Cutler, 1989). That said, there has been some research describing characteristics of the rural older adult population, as well as the older consumer in general. A number of relevant points will be discussed in this section, but readers should consider this information as only a guideline to the type of information they should gather about specific older consumers and/or their significant others in their own service provision area.

Older consumers might be considered different from younger consumers in some predictable ways. On the one hand, older consumers are more sophisticated consumers in general (Kaye, 1995b). This is because they have had a lifetime of consumption experience, including product and service experience, viewing of advertisements, retail experiences, etc. As Vesperi (2001) notes, elders are "less vulnerable to suggestion than advertisers might like" (p. 9). Yet at the same time, older consumers *can* be vulnerable. They may be experiencing life shifts, such as health deterioration, restricted social interaction, or loss of income, that make it more difficult to deal with consumption situations and dilemmas. For example, one way consumers find out about the value of new products and services is to listen to other consumers who have already tried them. If the consumer's social circle shrinks dramatically, he or she will not have access to this valuable marketplace information, and may have to rely on more marketer-dominated sources of information (such as advertisements). Of course, such information may or may not be accurate, and it will quite probably not be delivered by a trusted relative, friend or significant other, all of whom are increasingly difficult to locate in one's contracting social network.

Rural consumers also may differ from consumers in general. Yasin and Green (1995) note that the "subjective culture" of a region (p. 80) is very important. "'Rural' actually reflects a state of mind" (Boyd, 1986). Consumption takes place within a culture which shapes the attitudes and values of its members. This means that "marketing theory cannot be applied universally without taking account of context" (Anderson and McAuley, 1999, p. 176). Consumption behavior takes place in the context of broader social patterns and connections (Miller, Kim, and Schofield-Tomschin, 1998). This is referred to as embeddedness (Granovetter, 1990; Miller and Kim, 1999).

One way in which rural older consumers can be distinguished from the general population is through their value system. For example, a number of studies have cited the independent, 'take care of yourself' (Smith et al., 1993, p. 2; Rosel, 2001) attitude of rural elders. This attitude leads these consumers to eschew help, especially low-cost or free help that suggests charity. They also often have a strong sense of community and tend to distrust outsiders (Franzak et al., 1995), another reason they may refuse help. "Rural values" (Quandt and Rao, 1999) include self-reliance and stoicism. In many cases, these values fit well into those expressed among wider (both rural and non-rural) groups of older consumers–autonomy, personal growth, connectedness, altruism and revitalization (Bradley and Longino, 2001; Kaye and Sherman, 2002). This is important to note in adapting communications from a wider audience for rural elders. In general, tapping into these core values, as well as traditions and aspirations, may be the most effective means of constructing a meaningful service delivery message (Bradley and Longino, 2001).

Another manifestation of the importance of context is the growth in the relationship marketing orientation that seeks to build long-term, ongoing relationships with consumers, and the attendant importance on communication with customers (Anderson and McAuley, 1999). This type of context already operates in rural communities. Compared to consumers in general, rural older consumers tend to have long-term relationships with institutions (banks, stores, etc.) in the community (Quandt and Rao, 1999; Miller and Kean, 1997b). They have equally strong and lasting affiliations with local groups and organizations (social groups, churches, synagogues, Rotary, etc.). Compared to younger consumers, elders tend to shop more frequently in stores where they are known, and they rely more on help from store employees (Miller, Kim, and Schofield-Tomschin, 1998). They are also fiercely loyal to long-term and smaller- scale community businesses and organizations compared to recently established enterprises. Older consumers will even eschew lower prices or brand selection in favor of the retailer's reputation (Miller, Kim, and Schofield-Tomschin, 1998). Retailers, conversely, try to position themselves based on high service levels and the consumer's local affinity, in order to compete with larger regional or national companies (Duff, 1990).

While these insights into rural elderly consumers are not necessarily surprising, not all assumptions about rural consumers are valid. For example, rural no longer means "farming"–more rural counties depend on manufacturing than on agriculture as their primary source of employment and income (Drabenstott, 1999). Nor are rural economies based primarily on natural resource extraction (Coates, Jarratt, and Radunas, 1992). Rural areas, like the rest of the developed areas of the globe, generally are moving toward service-based economies (Anderson and McAuley, 1999). Older consumers, with their increasingly intact pensions, social security, and savings, bring valuable cash inflows to these economies (Coates, Jarratt, and Radunas, 1992).

Consumers in remote areas also face problems that are not even considerations in urban centers. The technology revolution has not entirely pervaded rural areas–many rural communities still must make a long-distance phone call to log on to the Internet (Drabenstott, 1999). Low-income, rural elders are less likely to have Internet access than other elders (Leavengood, 2001), who are already very unlikely to have Internet access (*Wall Street Journal*, 2001). Rural areas also continue to experience difficulties in maintaining their health care services at a level sufficient for the needs of elderly residents (Coates, Jarratt, and Radunas, 1992; LaFleur, Taylor, and Sumrall, 1997). There are numerous barriers to consumption for the rural elderly (Quandt and Rao, 1999; Coward and Cutler, 1989) including financial, social, psychological, and physical (e.g., disability). Some of these, such as mobility difficulties, are exacerbated by residing in remote, rural locations.

Market Segmentation and Customer Management

One of the primary tools of marketing is Market Segmentation. Segmentation supposes that an organization's potential clients are not homogenous, but may have identifiably different needs or capacities. Furthermore, segmentation requires that the organization (whether it offers services or products) be able to group its clients into a manageable number of groups within which clients are as similar as possible, and between which clients are as different from other groups as possible. Then, service offerings are tailored to each group. This is the basis of market segmentation and positioning and should be seen as being just as relevant in serving older adults consuming social work services as those purchasing consumer products.

Marketers must be careful that segmentation does not lead to stereotyping and segregating elders (Vesperi, 2001). The way in which stereotypes have been manifest has changed over time. Initially, elders were portrayed as frail and poor. More recently, some older consumers have been identified as Woofies (well-off older folks, Vesperi, 2001, p. 6) and Zoomers[1] (Cutter, 2001). These images resonate with elders better than the previous ones, because people will react well to images portraying their aspirational clusters–what people want to be, rather than what they are (Vesperi, 2001). However, the images can also have a negative effect on perceptions of what aging people *should* be like. These active, well-off images become "a standard against which aging has come to be defined and measured" (Vesperi, 2001, p. 7). Yet they are still not the reality for most elders, who lie somewhere between this ideal and the negative stereotype of being decrepit, impoverished, and chronically frail (Vesperi, 2001). What we need is a true diversity of images and information presented in the media (Cutter, 2001). Proceed with caution.

Segmentation Variables–How We Understand Consumers

The program planner and administrator must consider which variables are useful in describing the organization's market segments. Numerous possibilities exist. One of the most useful segmentation bases is consumer need. A responsive health and human services network in a community should recognize that older adults are not homogeneous in their needs and should insure that a continuum of services to help older adults remain comfortably in their homes is available (e.g., visiting nurses, senior companions, homemakers, escort workers, etc.). Another useful segmentation basis is psychographics. Psychographics include attitudes, tastes, preferences, values, activities, etc. These variables tend to be motivations for clients to consume or prefer one service over another. They are often useful in formulating communications to older adults. One of the important considerations for older consumers is activities. Miller, Kim, and Schofield-Tomschin (1998) note that "understanding the individual's level of social activity in their particular community may explain as much or more about their consumer behavior than their chronological age" (p. 345). In addition, activities are taking on more complexity as we learn that simple measures are not adequate to capture the lived experiences of older people. For example, marketers can't just talk about "retired" consumers anymore, as there are various types and levels of retirement (Miller, Kim, and Schofield-Tomschin, 1998). Some consumers retire from one career and start another, some work part time for pay, and some retire from paid work and volunteer. The possible permutations are too numerous to list. Another example is values segmentation (Leinweber, 2001). Here, older consumers are clustered together based on configurations on dominant values that they express, such as "Hearth & Homemakers" who embrace family, belonging, and conformity, or "Liberal Loners" who value thinking, benevolence, and frugality (Leinweber, 2001, p. 23). Given that customer needs and psychographics are very useful, why bother with other characteristics to segment the social service marketplace? The biggest reason is that needs and psychographics are not always easy to measure on a consumer by consumer basis. It is often necessary to find some other variable, easily measured, to use to segment older consumers. In many cases, these other variables are demographics. If there is a good correlation between a set of demographic measures and dominant needs/psychographics, then the demographics can be used to assign consumers to segments and then those consumers can be targeted using the underlying psycho-social variables known to be characteristic of that group.

There are a number of demographic characteristics that should be considered as potentially useful when designing rural programs. These include age, income, marital status, gender, race/ethnicity, geographic location, and educational level. When considering older consumers, age is especially intriguing. First, age may turn out not to be a good segmentation variable at all–indeed, "age is not very central in defining who older people think they are" (Bradley and Longino, 2001, p. 17). Consumers seem to dislike being identified with a specific age-related market segment (Bradley and Longino, 2001). In addition, no longer do marketers lump all older consumers into one "over 65" group–there are the "old old" (85 years and older), for example, who have much different needs from those in their sixties. Even within a more narrow age range, other demographic characteristics (income, education, etc.) are likely to be quite varied, leading to the conclusion that age is potentially a very weak proxy for psychographic and needs-based variables.

Some demographics, such as income and educational level achieved, can be good proxies for social class, especially when used in combination. Since social class tends to have long-term effects on access to resources and wealth accumulation, it is an important variable to consider. Within a social class, rural consumers may have different experiences from urban residents. For example, Dubay (1993) notes that rural Medicare enrollees are different than urban older adults. They are slightly older, somewhat more likely to be male, and white. They are "more dependent in both activities of daily living (ADLs) and instrumental activities of daily living (IADLs)" than their urban counterparts (p. 27).

Customer Management

One of the recent permutations of the market segmentation approach is Customer Management. The idea behind this approach is that some consumers are more profitable (or less costly) than others. Some consumers are a better match to an organization's capabilities than others. The most efficient solution is that which matches customer needs and organizational capabilities the closest. This approach is growing in health care (Rohrer and Culica, 1999). Marketers are identifying potential heavy users and targeting them for prevention and disease management programs, as well as designing less expensive services that can meet some of their needs (such as follow up care programs to make sure they get their prescriptions refilled). The use of case managers to target services to the elderly is another type of customer management. Here, case managers can increase the efficiency with which services are allocated throughout the client base (Davidson, Moscovice, and McCaffrey, 1989) at the same time that they insure older adults are aware of and accessing the services and entitlements that they can most benefit from.

In order to gain the efficiencies sought, program planners must undertake market segmentation and customer management activities within their specific markets. In each case, local context must be considered. Rural consumers will have different needs and risk factors than urban, and those located in one rural community (such as a mining community) may have different profiles than consumers in another rural community (such as a farm-based one).

Reference Groups

Another important element in the experience of consumers that has particular importance for the social services program planner is family and group consumption patterns. In any circumstance where more than one person may be involved in the service utilization decision, group influences must be considered. The groups can be family groups or others, such as church or social groups. In marketing, these influences are treated under the rubric of reference groups (McKee, Wall, and Luther, 1997). In general, people trust people they know, and these personal sources (family, friends) are generally considered more trustworthy than others, especially salespeople or other marketers. In many cases, family members are involved in caring for elders (Coward and Cutler, 1989), and these caregivers will have an enormous influence on the elders' service consumption choices.

In addition to the dynamic of interpersonal influence, in any situation where more than one person is involved, the service provider must mediate between multiple perspectives and, perhaps, diverse needs among consumers. Doing so is, to some extent, another part of the service offering, and may even approach formalized conflict resolution. On the other hand, the network of family involvement in elder care also creates situations where marketers can meet the needs of more than one member of the network. For example, caregivers for older relatives may need support or respite services for themselves (Coward and Cutler, 1989). Thus, friends and family members become a secondary market for many services aimed toward the elderly (Kaye, 1996).

UNDERSTANDING YOUR COMPETITION

Because of the less-developed markets (for almost everything) that exist in rural areas, there are often fewer direct competitors for any particular service offering. That does not mean there are no competitors. Home care agencies, for example, might be competing with health-care facilities, continuing care retirement communities, or congregate housing (Kaye, 1995b). Yasin and Green (1995) note that many health care providers incorrectly assumed that they were in a unique position and not subject to competitive dynamics, and they are paying the price for that now, sometimes even closing. However, the competition may be more indirect (such as moving in with a relative, rather than going to an assisted-living facility) and may suggest opportunities to provide better services to customers. Even more commonly, rather than competition being an issue at all, a weak and incomplete service network, with attendant lack of service availability, may be the big market issue (Boyd, 1986).

The focus is sometimes not even on lack of competition but rather lack of complementary services. In rural areas, some agencies may not provide the same level of service they would in urban areas. For example, not only are home health agencies (HHAs) less commonly found in rural communities, but they are less likely to provide medical social services and occupational, speech, and physical therapy in rural areas than in urban ones (Dubay, 1993, p. 25). This may leave other agencies and providers in the system to pick up the slack. The market, then, may offer more opportunities for cooperation than for competition.

Indeed, there has been a general trend toward the formation of networks of firms coordinating their efforts (Anderson and McAuley, 1999; Kaye, 1996). In 1996, Kaye noted that "59.8% of those who market elder services (in both rural and urban communities) have collaborated with other organizations" (p. 41). This often includes building networks of service providers, and policy makers are encouraging these efforts. The Coming Home program of the Robert Wood Johnson Foundation was designed to promote systems that included health, social, and personal care services along with housing services (*Health Care Financing Review*, 1994). Similarly, government initiatives such as the National Rural Health Care Act of 1988, the Health Care Financing Administration, and the Department of Health and Human Services (Christianson, Moscovice, Johnson, Kralewski, and Grogan, 1990) encouraged formation of rural cooperatives among health care providers. One idea that can work is exemplified by the Rural Cancer Outreach Program (RCOP) where cancer specialists (physicians and nurses) travel from an academic medical center to rural areas and provide cancer care services *in situ* (Franzak et al., 1995). This program has been successful because it deals with the geographic issue that has worked against programs in the past. It has also reduced costs! These networks can be a strong structure for providing integrated services to older consumers with a complex configuration of needs. However, program planners and administrators should enter into these alliances with one caveat. If one agency is seen as a 'free resource,' then that particular agency may be over-utilized and, ultimately, burn out or be unable to sustain its service quality level (Smith et al., 1993, p. 5).

Outshopping

The geographic issue mentioned above is not a minor consideration. Vertical integration and strategic alliances have not necessarily solved the problems of rural health care. In large part this is because such solutions tend to result in concentration of service offerings in more urban areas to which rural elders do not have geographic access (Franzak et al., 1995). This urban concentration only encourages outshopping behavior.

A serious problem that rural programmers face is outshopping, the propensity to go outside one's local trading area to procure goods or services. This is a particular problem for health care providers and for retailers of certain items, such as apparel and home furnishings. In both cases, consumers' motivations for outshopping center around quality concerns and perceptions of the availability of goods or services locally (Gooding, 1994; Wright, 1995; Yasin and Green, 1995; Miller and Kean, 1997a). The good news is that rural elders are generally more satisfied with their local community and less likely to outshop than younger consumers (McDaniel, Gates, and Lamb, 1992; Miller, Kim, and Schofield-Tomschin, 1998; Taylor, 1997). Rural older consumers tend to be "regular shopper[s] at regular venue[s]" (Rosel, 2001, p. 49). The bad news is that outshopping can create a spiral of lost revenues and organizational failures, leaving rural elders with even fewer local options, particularly in health care and specialized social service provision (Gooding, 1994; Franzak, Smith, and Desch, 1995; Miller and Kean, 1997a; Miller and Kim, 1999).

Outshopping can dominate a local market. When there is a high tendency to outshop, competition comes not only from within the local market, but from a distance. The geographic isolation that may protect some services from direct competition becomes null and void when consumers are willing and able to shop outside the local economy. One strength of cooperative health and social service systems is that they can strengthen each member of the network and encourage inshopping by sharing information through the network about locally available options.

STRUCTURING THE SERVICE SYSTEM

Once the service provider has an understanding of his or her consumers and recognizes the special characteristics of services marketing, it is time to design the "offerings" that will be provided to consumers. That is, it is time to design a service system. The system is comprised of the Four P's of marketing, Product, Place, Price, and Promotion, as well as a consideration of the role of employees.

Product

The first question the service provider must ask is "What is the product?" While this often seems like a simple enough question, it is deceptive. Often, human service providers tend to characterize the product they offer in terms of what they do rather than what the client receives–so they might say that their product is "providing advice on living options to elderly couples." However, it is quite possible that the couples mentioned see the service as maintaining their independent living situation as long as possible or finding the housing option that will best preserve their capital investment. Family members might see a mediation service that tries to convince older parents to select one option (that the family prefers) over other options. Being aware of these dynamics helps the service provider focus on what is truly important.

Focus is critical for the services marketer. It is very tempting to try to be all things to all people, but that is a quick way to get into trouble (Cooper, 1995). Limited resources and the need to strategically target markets to serve mean that organizations must be careful in deciding what they can and cannot provide in the marketplace. Sometimes, the marketer must completely reconceptualize the service offering. For example, since the mid-1980s rural hospitals and health care providers have begun to think of themselves as wellness centers rather than simply acute care facilities, a major conceptual shift (Boyd, 1986).

Product quality is particularly difficult to manage in services marketing. Products are assessed in the mind of the consumer, and so is product quality. Because of Intangibility, it is difficult to make verifiable assertions about quality. One way we deal with this is to focus on the tangible aspects of the service and use those to signal quality. An example of this is the physician's office decorated in wood tones and earthy hues, with quality wooden furniture and carpets. All accoutrements are designed to convey quality. Contrast that with a government agency where the floors are linoleum, walls are painted a stark white, and furniture is institutional, plastic, and uncomfortable.

Not only do social services planners need to manage their existing products, they also need to plan new service offerings. These can either be to serve new clients who are not being attracted by current services, to respond to the changing needs of clients, to respond to competitive offerings, or to respond to external factors, such as new regulations or technology. The planner often offers bundles of services. In rural settings, often you cannot just offer one service and be done with it. Once you start interacting with the older consumer, you may identify a constellation of needs that are not being met (Smith et al., 1993; Coward and Cutler, 1989). The program planner must be prepared to expand the idea of the service offering, and also to consider the limits of the organization's ability to provide a holistic service package. Given some flexibility in organizational mission and design, the managers and marketers can develop additional services in response to emergent consumer needs. Strategic alliances and confidence in the ability to refer consumers to other service providers are also helpful.

One example of this type of product development is the use of geriatric technicians as adjuncts to rural physicians. These employees schedule appointments, monitor compliance with treatment regimens, arrange for other social services, and call and keep in touch with patients between visits (Anderson, Brewer, and Stein, 1998). In one study, patients who were served by these technicians rated the quality of their care higher than those who did not (Anderson, Brewer, and Stein, 1998).

The key here is that the service planner cannot rest assured that all is well once the service is designed and operating effectively. Rather, he or she must constantly be scanning the environment for threats and new opportunities.

Place

The key concept in service provision to the rural older adult is *access*. This is especially true with health care services (Watt, 1992) but impacts use of social services as well. With many services, the first issue is whether the service is delivered in the client's home or in the establishment of the service provider. One aspect of this question is that of convenience. If it is desirable that a consumer use the service, the degree of consumer motivation must be assessed. The lower the inherent motivation, the more important accessibility and convenience become. For example, attempts to get local citizens to recycle often include tactics to make drop off as easy as possible (Carter, 1994). Because some rural elders have very limited mobility, locational convenience can become the critical factor in whether services are utilized or not (Smith, Buckwalter, Zevenbergen, and Kudart, 1993).

Terrain is very important (see Quandt and Rao, 1999; Coward and Cutler, 1989). If you are providing services in terrain that is rugged or difficult to navigate (even seasonally, as in winter), you have to consider your consumer base to have geographic access problems that would not be an issue in other locales.

Another important issue that comes under place is space design. More and more, marketers are understanding the importance of creating visually appealing facilities that complement the goals of the service. For example, in the area of health care, marketers and architects are designing spaces that meet patients' physical, psychological, and social needs in order to foster better recovery. These spaces also reduce stress for the patients' families and friends. Some examples are the North Pavilion at Northwest Community Hospital in Arlington Heights, IL and HealthPark Florida–Lee Memorial Hospital in Fort Meyers, FL (Hair, 1998). North Pavilion's "welcoming center" includes a fountain, piano, greenery, and artwork (Hair, 1998, p. 4). HealthPark was built in an orange grove and has an atrium lovely enough to be used for weddings (Hair, 1998)! Especially for elders, who may find a highly technological environment somewhat offputting, humanizing the physical environment of the service can create immense benefit.

Two emergent issues in place are destination marketing and virtual places. These are specialized concerns, and are discussed separately in the next two sections.

Destination Marketing

In marketing to elders, sometimes place is the service itself. A good example of this is when "community" is the ideal that is marketed, including a sense of attachment and community spirit (McKee, Wall, and Luther, 1997). On a broader level, this would include town festivals. On a narrower level, an example is a pool exercise program for health and socialization. In this case, going to the pool is an integral part of the service. Clients could undertake alternative exercise programs, or could swim in different places. They could also meet friends and socialize elsewhere. But having a suitable indoor pool allows for the development of year-round programs and may encourage clients to think of the pool as "their place"–the destination takes on meaning above and beyond the basic services provided.

Virtual Servicescapes

With the advent of the Internet and increasing rates of Internet access and usage, service providers must consider the role of virtual space in the provision of their services. One clear implication of the growth of the Internet is that traditional channels of distribution for both goods and services are challenged by the increased competition that the Internet brings. One benefit that online competitors bring to consumers is increased selection and variety. For example, if you want to buy a wheelchair, no longer are you restricted to those available at your local medical equipment supplier. The Internet can quickly place a variety of manufacturers and models within the consumer's reach. Another benefit, which may be particularly appealing to elderly consumers, is the safety and security of shopping from home rather than venturing out to stores. Due to increasing crime rates at shopping centers (Claxton, 1995) as well as poor weather conditions in some rural areas (Coward and Cutler, 1989), some older consumers may be afraid to venture out.

In addition, a number of services can be provided via technology. For example, rather than just setting up the Internet as a method of shopping (a service itself), services (such as order tracking, information dissemination) can be provided. The Department of Health and Human Services developed its *Computers for Seniors* program, and AARP (www.aarp.org) includes a listing of online resources for elders (Leavengood, 2001). With many e-marketers, a consumer can email a question or problem (or discuss it via live chat rooms) and get an answer back online. Telemedicine is expanding the ability to offer medical services to remote consumers (Franzak et al., 1995).

While the degree of acceptance of this technology among older rural consumers may initially be low, tech savvy Baby-Boomers are more likely to embrace this technology as they transition into the ranks of consumers 65 and older (Leavengood, 2001). A 1999 study found that about 30 percent of older people (over 50) in the US own and use a computer, and computer buyers over the age of 55 are a growing segment (Leavengood, 2001, p. 69).

Promotion

One of the most fundamental questions the service provider must ask, with regard to promotion, is the overall goal of the communication. Generally, social service providers will fall into two broad categories–those with more capacity than demand, and those with more demand than capacity. The promotional goals are very different for these two types of firms (Kaye, 1995a). The goals for a firm with excess capacity are fairly self-evident and familiar–increase demand through letting customers know of your service and by positioning your offering in a way that is appealing. However, there is also a valid role for promotion in the latter case of excess demand, although social service agencies may not have considered it as thoroughly as they have the former (Kaye, 1995a). The approach, Customer Management, was discussed in the section on Market Segmentation. The idea is to more closely align the interests and expectations of the consumer with the offerings and capabilities of the organization.

Additional areas of concern in promotion are the media and the message. Each of these is discussed in the following sections.

Media

There are a variety of communication outlets service providers can use to get their message out to prospective clients. Each of these has their own strengths and weaknesses, and a detailed discussion of each media is beyond the scope of this chapter. In many cases, the organizations that sell media access will be willing to help the service provider to construct the content and style of the communication as part of the media package. Unfortunately, it is harder to get accurate information on how effective your chosen media outlet is, especially in rural markets (Harmeson and Dennis, 1996).

Elders consume a lot of mass media. For example, Vesperi (2001) notes that "older people are the most loyal readers of newspapers" (p. 8). They are also used to having a news hour and viewing it faithfully. This sets them apart from younger, media-demanding consumers who want their news and entertainment where and when they want it (often on CNN Headline news and on the Internet; Vesperi, 2001, p. 8). In addition, children and elders are the biggest consumers of television (Signorielli, 2001, p. 34). One trend in magazines is the development of age-segmented publications–such as AARP's *Modern Maturity* (two versions, for 55-65 and 65+) and their *My Generation* for consumers 45-55 (Cutter, 2001). Another is the inclusion of special sections devoted to older readers' interests in newspapers (Cutter, 2001).

Despite these media consumption habits, the rural elderly can be difficult to reach and influence with advertising and other mass media communications. This may stem from a distrust of media images and intentions. Aside from the trend toward age-targeted magazines, general-audience publications tend to ignore older consumers (de Luce, 2001). No wonder these consumers tend to place more trust in personal communications (Franzak et al., 1995).

Rural customers especially are not impressed by slick ads. Elders have firm opinions about the marketing efforts that agencies engage in, both positive and negative (Kaye, 1996). Direct, face-to-face communications with customers and excellent service over time are much more likely to build loyal, committed customers among rural older adults (Taylor, 2001; Kaye, 1995b). Local newspapers, local bulletin boards, and especially word of mouth (WOM) are more likely to be effective promotional media. Being active in community events is also effective.

For some services, "non-traditional" referral sources–television coverage of the program, clergy, veterinarians, bankers, grain and feed dealers, senior health fairs, trained community agency staff–are usually more effective than traditional media outlets (Smith et al., 1993). Note that some of these may seem "traditional" to marketers, but are not (television) for social service agencies.

Message

The message also must be tailored to the interests of the older consumer. This recommendation refers to both the verbal message and the images shown in advertisements. In general, older consumers prefer informational to persuasive communications (Kaye and Reisman, 1993). They like realistic images that are slightly aspirational but not ridiculous. Older consumers are more likely than younger ones to report being offended by an ad and not buying something based on stereotypical advertisements (Bradley and Longino, 2001). Yet that is exactly what continues to be presented to older customers–images that are very unrealistic, either over-glamorized or under-capable, and not representative of even the basic demographic patterns (in terms of gender, occupational status, etc.) found in the actual population (Signorielli, 2001). Discussing a content analysis of ads in wide-circulation magazines, de Luce (2001) notes:

> If we were to draw a picture of American life exclusively from evidence derived from these thirty-one magazines, we would have to conclude that the consuming population consists primarily of people 18 to 49 years old. We would also have to conclude that there are almost no people of color in the United States [and that] this cohort of people . . . has substantial discretionary income. (p. 41)

This obviously won't do. The programmer must find a middle ground that presents a realistic and diverse picture of the older population to media consumers. We must keep in mind that "unless they are ill or depressed, older people do not feel 'old.' Furthermore, older people tend to associate old age with the residents of nursing homes, an image from which they want to distance themselves" (Bradley and Longino, 2001, p. 18). Some slight modifications to our models can yield an image that is more nearly representative. For example, Moschis (1994) recommends that advertisers use models ten to fifteen years younger than the target audience when advertising to elders, at least when the product is related to self-image.

In addition to modifying visual images, marketers should be careful about their verbal messages as well. Rural consumers may use a different "language" of commerce that is embedded in their local culture (Anderson and McAuley, 1999). In addition, rural older consumers tend to look to their peers as role models, rather than to media-generated images (Rosel, 2001). For these reasons, WOM may be one of the most effective means of communication–messages will travel in words and media (through local role models) that are seen as more authentic by local residents (Kaye and Reisman, 1993).

Costs and Measures of Effectiveness

When considering what types of communication to utilize, a service marketer must consider the cost and effectiveness of the media under consideration. There are some standard metrics that can help the marketer assess and compare different media, including reach, frequency, hits, and CPM.

Reach means how many different consumers will be exposed to the communication one time. All things considered, the higher the reach the better when comparing communications having the same cost. In many cases, though, communications in different media (and even in the same media) will not have the same cost. One way to equalize the figures for cost and reach is to look at the CPM, or cost per thousand. Media suppliers should be able to provide this figure, and it is a handy shortcut to compare different media.

In many cases, one exposure to a communication is not enough to achieve the desired results with consumers. The service marketer must also consider frequency, which is the number of times a given consumer should be exposed to a communication. In many cases, repeated exposure over some period of time is necessary to gain trial, purchase, or ongoing usage of a service. The difference between reach and frequency can be thought of using newspaper advertising. Reach is the number of people who will read the paper. Frequency is the number of times the ad is placed in subsequent editions. Generally you want to reach your audience, but you also need to reach consumers more than once for any message to take hold.

In marketing on the Internet, the idea of reach and frequency is translated into hits. A hit is any time that a consumer accesses a particular page. Given that e-marketers can track how many times a particular consumer accesses a page, frequency can also be calculated.

Price

The basic idea in setting prices is cost/benefit analysis. Costs are all the monetary and non-monetary resources that must be sacrificed to offer a particular program or service. Benefits are all the monetary and non-monetary gains that will be realized from the program or service. These generally fall into the two categories of monetary revenue and non-monetary contributions to meeting the mission of the organization (Kotler and Andreasen, 1991). Note that financial resources that rely on local tax bases can be limited in rural areas, which tend to be more impoverished generally (Quandt and Rao, 1999).

Pricing for For-Profit Services

For-profit services should consider the costs of their services, the market prices for competitive services, and their own profit objectives. While a detailed explanation of cost-volume-profit analysis is beyond the scope of this chapter, it is worth noting that service providers must consider a couple of issues that are different from experiences with goods marketing.

First, cost structures may be very different in services marketing than for goods marketing. Typically, fixed costs are much higher for service providers and variable costs are lower. Thus the incremental cost of bringing in one additional consumer is quite low, and the benefits are very high. This is why capacity is such a consideration for service marketers–over some reasonable range of demand, costs will not vary considerably.

Second, because of this cost structure, it is difficult to trace costs directly to specific services rendered. Basing prices directly on costs may be more difficult for services than for many goods. Faced with a lack of accurate cost data, the marketer must turn to another arena for pricing information. The most useful information often comes from the competitive arena–what are the competing products and services that consumers could use to meet this need, and what are their costs? In the absence of good competitive market data, market research can be undertaken to ask consumers about the prices they are likely to pay for particular services. This issue is especially significant when planning a new service that requires a significant expenditure of resources.

Not-for-Profits

In the resource scarce environment that usually characterizes rural communities, cost containment is obviously a large issue for non-profit human services organizations. Again, the basic equation is how to get the most (and best quality) services out of a given level of funding. Government agencies in the past have not necessarily understood the cost structure of rural service providers. The dispersed population and remote geography often leads to lower patronage volume for a given service than would be achieved in urban areas (Franzak et al., 1995). This is inefficient, and results in higher per-service costs because economies of scale are not achieved (Watt, 1992). In addition, rural delivery costs tend to be higher due to additional travel and transportation costs, telecommunications costs, and the extra costs of providing mobile services and training and supporting service providers (Watt, 1992).

One of the considerations for not-for-profits is transitioning from grant-based to fee-for-service funding (Smith et al., 1993). It is difficult to predict how many consumers may choose to turn elsewhere when they are asked to pay for a service that was previously free. However, as long as the fees are not exorbitant, the program planner in this circumstance is in the best position to make a good case for continued patronage–to whit, the consumer has already received the service and experienced satisfaction with it. In the case of the Elderly Outreach Program described by Smith et al. (1993), the defection rate was very low. Of course charging for services rendered may not need to be a consideration for certain social services that remain available because of federal or state statutory mandate, or for whom alternative sources of external support remain available. Rather, the point here is that fee-for-service is frequently a legitimate consideration that social workers and others need to be willing to consider.

EMPLOYEES AS SERVICE PROVIDERS

Unlike product manufacturing, service provision is inexorably tied to the performance of employees. In automated services, such as ATM machines, the physical machine stands in place of the employee–but it is not the 'product' of interest. Because of this aspect of inseparability, employees such as social workers are of paramount importance to service delivery. They must understand the importance of their own service orientation to a much greater extent than, say, a production line worker building a car. Because service systems are so complex and interdependent, every employee of the service system matters. Not only frontline employees, but those who are behind the scenes helping deliver the service are critical to the ultimate 'product' that the consumer will see. These general rules are just as true of a social service agency as they are of any other service (Kaye, 1995b).

There is some evidence that service employees may be even more crucial to the service experience and satisfaction therewith for rural elders. In a comparison of rural and urban consumers, Yasin and Green (1995) found that friendly and courteous providers seemed even more important in rural settings than in urban ones. Miller, Kim, and Schofield-Tomschin (1998) examined retail settings and found that, compared with younger consumers, older consumers express a desire for retail employees to behave with more courtesy and patience and to offer more assistance locating products. Because they tend to be socially imbedded, rural elders may be particularly sensitive to the role of personnel in providing services.

While every employee of the human service organization is important in developing and delivering the service, frontline personnel who interact with older adults are in a critical position due to the boundary spanning nature of their responsibilities. For example, a number of studies have found that employees were important factors in determining consumers' perceptions of health care, including how concerned, courteous, competent, attentive, caring, and helpful hospital employees were, the behavior of office personnel in a medical practice, and whether physicians take a personal interest in patients (Gooding, 1994; Bart, 1990; MacStravic, 1987/88; Rushinek and Rushinek, 1986). Lovdal and Pearson (1989) noted that patients care very much about how their doctors treat them. They seem to assume technical competence, and make their judgments about the medical profession and hospitals, as well as their ultimate satisfaction, based on more affective aspects of the physician's behavior–what we traditionally called bedside manner. Bart (1990) found that many patients noted that they would "prefer the comforts of their hometown doctor and hospital if they really felt that their needs could be met" (p. 224). In these cases, the physician's role mediates the patient's relationship with the facility and the technical aspects of care.

Boundary spanning employees, including social workers, are those who mediate between the expectations and demands of multiple parties. In this case, frontline employees mediate the boundary between the organization (the "inside") and the consumer (the "outside"). Boundary spanning employees thus often experience multiple, potentially conflicting demands and must mediate between the expectations of the organization and customers. When these expectations are not perfectly aligned (which happens frequently), it is the frontline employee who is responsible for providing the service in such a way that both the customer and the organization are satisfied. Social workers are well aware of this particular feature of employment and grapple with it on a regular basis. In rural communities, tight social service budgets and the expectations of older adults concerning high service customization can be expected to create even more frequent confrontations for social workers with conflicting organizational and client expectations.

Additional Considerations

One additional consideration that deserves mention is the role of the employee in home-care situations. Social services share a characteristic of place with other services, that is, they are sometimes delivered in the client's home rather than in the organization's location. This is expected to be more common in rural communities. When the service provider is in the home, the employee has less control than he or she would when the consumer is on the employee's "turf." Because of this, managers should be particularly attuned to the need to train service providers about how to deal with stresses and ambiguity in situations where they are working remotely. In addition, the service organization needs to ensure that service providers can carry with them all the tools they will need to enact the proper service script in the older adult's home.

Another aspect of employees that deserves mention is the role they play in informing the organization about the service consumer of that organization. This can occur in two ways. One is by explicitly passing information back up the organization to higher-level administrators who need to understand consumers but do not regularly interact with them. The information provided by those on the "front lines" is invaluable in this case and certainly contributes in critical ways to developing an informed marketing program.

The second way that employees can be informative sources of consumer information is when they are like the clients they serve. Kaye (1996) noted that "in the case of several organizations, the fact that older adults occupied the majority of staff and/or volunteer slots appears to have increased the likelihood of older adult involvement in market planning" (p. 36). In any case where elders can be recruited to be part of the organization, they bring not only their skills but also their insiders' perspectives on the organization's clients. While the marketer must be careful not to over-rely on idiosyncratic information, the insights of older employees can be valuable in refining or lending richness to our understanding of older consumers.

ASSESSING SATISFACTION AND EFFECTIVENESS

One of the first issues the social services marketer must confront is the Quantity/Quality trade off (see Smith et al., 1993). It is often tempting to provide as many services as possible to as many people as possible. At some point, though, quality may be compromised. Which is more important? The answer will depend on the particular situation the agency faces as well as the resources at hand.

Traditionally, social service providers have been more proficient at documenting quantity as compared to the quality or effectiveness of services provided. Responsible programs should include ongoing assessment as part of their overall philosophy of service provision and should employ specific measures suitable to their purposes. It is important to include measures of the degree to which services provided and outcomes meet the expectations and needs of clients. Such assessments are critical to maintaining a program of sound service provision. This feedback should also lend itself to continuous refinement of services provided. A continuous process of service evaluation and refinement helps assure that service quality levels remain high.

CONCLUSION

A cautionary note is offered in bringing this discussion to a close. Be careful in translating the principles of corporate marketing to rural services delivery. Not all models and methods work well in all settings. Caution is recommended not because rural health and social service providers do not need to be market-oriented (indeed they do), but rather because different strategies of service design and delivery may lend themselves to nonmetropolitan communities than to the inner city metropolis. Often this is because the underlying market structure is different in urban and rural areas (Boyd, 1986). As one example, the use of a product-line management approach for hospitals was touted as a way to attract new patients and develop centers of excellence (MacStravic, 1986). However, when Naidu, Kleimenhagen, and Pillari (1993) studied the usefulness of the approach, they concluded that it was not as effective for small, rural hospitals as for larger, urban ones. The limited number of beds in small hospitals (generally, under 100) contraindicates specialization to the degree necessary to implement product-line management. Indeed, these small hospitals are more likely to have a capacity utilization problem, and to undertake activities such as swing bed programs that will allow them to utilize the capacity they have more fully (Grimaldi, 1988).

Maintaining an explicit marketing program in rural health and human service agencies and engaging social workers at all levels of the organization in the various stages and dimensions of the marketing process is essential in today's world. Informed consumers, scarce resources, ongoing competition, and complex and evolving consumer need require that services be delivered strategically and that their quality be maximized. Thinking from a marketing perspective increases the likelihood that social workers and other allied health professionals will remain responsive and accountable to the older adults they serve and the sources of support that make service delivery possible in the first place.

NOTE

1. A Zoomer is a 'no limits baby boomer who sees retirement as the fast lane to a more energetic, new life characterized by healthy living, a high level of physical activity, and quest for further education, and who possesses technological and financial saavy' (Cutter, 2001, p. 14). Xtreme Aging, if you will.

REFERENCES

Anderson, A.R., & McAuley, A. (1999). Marketing landscapes: The social context. *Qualitative Market Research, 3* (2), 176-188.

Anderson, S.E., Brewer, B., & Stein, M. (1998). Closing the distance. *Nursing Management, 29* (11), 44-48.

Bart, B.D. (1990). Evaluating the effectiveness of wellness programs: Urban and rural hospital experience. *Health Marketing Quarterly*, *7* (3/4), 219-227.
Boyd, S.H. (1986). Marketing 'Dary Queenland,' U.S.A.: Rural America's health care challenge. *Health Marketing Quarterly*, *3* (4), 59-71.
Bradley, D.E., & Longino, Jr., C.F. (2001). How older people think about images of aging in advertising and the media. *Generations: Journal of the American Society on Aging*, *25* (3), 17-21.
Carter, B. (1994). Recycling strategies in remote regions. *BioCycle*, *35* (11), 52-53.
Christianson, J.B., Moscovice, I.S., Johnson, J., Kralewski, J., & Grogan, C. (1990). Evaluating rural hospital consortia. *Health Affairs*, 135-147.
Claxton, R.P. (1995). Customer safety: Direct marketing's undermarketed advantage. *Journal of Direct Marketing*, *9* (1), 67-78.
Coates, J.F., Jarratt J., & Ragunas, L. (1992). Reviving rural life. *The Futurist*, *25* (2), 21-27.
Cooper, P.D. (1995). Managed care positives and negatives for health care marketing. *Health Marketing Quarterly*, *13* (2), 55-60.
Coward, R.T., & Cutler, S.J. (1989). Informal and formal health care systems for the rural elderly. *HSR: Health Services Research*, *23* (6), 785-806.
Cutter, J.A. (2001). Specialty magazines and the older reader. *Generations: Journal of the American Society on Aging*, *25* (3), 13-15.
Davidson, G., Moscovice, I., & McCaffrey, D. (1989). Allocative efficiency of case managers for the elderly. *HSR: Health Services Research*, *24* (4), 539-554.
de Luce, J. (2001). Silence at the newsstands. *Generations: Journal of the American Society on Aging*, *25* (3), 39-43.
Drabenstott, M. (1999). Meeting a new century of challenges in rural America. *The Region*, *13* (4), 16-19.
Dubay, L.C. (1993). Comparison of rural and urban skilled nursing facility benefit use. *Health Care Financing Review*, *14* (4), 25-29.
Duff, M. (1990). Home cooking keeps them home at the store. *Supermarket Business*, *18* (March), 19A-20A, 29A.
Franzak, F.J., Smith T.J., & Desch, C.E. (1995). Marketing cancer care to rural residents. *Journal of Public Policy and Marketing*, *14* (1), 76-82.
Gooding, S.K.S. (1994). Hospital outshopping and perceptions of quality: Implications for public policy. *Journal of Public Policy and Marketing*, *13* (2), 271-280.
Granovetter, M. (1990). The old and the new economic sociology: A history and an agenda. In B. Friedland, & A.E. Robertson (Eds.) *Beyond the Marketplace*. New York: Aldine de Gruyter.
Grimaldi, P.L. (1988). More hospitals likely to swing beds. *Nursing Management*, *19* (3), 24-25.
Hair, L.P. (1998). Satisfaction by design. *Marketing Health Services*, *18* (3), 4-8.
Harmeson, P., & Dennis, E. (1996). Targeting the media message. *Journal of Professional Services Marketing*, *14* (1), 3-5.
Health Care Financing Review. (1994). New program being formed to aid rural elderly. *Health Care Financing Review*, *15* (3), 198.
Kaye, L.W. (1995a). An analysis of promotional materials used by health and social service programs for older adults. *Journal of Nonprofit & Public Sector Marketing*, *3* (1), 17-31.

Kaye, L.W. (1995b). Marketing techniques for home care programs. *Journal of Gerontological Social Work*, *24* (3/4), 133-156.

Kaye, L.W. (1996). Patterns of targeting and encouraging participation of elder consumers in human services marketing. *Health Marketing Quarterly*, *13* (3), 27-46.

Kaye, L.W., & Reisman, S.I. (1993). Elder consumer preferences of marketing strategies in the human services. *Health Marketing Quarterly*, *10* (3/4), 195-220.

Kotler, P., & Andreasen, A. (1991). *Strategic Marketing for Nonprofit Organizations*, Englewood Cliffs, NJ: Prentice Hall.

LaFlaur, E.K., Taylor, S.L., & Sumrall, D.A. (1997). Assessing the health care needs of a rural community. *Marketing Health Services*, *17* (4), 12-19.

Leavengood, L.B. (2001). Older people and internet use. *Generations: Journal of the American Society on Aging*, *25* (3), 69-71.

Leinweber, F. (2001). The older adult market: New research highlights 'key values.' *Generations: Journal of the American Society on Aging*, *25* (3), 22-23.

Lovdal, L.T., & Pearson, R. (1989). Wanted–doctors who care. *Journal of Health Care Marketing*, *9* (1), 37-41.

MacStravic, R.S. (1986). Product-line administration in hospitals. *Health Care Management Review*, *11* (2), 35-43.

MacStravic, R.S. (1987/88). Professional and personal quality of care in health care delivery. *Health Marketing Quarterly*, *5* (1/2), 75-87.

McDaniel, C., Gates, R., & Lamb, Jr., C.W. (1992). Who leaves the service area?: Profiling the hospital outshopper. *Journal of Health Care Marketing*, *12* (3), 2-9.

McKee, D., Wall, M., & Luther, V. (1997). Community culture and marketing strategy as sources of economic development competitive advantage: A study among rural U.S. communities. *Journal of Macromarketing*, *17* (1), 68-87.

Miller, N.J., & Kean, R.C. (1997a). Factors contributing to inshopping behavior in rural trade areas: Implications for local retailers. *Journal of Small Business Management*, *35* (2), 80-94.

Miller, N.J., & Kean, R.C. (1997b). Reciprocal exchange in rural communities: Consumers' inducements to inshop. *Psychology & Marketing*, *14* (7), 637-661.

Miller, N.J., & Kim, S. (1999). The importance of older consumers to small business survival: Evidence from rural Iowa. *Journal of Small Business Management*, *37* (4), 1-15.

Miller, N.J., Kim, S., & Schofield-Tomschin, S. (1999). The effects of activity and aging on rural community living and consuming. *The Journal of Consumer Affairs*, *32* (2), 343-368.

Moschis, G.P. (1994). *Marketing Strategies of the Mature Market*, Westport, CT: Quorum Books.

Naidu, G.M., Kleimenhagen, A., & Pillari, G.D. (1993). Is product-line management appropriate for your health care? *Journal of Health Care Marketing*, *13* (3), 6-18.

Quandt, S.A., & Rao, P. (1999). Hunger and food security among older adults in a rural community. *Human Organization*, *58* (1), 28-35.

Rohrer, J.E., & Culica, D.V. (1999). Identifying high-users of medical care in a farming-dependent county. *Health Care Management Review*, *24* (4), 28-34.

Rosel, N. (2001). Inconspicuous consumption: How a small sample of rural elders see images in the media. *Generations: Journal of the American Society on Aging*, *25* (3), 47-51.

Rushinek, A., & Rushinek, S.F. (1986). Factors affecting rural consumers' satisfaction with medical care. *Health Marketing Quarterly, 3* (4), 37-57.

Signorielli, N. (2001). Aging on television: The picture in the nineties. *Generations: Journal of the American Society on Aging, 25* (3), 34-38.

Smith, M., Buckwalter, K.C., Zevenbergen, P.W., & Kudart, P. (1993). An administrator's dilemma: Keeping the innovative mental health and aging programs alive after the grant funds end. *Journal of Mental Health Administration, 20* (3), 212-217.

Taylor, D.L. (2001). Telling it like it is: Marketing maneuvers for rural telcos. *Rural Telecommunications, 20* (5), 52-57.

Taylor, S.L. (1997). Outshopping: The battle between rural and urban medical services. *Marketing Health Services, 17* (3), 42-44.

Vesperi, M.D. (2001). Media, marketing, and images of the older person in the information age. *Generations: Journal of the American Society on Aging, 25* (3), 5-9.

Wall Street Journal. (2001). Simple PCs can help speed elderly onto net. *Wall Street Journal*, July 16, p. B5.

Watt, I.S. (1992). Perceptions of quality: The rural dimension. *Journal of Management in Medicine, 6* (4), 30-37.

Wright, R.A. (1995). Equal access will shift marketing focus to consumers. *Journal of Health Care Marketing, 15* (3), 9-12.

Yasin, M.M., & Green, R.F. (1995). A strategic approach to service quality: A field study in a rural health care setting. *Health Marketing Quarterly, 13* (1), 75-82.

SECTION III
SPECIAL POPULATIONS

Chapter 7

Indigenous Elders in Rural America

Amanda Barusch, PhD
Christine TenBarge, PhD

SUMMARY. Using figures from the most recent census as well as available literature, this chapter considers the status of Indigenous elders in rural areas of the United States. Following a review of basic demographic indicators, we examine history of forced assimilation and colonization, and the impact of that history on Indigenous elders. We note the common belief that the status of Indigenous elders is less than historical and contemporary cultural norms would dictate. Discussion at a public meeting about the return of artifacts is offered as an illustrative example. We then consider service approaches that can both empower elders and improve their quality of life–suggesting that the pursuit of culturally ap-

[Haworth co-indexing entry note]: "Indigenous Elders in Rural America." Barusch, Amanda, and Christine TenBarge. Co-published simultaneously in *Journal of Gerontological Social Work* (The Haworth Social Work Practice Press, an imprint of The Haworth Press, Inc.) Vol. 41, No. 1/2, 2003, pp. 121-136; and: *Gerontological Social Work in Small Towns and Rural Communities* (ed: Sandra S. Butler, and Lenard W. Kaye) The Haworth Social Work Practice Press, an imprint of The Haworth Press, Inc., 2003, pp. 121-136. Single or multiple copies of this article are available for a fee from The Haworth Document Delivery Service [1-800-HAWORTH, 9:00 a.m. - 5:00 p.m. (EST). E-mail address: docdelivery@haworth press.com].

http://www.haworthpress.com/web/JGSW
© 2003 by The Haworth Press, Inc. All rights reserved.
Digital Object Identifier: 10.1300/J083v41n01_07

propriate interventions should begin with the employment of Indigenous service providers. *[Article copies available for a fee from The Haworth Document Delivery Service: 1-800-HAWORTH. E-mail address: <docdelivery@haworthpress.com> Website: <http://www.HaworthPress.com> © 2003 by The Haworth Press, Inc. All rights reserved.]*

KEYWORDS. Indigenous elders, rural Native Americans, culturally appropriate practice

INTRODUCTION: DEMOGRAPHICS

Prior to the 2000 Census, the last careful count of the nation's Indigenous[1] population was that mandated by the Dawes Act in 1887. Census counts during the interim under-counted the Indigenous population, and as a result much was written about the so-called "vanishing race" (Churchill, 1999; Johansen, 2002; Thornton, 1987, 1996). Using a strategy familiar to social work since the Settlement House days, the Census Bureau hired Indigenous people to collect data for the 2000 Census. The need to cooperate with Census personnel was advertised, and Indigenous People were encouraged to participate in the Census at PowWows and other cultural events, urban Indian centers and clinics, schools and universities, and other settings where Indigenous Peoples are known to gather. Images of famous Indigenous figures–Sitting Bull, Chief Joseph, Geronimo–were imposed on huge posters exhorting people to "stand up and be counted," and Census personnel offered free gifts–key chains, flashlights, pens, notepads, mirrors, posters, and t-shirts–respecting a universal Indigenous tradition.

And they did a better job than usual with the count. In the 2000 Census, more than 4.1 million people said they were at least partially Native American, which is double the 2 million reporting Native ancestry in the 1990 census and 14 times the official figure of about 300,000 a century ago (Johansen, 2002; Thornton, 1987, 1996; U.S. Census Bureau, 2002). By comparison, the total U.S. population grew by 13% during the same interval (U.S. Census Bureau, 2002). Most of this growth was due to a change in the Census procedures. Census 2000 was also the first in which respondents were allowed to choose more than one race. A total of 1.6 million Americans identified themselves as part American Indian/Alaska Native, which accounted for most of the increase. Even when those identifying as part-American Indian/Alaska Native are not included, Census 2000 documented a 25% increase in the number of Americans identified as Indigenous Peoples since the 1990 Census.

Federal recognition is critical for tribes seeking to establish services and provide benefits to their people. There are 562 federally-recognized tribes in the U.S., and about 148 groups seeking federal recognition. Thirty-six tribes are recognized by states (U.S. Census, 2002). The process of attaining federal recognition is difficult and arbitrary. During the 1950s and 1960s the federal government pursued a policy of "termination," discontinuing recognition of several tribes (Churchill, 1998; Yellow Bird, 2001a). At the same time, a program of relocation dispatched Indigenous Peoples from reservations to cities with the goal of forcing them to assimilate into mainstream society.

A direct result of this policy is seen today in the greater numbers of Indigenous Peoples living off reservations. In 1900, 99.6% of federally recognized Indigenous Peoples lived on reservations. By 1970, nearly half (44.5%) lived off reservations. Current estimates suggest that over half of Indigenous peoples–from 55 to 70%–live off the reservation (Churchill, 1998; Walters, 1999).

Still, Indigenous elders are significantly more likely than Whites to live in a rural setting. According to the 2000 Census, only one in four non-Hispanic whites lived in rural locations. This led Share DeCroix Bane to observe that "Native American elderly are the most rural of the minorities . . . " (p. 63).

The 2000 Census also indicted that California and Oklahoma were home to one in four American Indian/Alaska Natives. Nearly half of Indigenous elders aged 55 and older live in just five states: Oklahoma, California, Arizona, New Mexico, and North Carolina (Ogunwole, 2002). Although we focus on elders in rural settings here, we should note that many Indigenous elders live in urban centers, such as New York and Los Angeles (Ogunwole, 2002). Urban elders generally enjoy greater income and better health than those living on reservations, although urban settings do not allow for access to Indian Health Service facilities. As the National Indian Council on Aging (NICOA) noted, Indigenous elders live in diverse settings–in *hogans* in the deserts of Arizona, Utah, and Nevada, in concrete block houses on reservations, in urban apartments, and in suburban homes (NICOA, 2003). Most Indigenous elders, both rural and urban, do not live on reservations.

Reservation-based elders live on treaty-based, executive ordered, and state-created reservations, as well as in bands not federally recognized. Although reservations offer greater access to tribal community and Indian Health Services, living conditions are extremely difficult.

The most recent information available comes from the 1980 Census, which reported that 16% of homes on the reservation had no electricity; 17% had no refrigerators; and 21% had no indoor toilets (National Indian Council on Aging, 2003). Transportation is also difficult on reservations, where many rely on poorly maintained dirt roads that become impassable in rain or show. Finally, communication is a challenge, as most elders do not have telephones, receive newspapers or have television sets (Bane, 1991).

Harsh, impoverished living conditions contribute to lower life expectancies for Indigenous Peoples. In the mid 1990s, life expectancy for American Indian/Alaska Native men was estimated at 66.1 years, while life expectancy for women was 74.4 years. This compares to life expectancies of 73.2 years for white men, and 79.6 years for white women. Indigenous men are second only to African-American men in the shortness of their life expectancies (U.S. Department of Health and Human Services, 1998). The life expectancies of Indigenous Peoples have, however, improved dramatically in recent decades. For example, John (1980) estimated the average life expectancy for Indigenous Peoples at 45 years.

Despite this improvement, shorter life expectancy continues to limit the number of years that elders can access benefits widely available to older non-Indigenous Americans. If full Social Security benefits begin at age 65, a person with a 66-year life expectancy has fewer years to collect, even though s/he contributed to the system for as many years as someone who enjoys a longer life expectancy.

FORCED ASSIMILATION AND COLONIZATION

Any understanding of the lives of Indigenous elders must be informed by knowledge of the historical trauma imposed by forced assimilation and colonization. Assimilation refers to the process of absorbing or being absorbed into the cultural tradition of a population or group. It is frequently used to describe the degree of acculturation achieved by immigrants. But in the case of Indigenous Peoples, forced assimilation was the result of systematic policies designed to eradicate the Indigenous culture.[2]

For example, the U.S. government set out to "kill the Indian in every child" by removing Indigenous children from their homes and placing them in government-run boarding schools (George, 1997; Churchill, 1998). These schools forced the children to wear the clothes, eat the food, speak the language, and practice the customs of the dominant culture. In the U.S., this practice continued from the late 19th century until the middle years of the 20th century (George, 1997). Most boarding schools were closed by the 1960s and 1970s, although a number continue to operate.

Boarding schools were replaced by perhaps a more insidious form of repression, the Indian Adoption Program. A joint venture of the Bureau of Indian Affairs and the Child Welfare League of America, this program placed Indigenous children in White adoptive homes located as far as geographically possible from their families of origin. Between the 1950s and the 1970s, an estimated 395 Indigenous children were adopted through this program (George, 1997). The general practice of placing Indigenous children in white homes was slowed by the passage of the Indian Child Welfare Act in 1978.

Another policy designed to force assimilation was the Indian Relocation Act of 1953, put forward in House Concurrent Resolution 108. This policy, couched in the concept of "entitling [Indigenous Peoples] to the same privileges and responsibilities as are applicable to other citizens of the United States" is commonly referred to as "termination policy." The purpose of the Resolution was to end protected trust status of Indigenous land and to withdraw the federal support of educational, health, and social programs promised in exchange for lands when treaties were signed. The Resolution included plans for the immediate termination of tribes in California, Florida, New York, and Texas (Bonvillain, 2001).

Christian religious sects were willing partners in government efforts to force Indigenous Peoples to adopt the majority culture. Churches were given federal funds to establish and operate schools on reservations, and some engaged in aggressive proselytizing (Linn, Berardo, & Yamamoto, 1998; McCarty, 1998). Religious conversion meant abdication, not only of traditional religious practices, but also of health practices, which in Indigenous cultures have a strong spiritual component.

Pivotal to the process of forced assimilation is the eradication of Indigenous languages. As Fillmore (1994) pointed out, "the question of cultural identity is synonymous with the question of language" (p. 1; as cited in Linn, Berardo, & Yamamoto, 1998). The U.S. government has long recognized the importance of language. In the boarding schools children were severely punished for using their native tongue. This policy was also pursued by the Kennedy administration during the Americanization of the Western Pacific (Barusch & Spaulding, 1989). The result is what some linguists call "language extermination." Roughly half of the Indigenous languages of California have no fluent speakers left at all (Hinton, 1998). As Teresa McCarty explained:

> Indigenous languages in the United States are under siege . . . of the 175 indigenous languages still extant in the USA, only 20 are being transmitted as child languages. The remainder are spoken by parental or grandparental generations, and over a third are spoken only by the most elderly members of the community, often fewer than ten individuals. (McCarty, 1998, p. 27)

COLONIZATION

What assimilation does to culture, colonization does to political and economic power. Through the process of colonization, Indigenous people become second-class citizens and lose control of their land and other sources of wealth. The result of this process is seen in the financial poverty of Indigenous people. In 1999, for example, American Indian/Alaska Natives had the highest poverty rate of any ethnic group in the United States. Whereas 7% of non-Hispanic Whites lived with incomes below the federal poverty threshold, 25.9% of Indigenous Peoples lived in poverty. Thus, in this country, Indigenous people have *over three times* the risk of poverty of the white majority (U.S. Census Bureau, 2000). Indigenous elders experience higher rates of poverty. The Indian Health Service (IHS) reported that 31.6% of Indigenous elders had incomes below the poverty threshold, compared to 9.8% of whites aged 60 or older (IHS, 1996).

The association between poverty and ill health[3] is evident in the health and functional status of Indigenous elders. Assessments of functional status and need for long-term care consistently suggest that Indigenous elders suffer from more activity limitations than the general population (McFall, Solomon, & Smith, 2000). For example, Share DeCroix Bane (1991) reported that "Native Americans experience the same limitations in their activities of daily living at age 45 as do non-Indian people at age 65" (p. 64).

In addition to greater functional impairments, Indigenous peoples experience high rates of many diseases. These include phenomenal rates of diabetes, with experts suggesting that 40 to 50% of Indigenous adults have the disease (Roubideaux, 2002). Indeed, the Pima tribe in Arizona reports the highest recorded prevalence of diabetes in the world (Acton, Burrows, Moore, Querec, Geiss, & Engelgau, 2002). This led one IHS doctor to remark, "I was often surprised to see a patient *without* diabetes" (italics added, Roubideaux, p. 1401). Indigenous Peoples are more likely than others to die of tuberculosis, influenza, and pneumonia (Harris, 2002).

In addition to health problems, practitioners who work with Indigenous Peoples see the legacy of forced assimilation and colonization in the behavioral and emotional problems they confront each day. In 1992, Maxwell and Maxwell conducted an ethnographic study of elder abuse on two reservations. The reservation with the highest rate of poverty and isolation also had the highest rate of elder abuse. Their findings underscored the role of social conditions in producing what some perceive as individual dysfunction. As they explained, "We attribute differences in prevalence of mistreatment of elders to variations in economic opportunities for younger residents" (p. 3). Like the tribal respondents they interviewed, these researchers concluded that mistreatment of elders was the explosive result of perceived powerlessness, "a dysfunction in community health" (p. 3). As two leading Indigenous scholars write:

> Historical trauma refers to cumulative wounding across generations as well as during one's current life span. For Native people, the legacy of genocide includes distortions of Indigenous identity, self-concept and values. The process of colonization and varying degrees of assimilation into the dominant cultural value system have resulted in altered states of an Indian sense of self. (Weaver & Yellow Horse Brave Heart, 1999, p. 22)

Similarly, Yellow Bird (2001b) argued that:

> Today, more than ever, I am convinced that the disproportionate amount of substance abuse, family violence, and suffering within First Nations communities is a result of the continuing effects of European American colonialism. First Nations Peoples are the survivors of a massive and prolonged campaign of racial and cultural terrorism perpetuated by the United States of America. (p. 2)

A young person's history is an old person's lived experience. Many of today's elders had direct experience in boarding schools and White foster homes. They carry the memory of having their mouths washed out with soap for speaking a language some considered "primitive." Many have had to re-learn their cultural practices late in life because they were unable to do so as children. Still others have had to learn to parent, having spent years moving from foster home to foster home. So Indigenous elders are especially sensitive to the effects of historical trauma and those who work with them must be as well. Some of the more subtle effects relate to changes in the role and status of elders within the community.

THE STATUS OF ELDERS

There is no way to empirically demonstrate that Indigenous elders today have less power and status than they did prior to the arrival of Euro-Americans. Within the field of aging we refer to the "myth of the golden age," suggesting that it is popular to believe that elders were once treated better than they are now. With that caution in mind, we can note that many believe the current status of Indigenous elders is not consistent with either historical or contemporary cultural norms.

In the early years following the arrival of Europeans, some elders did live to advanced ages. Although life expectancy was short, there are recorded cases among Indigenous tribes of individuals who reached 95 to 103 years (Simmons, 1945).

Respect for advanced age has always been an integral part of many Indigenous cultures. Elders were central figures in many stories of creation. Among the Hopi two aged goddesses were believed to have created all living things, and old Spider Woman is said to have invented arts and crafts (Simmons, 1945). The Menomini, Creek, and Omaha all have held that old men were the first recipients of magic powers and healing arts. Among some tribes, like the Omaha, elders retained leadership positions long after they began to physically fail.

Today respect for elders remains an important value among various Indigenous groups. Yet several forces operate to undermine that respect. Generational differences in education and language can create barriers. Poverty can undermine dignity, even as it reduces the material resources an elder can share. Finally, television, the Internet, and other mass media devices may succeed where government programs failed: "taking the Indian out" of Indigenous children. As young people strive for the material wealth promised by the mass media, they lose appreciation for the knowledge and support offered by their elders (Barusch & Steen, 1996). As they rattle on in their first language, English, young people may think their elders are ignorant or uneducated because their English is less fluent.

Perhaps a more distressing aspect of the lack of honor occurs when the dominant culture treats Indigenous elders as if their requests have little or no value, or worse, dismissed out of hand. Such an event occurred during a Native American Graves Protection & Repatriation Act (NAGPRA) review committee meeting.

The Native American Graves Protection & Repatriation Act of 1990 (NAGPRA) is, like the Indigenous Peoples, interests that it represents, unique and largely ignored. Meant to protect the human remains, funerary and sacred objects of the ancestors of Indigenous Peoples, many tribal nations expend vast amounts of time, energy and money to ensure that provisions of the federal law are enforced. They do this because, as was admitted during a recent NAGPRA review committee meeting, many federal agencies do not comply, and the Department of Justice does not enforce the federal law.

During a recent NAGPRA oversight review committee, which Christine TenBarge attended, a dispute for ownership of a ceremonial mask in possession of the Denver Art Museum (DAM) was before the committee. According to White Mountain Apache tribal leaders and elders, the artifacts in question were sacred objects and were needed by the tribe for healing the intergenerational trauma from which the tribe suffered. The DAM representatives, as they were called, were concerned that a particular mask, culled from the White Mountain Apache Tribe in the 1930s and given to the museum by a donor, was not culturally significant or relevant to the tribe. The DAM representatives were disputing the demand by the tribal community that the mask be returned along with undisputed human remains. The principal voice against returning the artifact to the White Mountain Apache Tribe came from a non-Native review committee member, an anthropologist, and was supported by another of the non-Indigenous members. Those who supported returning the artifacts were White Mountain Apache representatives, including tribal leaders and elders who made the long journey from Colorado to Oklahoma by car.

A respected elder stood to address the committee and offered this plea: "We have come to ask that you return all the objects that belong to us. We need them to perform the ceremony necessary for our tribe to get back on the path to healing. Our tribe has too many problems, too much pain, and we will continue to suffer as long as those things we need to heal are in the hands of others."

"These artifacts are not sacred, nor can they be considered cultural patrimonial objects," said the anthropologist dismissively, "Especially that mask. That mask is probably a fake. I can take you down to the most popular Indian store in Tulsa, where no doubt many of you have been, and show you one just like it. It was common practice for Indians to sell, quote, authentic unquote, ceremonial masks to unsuspecting collectors that had no cultural value or significance whatsoever." (Quotes are from Christine TenBarge's notes of the meeting. A summary of the meeting is available at: http://www.cast.uark.edu/other/nps/nagpra/DOCS/rms023.html.) The Indigenous elders were not only disrespected before the committee and mostly Indigenous audience, but were discounted as experts in their own tribal customs and lore. Such disregard perpetuates this nation's legacy of racism and destroys hope for inter-ethnic reconciliation.

STRATEGIES TO SUPPORT AND EMPOWER INDIGENOUS ELDERS

Observing that interventions designed to reduce elder abuse by treating individuals have proven ineffective, Maxwell and Maxwell (1992) argued for the potential efficacy of community-based interventions. They acknowledge that we tend to "slight trauma suffered by the community as a whole" and note that "police do not arrest 'conditions,' they arrest someone naïve or unlucky enough to have drawn attention to himself by doing something disapproved of" (p. 20). Further, interventions that target social conditions risk alienating those currently privileged as they inevitably require the re-allocation of resources. Nonetheless, our survey of emerging interventions highlights several promising community-based interventions.

Several interventions address the health needs of Indigenous Peoples. The Indian Self-Determination and Educational Assistance Act of 1975 set the stage for tribes to manage health programs that had been under the Indian Health Service. Many tribes have taken advantage of this opportunity, and Yvette Roubideaux (2002) reported that "approximately half of the IHS budget is now managed by tribes" (p. 1402). Recognizing the growing need for long-term care, several tribes have, in collaboration with the Indian Health Service, and on their own, established nursing homes and home-health agencies on their reservations. Noting "Most elderly Indians who require nursing home care must leave the reservation and their families" (p. 181), Susan Mercer (1996) described the culturally sensitive care provided by a nursing home operated by the Navajo nation, with primarily Navajo staff. Similar care is provided by the Navajo Area Home Health Agency (McCabe, 1988). The Alaska Native Women's Wellness Project has successfully increased cancer prevention screening rates among Indigenous elders in its catchment area through respect of the individual and her culture (Stillwater, 1999).

To address the weakening of intergenerational bonds, activists in New York established ELDERS (Encouraging Leaders Dedicated to Enriching Respect and Spirituality), a week-long gathering where elders teach youth the traditional ways of the Iroquois. Although primarily intended as a substance abuse prevention program for youth, this effort has the secondary benefit of offering meaningful activity and connection to local elders (Skye, 2002).

Language revival and restoration efforts have the dual benefits of salvaging language and empowering elders. The 1990 Native American Languages Act (PL 101-477) reflected the discovery that hundreds of native languages in this country were endangered. That is, they were spoken by only a handful of elders. Linguists have pointed out the importance of language diversity, not only for minority language speakers themselves, but for the nation as a whole, noting that "language loss is part of a much larger process of loss of cultural and intellectual diversity in which politically dominant languages and cultures simply overwhelm Indigenous local ones . . . " (Linn, Berardo, & Yamamoto, 1998, p. 63).

Several community-based interventions have been initiated to salvage the nation's Indigenous languages. Christine Sims (1998) described one such intervention, designed to preserve and restore the native language of the Karuk Tribe in Northern California. Using tribal funds, a language-immersion camp was offered in 1992 for children, parents, and fluent-speaking elders. Both overnight and day-camp experiences were offered, in which children learn the language of their elders in highly structured sessions. Sims reported that " . . . language support and interaction that elders provide is a key element . . . " of the program, establishing " . . . the crucial intergenerational linkages necessary for language vitality" (p. 103-104). The tribe also established "master-apprentice language teams," who devote at least 20 hours each week to language learning. Language interventions like these not only help to restore cultural diversity to the USA, they add meaning and power to the lives of Indigenous elders.

THE NEED FOR INDIGENOUS SOCIAL WORKERS

While laudable, efforts to develop cultural competency fall short of the mark if the goal is to meet the needs of Indigenous elders in ways that are personally satisfying and culturally appropriate. Certainly, the White social worker needs cultural knowledge and skills to even begin to provide support to an Indigenous elder, and certainly that support will be better than nothing. But it would be more effective and more efficient to recruit and train Indigenous social workers.

It is almost comic to consider advice that has been given to White practitioners (and researchers) seeking to work with Indigenous elders. For example, Ferraro (2001) identified "hurdles" faced by researchers seeking to collect information on elders in "Indian Country." The first such hurdle "is gaining the trust of the native elder to actually want to participate in your study" (p. 314). He suggests that a "gift of tobacco" might be offered, and warns the potential researcher "in some Native cultures it is considered disrespectful to look someone in the eyes." Similarly, McDonald, Morton, and Stewart (1992) offered suggestions for clinical practice with Indigenous Peoples. The first piece of advice: "Begin and end each session with a handshake" will poorly serve a practitioner working with the Navajo, for example, for whom such physical contact can be uncomfortable, especially the Euro-American tendency to pump the hand hard and vigorously. A more common Indigenous handshake involves the brief and gentle pressure of fingers to fingers.

Indeed, most tribal people do not use the handshake as a greeting between strangers. It was thought (and still is to some extent, though now it seems more a custom than absolute belief), that in a handshake the other person might be trying to steal your soul and zap your energies. One didn't know if that person was friend or foe, especially in the case of the White man. So physical contact involved risk of loss. The same thing applies, although to a lesser extent, to the reluctance to engage in eye contact with an unfamiliar person. That person could be an enemy, or in Navajo stories, a witch, and horrible things could happen if a witch puts an eye on you.

CONCLUSION

Today's Indigenous elders experience the consequences of yesterday's efforts to eradicate Indigenous cultures (assimilation) and appropriate the resources of Indigenous Peoples (colonization). They were victimized by policies that have since been abandoned: boarding schools, adoption by Whites, and language suppression. Many live in harsh and impoverished conditions–the direct result of colonization. Perhaps more subtle, many experience insults to their dignity and do not enjoy the stature to which they should be entitled under Indigenous cultural norms. A few are neglected and abused by family members.

Recognition of these devastating experiences yields a difficult conclusion: non-Indigenous social workers do not effectively meet the needs of indigenous elders. Asking an elder to "trust" a White person who offers a gift of tobacco and a hearty handshake adds insult to injury. Indigenous elders deserve to receive care from someone who does not remind them of past oppression and current humiliations. There is a crying need for Indigenous practitioners from all professions (doctors, teachers, social workers, counselors, rehabilitation specialists, administrators) to serve elders in rural areas. The Census Bureau figured this out, and in a masterful stroke hired Indigenous staff to count the nation's Indigenous people. Non-Indigenous social workers should be considered a second choice for direct service (on the dubious principle that "something is better than nothing"). First choice would be a well-trained, highly skilled Indigenous social worker.

We also note the limited impact of interventions that punish individual perpetrators, and recommend expansion of community-based programs designed to empower elders and enhance the quality of their lives. No doubt, the interested reader will add to our list of examples, which includes health services for Indigenous elders, as well as language restoration efforts in which the elders play a vital role. At the policy level, it is way past time for federal, state, and local governments to defer to tribal authority on matters affecting Indigenous peoples.

NOTES

1. According to Michael Yellow Bird, of the Sahnish/Hidatsa Nation, the terms "Indian," "American Indian," and "Native American" are "counterfeit identities" imposed on indigenous people by Euro-American colonizers. To show respect and agreement, this paper uses "First Nations" and "Indigenous Peoples." As Yellow Bird explained, "The change in terminology is a matter of social justice because Indigenous Peoples have, and continue to, struggle against the oppressive paradigms of American linguistic colonialism that ignores individual tribal identities and falsely names Indigenous Peoples to serve the needs and history of the colonizer" (Yellow Bird, 1999, p. 86).

2. As evidence of the tenacity of Indigenous culture, Vira Kivett observed in 1993, "In many ways, they [Indigenous Peoples] are the least assimilated of the ethnic groups" (p. 211).

3. The exact mechanism responsible for the association between poverty and ill-health is unclear. Some people have suggested that ill health *causes* poverty. Others suggest that the genetic make-up of Indigenous Peoples predisposes them to some diseases. One case study clearly illustrates the causal role of economic disadvantage. Lacking access to other jobs, Navajo men gravitated to Uranium mines in the 1940s. The combination of radiation

and radon in the mines exposed these men to increased risk of lung cancer, and indeed became the cause of most lung cancer deaths among Navajo (Brugge & Goble, 2002).

REFERENCES

Acton, K.J., Burrows, N.R., Moore, K., Querec, L., Geiss, L.S., & Engelgau, M.M. (2002). Trends in diabetes prevalence among American Indian and Alaska Native children, adolescents, and young adults. *American Journal of Public Health, 92*(9), 1485-1490.

Bane, Share Decroix. (1991). Rural minority populations. *Generations, Fall/Winter*, 63-65.

Barusch, A.S., & Spaulding, M.L. (1989). The impact of Americanization on intergenerational relations: An exploratory study on the US territory of Guam. *Journal of Sociology and Social Welfare, 16*(3), 61-79.

Barusch, A.S., & Steen, P. (1996). Keepers of community in a changing world. *Generations, 20*(1), 49-52.

Bernard, M.A., Lampley-Dallas, V., & Smith, L. (1997). Common health problems among minority elders. *Journal of the American Dietetic Association, 97*(7), 771-777.

Bonvillain, N. (2001). *Native nations: Cultures and histories of Native North America.* Upper Saddle River, NJ: Prentice-Hall, Inc.

Brugge, D., & Goble, R. (2002). The history of uranium mining and the Navajo people. *American Journal of Public Health, 92*(9), 1410-1419.

Buchwald, D., Sheffield, J., Furman, R., Hartman, Dudden, M., & Manson, S. (2000). *Archives of Internal Medicine, 160*(10), 1443-1455.

Churchill, W. (1998). *A little matter of genocide: Holocaust and denial in the Americas, 1492 to the present.* San Francisco: City Lights Books.

Ferraro, F.R. (2001). Assessment and evaluation issues regarding Native American elderly adults. *Journal of Clinical Geropsychology, 7*(4), 311-318.

Fillmore, L.W. (1994). Language and cultural identity: What happens when languages are lost? Paper presented at the 1994 Alaska bilingual Education Conference, Anchorage (cited by Linn et al., 1998).

George, L.J. (1997). Why the need for the Indian Child Welfare Act? *Journal of Multicultural Social Work, 5*(3/4), 165-175.

Harris, C. (2992). Indigenous health: Fulfilling our obligation to future generations. *American Journal of Public Health, 92*(9), 1990.

Hinton, L. (1998). Language loss and revitalization in California: Overview. *International Journal of the Sociology of Language, 132*, 83-93.

Indian Health Service (IHS). (1996). *Regional Differences in Indian Health–1996.* Rockville, MD: Public Health Service, US Department of Health and Human Services.

Johansen, B. (2002). Native Americans in the 2000 census: Far from the "vanishing race." *Native Americas, 19*(1/2), 42-45.

John, R. (1980). The Older American Act and the elderly Native American. *Journal of Minority Aging, 5* (2-4), 293-298.

Kivett, V.R. (1993). Informal Supports Among Rural Minorities. In Bull, N.C. (Ed). *Aging in Rural America* (pp. 204-215), Newbury Park: Sage Publications.

Linn, M., Berardo, M., & Yamamoto, A.Y. (1998). Creating language teams in Oklahoma Native American communities. *International Journal of the Sociology of Language, 132*, 61-78.

Maxwell, E.K., & Maxwell, R.J. (1992). Insults to the body civil: Mistreatment of elderly in two plains Indian tribes. *Journal of Cross-Cultural Gerontology, 7*, 3-23.

McCabe, M.L. (1988). Health care accessibility for the elderly on the Navajo Reservation. *Pride Institute Journal of Long Term Home Health Care, 7*(4), 22-26.

McCarty, T.L. (1998). Schooling, resistance, and American Indian languages. *International Journal of the Sociology of Language, 132*, 27-41.

McDonald, J.D., Morton, R., & Stewart, C. (1992). Clinical concerns with American Indian patients. *Innovations in Clinical Practice, 12*, 437-454.

McFall, S.I., Solomon, T.G.A., & Smith, D.W. (2000). Health-related quality of life of older Native American primary care patients. *Research on Aging, 22*(6), 692-714.

Mercer, S.O. (1996). Navajo elderly people in a reservation nursing home: Admission predictors and culture care practices. *Social Work, 41*(2), 181-189.

National Indian Council on Aging (NICOA). (2003). Retrieved Feb. 24, 2003 from *http://www.nicoa.org/*.

Ogunwole, S.U. (2002). *The American Indian and Alaska Native population: 2000. Census 2000 brief*. Washington DC: US Bureau of the Census. pp. 1-12. (*http://www.census.gov/prod/2002pubs/c2kbr01-15.pdf*).

Roubideaux, Y. (2002). Perspectives on American Indian Health. *American Journal of Public Health, 92*(9), 1401-1403.

Simmons, L.W. (1945). *The Role of the Aged in Primitive Societies*. New Haven, CT: Yale University Press.

Sims, C.P. (1998). Community-based efforts to preserve native languages: A descriptive study of the Karuk Tribe of northern California. *International Journal of the Sociology of Language, 132*, 95-113.

Skye, W. (2002). ELDERS gathering for Native American youth: Continuing Native American traditions and curbing substance abuse in Native American youth. *Journal of Sociology and Social Welfare, March, 29*(1), 117-135.

Stillwater, B. (1999). The Alaska Native Women's Wellness Project. *Health Care for Women International, 20*, 487-492.

Thornton, R. (1987). *American Indian holocaust and survival: A population history since 1492*. Norman, OK: University of Oklahoma Press.

Thornton, R. (1996). Tribal membership requirements and the demography of "old" and "new" Native Americans. In G.D. Sandefur, R.R. Rindfuss, & B. Cohen (Eds.), *Changing numbers, changing needs: American Indian demography and Public health* (pp. 103-112). Washington, DC: National Academy Press.

U.S. Bureau of the Census. (2002). *Statistical Abstract of the United States* (1116th Ed.), Washington, DC (*www.census.gov/population/www/socdemo/race/indian.html*).

U.S. Census Bureau (2000). *Poverty Rate Lowest in 20 Years, Household Income at Record High*. Department of Commerce News Release (*http://www.census.gov/Press-Release/www.2000/cb00-158.html*).

U.S. Department of Health and Human Services. (2002). Grants awarded for Native American elders and caregivers. *Health Care Financing Review, 23*(4), 208-210.

U.S. Department of Health and Human Services (1998). Office on Women's Health. *Women of Color Health Data Book.* (*http://www.4woman.gov/owh/pub/woc/figure1.htm*).

Walters, K.L. (1999). Urban American Indian identity attitudes and acculturation styles. *Journal of Human Behavior and the Social Environment*, *2*(1/2), 163-178.

Weaver, H.N., & Brave Heart, M.Y. (1999). Examining two facets of American Indian identity: Exposure to other cultures and the influence of historical trauma. *Journal of Human Behavior and the Social Environment*, *2*(1/2), 19-33.

Yellow Bird, M.J. (1999). Indian, American Indian, and Native Americans: Counterfeit identities. *Winds of Change: A Magazine for American Indian Education and Opportunity*, *14*(1), 86.

Yellow Bird, M.J. (2001a). Critical values and First Nations Peoples. In R. Fong, & S. Furuto (Eds.), *Culturally competent social work practice: Practice skills, interventions, and evaluation.* (pp. 61-74). Boston: Allyn & Bacon.

Yellow Bird, M.J. (2001b, February). *Substance abuse and family violence affecting First Nations Peoples: The continuing effects of European American colonialism.* Paper presented at the Task Force Meeting of Cultural Competence in Child Welfare Practice: A Collaboration Between Practitioners and Academicians.

Chapter 8

Rural African American Older Adults and the Black Helping Tradition

Mikal N. Rasheed, PhD
Janice Matthews Rasheed, DSW

SUMMARY. By the year 2050, 21 percent of all Americans over 65 will be members of a minority group with African Americans being the largest subgroup. What is critical is that there are great disparities in the physical and mental health status, service availability, service access, and socioeconomic factors between elderly African Americans and elderly whites. These disparities are even more evident with older African Americans in rural communities. Along with these disparities, coupled with the "helping tradition" in the African American community, there has been a great reliance on community-based informal care systems for elderly African Americans.

This chapter will examine the informal care systems in rural African American communities within the context of the helping tradition found within the African American cultural history. In this examination there will be a discussion of how the gaps in the social services delivery system in rural communities reinforce this helping tradition. *[Article copies available for a fee from The Haworth Document Delivery Service: 1-800-HAWORTH. E-mail address: <docdelivery@haworthpress.com> Website: <http://www.HaworthPress.com> © 2003 by The Haworth Press, Inc. All rights reserved.]*

[Haworth co-indexing entry note]: "Rural African American Older Adults and the Black Helping Tradition." Rasheed, Mikal N., and Janice Matthews Rasheed. Co-published simultaneously in *Journal of Gerontological Social Work* (The Haworth Social Work Practice Press, an imprint of The Haworth Press, Inc.) Vol. 41, No. 1/2, 2003, pp. 137-150; and: *Gerontological Social Work in Small Towns and Rural Communities* (ed: Sandra S. Butler, and Lenard W. Kaye) The Haworth Social Work Practice Press, an imprint of The Haworth Press, Inc., 2003, pp. 137-150. Single or multiple copies of this article are available for a fee from The Haworth Document Delivery Service [1-800-HAWORTH, 9:00 a.m. - 5:00 p.m. (EST). E-mail address: docdelivery@haworthpress.com].

http://www.haworthpress.com/web/JGSW
© 2003 by The Haworth Press, Inc. All rights reserved.
Digital Object Identifier: 10.1300/J083v41n01_08

KEYWORDS. Black helping tradition, older African Americans, rural African Americans

INTRODUCTION

The dramatic growth of the aging population has created new challenges for the social work profession, calling for a growing demand for a variety of health, mental health, and social services (Rosen & Zlotnik, 2001). While social work has a long history in working with older adults in a variety of settings, the elderly population is increasing both in number and in diversity, thus reshaping the American demographic landscape (Torres-Gill & Moga, 2001). In the last century while the U.S. population tripled, the elderly population, including those over 65, increased 11 fold (U.S. Census, 1996). The U.S. 2000 Census found that 12.4 percent of the population was over 65. This percentage is expected to increase to 15.7 percent by 2020 and to 21 percent by 2040 (U.S. Census, 1996, 2000; Day, 1993; Torres-Gill & Moga, 2001). By the year 2050, 21 percent of all Americans over 65 will be members of a minority group, with African Americans being the largest subgroup (Ford & Hatchett, 2001). What is critical is that there are great disparities in the physical and mental health status, service availability, service access, and socioeconomic factors between elderly African Americans and elderly whites. These disparities are even more evident with older African Americans in rural communities. Along with these disparities, coupled with the "helping tradition" in the African American community, there has been a great reliance on community-based informal care systems for elderly African Americans.

This chapter will examine the informal care systems in rural African American communities within the context of the helping tradition found within the African American cultural history. In this examination there will be a discussion of how the gaps in the social services delivery system in rural communities reinforce this helping tradition. Finally, the authors will recommend ways in which social services might more effectively address some of the human service needs of older African Americans within the context of this helping tradition.

RURAL AFRICAN AMERICAN OLDER ADULTS AND INFORMAL CARE

Aging and the African American Experience

One of the most vulnerable populations within the African American community is older adults. There are in excess of two and one half million African Americans age 65 and older in the United States. This figure represents about 8% of the total African-American population (Barresi & Menon, 1990; Spence, Yogtiba, Perry, & Black, 1998). Elderly African Americans are increasing at a rate almost twice the rate of the African American population as a whole. By the year 2050 the projected number of African American older adults could reach 9 million or 15% of the total African American population (Cowgill, 1988). The vulnerability of this population is underscored by the following statistics:

1. African Americans have a shorter life expectancy than white Americans; 64.9 years for African American men compared to 73.2 years for white men; 74.1 years for African American women compared to 79.6 years for white women (Williams, Padgett, Blank, Guarini, Morton, Wilson, & Simmons, 2001). Curiously there is a cross-over phenomena in which African American males and females who reach the age of 73 and 85 respectively live longer that Whites (Greene & Seigler, 1984).
2. Older African Americans have a disproportional number of chronic health and health related problems, higher levels of functional dependence and a greater need for assistance than older Whites (Bane, 1991; Harper & Alexander, 1990; Hooyman & Kiyak, 2002). For example, older African Americans suffer disproportionately from hypertension, diabetes, and kidney problems (Spence, Yogtiba Perry, & Black, 1998).
3. Older African Americans experience greater disability and require more restricted days in bed that their older White counter parts (Hooyman & Kiyak, 2002).

In spite of these alarming statistics, Holmes and Holmes (1995) address ways in which the experience of aging are perceived differently and in some respects more positively, for African Americans as compared to whites. Holmes and Holmes (1995, pp. 188-189) state that it is possible to generalize that African Americans:

- See old age more as a reward than a disaster
- Have fewer anxieties about old age and therefore higher morale
- Are less likely to deny their actual age
- Tend to remain part of their family structure to a greater degree and consequently are more respected and better treated

- Are strongly supported by bonds of mutual assistance (with friends, neighbors and family)
- Are more likely to maintain useful and acceptable family functions
- Are more likely to be tolerated by their families in spite of behavioral peculiarities
- Are generally more religious but less involved in economic and political institutions
- Are considerably less prone to commit suicide.

These characteristics of the aging experience in African American communities may seem to suggest a more positive experience with the aging process among African Americans. Yet social problems such as poverty, lack of access to services, and racially or culturally insensitive services can mitigate against these seemingly positive orientations toward the aging process among African Americans. Additionally there are multiple factors in rural America that can contribute to the harshness of the aging experience for rural African Americans.

Rural African American Older Adults

In rural America the situation of African American elders reflects greater vulnerability than that of urban African American elders. The lack of appropriate senior services is indeed complicated by the lack of socioeconomic resources available to rural African American older adults. The lack of resources is compounded by the financial and physical realities of rural living–a reality where nearly 50% of all black elders live in poverty. Rural African American elders are additionally impacted by low literacy levels, poverty, poor and chronic health conditions, lack of transportation and housing (Wan, 1977; Wood & Wan, 1993). These factors contribute to the lack of knowledge of, access to, and ability to afford services.

Wood and Wan (1993) raise critical concerns about the nature of services that are available for rural elders, especially African American elders. The general network of formal community-based care for the elderly include: (1) in-home services, including skilled nursing, physical therapy, home health aide services and homemaker services; (2) geriatric day care and other support services such as home delivered meals, adult foster care and transportation; and (3) respite care, emergency lodging, or community housing options. In rural areas these facilities and services, other than institutional care in the form of nursing homes, are not as easily available.

One of the unique issues impacting social service development is the nature of community in a rural context which is scattered in terms of covering a large geographic area, with limited numbers of people. As Wood and Wan (1993) clearly point out, the social life of a rural community is usually centered on a general store, post office, or church. Patterns of interaction are informal and based on face-to-face contact. Much value is placed on knowing community residents personally. In such community settings, the chief providers of mental health services, especially to the aged, are likely to be the general practitioner and local minister.

Even though there is a paucity of elderly services in rural communities, there are certain practices and attitudes among elderly African Americans, particularly elderly rural African American women that shape their health protective behaviors (Wilson-Ford, 1992). Heath protective behavior are those behaviors performed by a person regardless of their perceived health status, in order to protect, promote or maintain their health regardless of whether that behavior is effective toward that end (Harris & Guten, 1979). These health protective behaviors among rural African American older adults include such practices as:

- Ignoring illness related symptoms until the condition becomes disabling
- Using prayer, living by religious principles, and using home remedies and self-medication as selective responses to symptoms and illnesses
- Denying the existence of health problems in order to maintain a sense of independence and self-reliance.

These health protective behaviors of elderly rural African Americans is grounded in a cultural ethos and belief system found in rural African American communities. These beliefs support the importance of using religious faith to protect health rather than traditional medicine or formal health care systems. Additionally there is the cultural belief that to be ambulatory is a sign of health in spite of biological and medical disturbances.

While there is the existence of a rural cultural ethos that relies on folk beliefs, self-help and self-care, there is also a reliance on a network of informal support and care systems that are family and/or community-based (Carlton-LaNey, 1992). Due to experiences with racism, discrimination, and personal histories of encountering injustices from formal support systems of care, older African Americans in rural communities have relied on a "helper network" (Chatters, Taylor, & Jackson, 1986) that includes spouses, children, siblings, friends, neighbors, and quasi-formal institutions such as the community church.

This helper network is the basis for informal caregiving for those older persons who find themselves unable to maintain complete self-care due to illness or physical infirmities. Informal caregiving for older persons is classified as instrumental and affective assistance (Barresi & Menon, 1990; Chatters, Taylor, & Jackson, 1986; George, 1988; Jackson, 1971, 1972). Instrumental assistance includes such support as grocery shopping, transportation, and meal preparation. Affective or expressive assistance includes emotional support, giving advice, encouragement, companionship, and prayer (Spence, Yogtiba Perry, & Black, 1998). Research does not support the idea that the family as such is the primary care giver. In fact there are a variety and range of significant informal supports including family, extended kin and non-kin, including church members, neighbors, and friends (Chatters, Taylor, & Jackson, 1986; Wood & Parham, 1990). This vast support network appears to perform functions that close relatives more likely perform in white families (Wood & Wan, 1993). Additionally within the support network is the concept of reciprocity that arises out of the African American sense of community and the African American helping tradition (Martin & Martin, 1985). Older adults, including frail elders, may provide child care, shared housing, or financial assistance to younger family members in need of aid. In return, health care and transportation services are provided informally by friends and relatives in order to allow the older individual to live out his/her life within the context of home and community (Wood & Wan, 1993). In spite of the fact that many of the caregivers are themselves likely to be in poverty or near poverty levels, the African American sense of community and the black helping traditions persist as the cultural foundation for providing informal care to African American older adults.

THE AFRICAN AMERICAN EXPERIENCE OF COMMUNITY AND THE AFRICAN AMERICAN HELPING TRADITION

The African American Sense of Community

Being a part of a unique community has long dominated the social consciousness of African Americans. This sense of "peoplehood" has emerged from a commonality of experience. These experiences result from a collective response to the forces of racism and oppression. Notwithstanding the debilitating impact of these forces, the African American community has contained a reservoir of strength and resources which often go untapped and/or unrecognized. Relying on this communal strength, African Americans have historically formed communal associations to pursue the attainment of civil rights, individual choice and legitimating claims for institutional and psychological liberation (Blackwell, 1975). These networks of community support have historically been the source of strength and resiliency for the African American community's most vulnerable members.

What are the factors that distinguish the African American community from other communities? Several social scientists have identified some distinctive characteristics of the African American community (Billingsley, 1992; Blackwell, 1975; Solomon, 1976). Geographically, many African Americans live in segregated neighborhoods in which most of their neighbors are also African Americans. These geographic communities, also known as "Black communities," although not always communities of choice, are often marked by a sense of personal intimacy and social cohesion. In many instances these geographic communities have also been marked by social, economic, and political isolation. This is especially the case within rural communities wherein ethnic minorities are sparsely populated. However, these communities have played an important role in shaping and reinforcing a sense of racial and cultural identity.

On a cultural level, the African American community can be described as representing multiple perspectives. Each perspective is shaped by the historical and traumatic experiences of enslavement. One perspective emphasizes a deep and rich cultural connection with an African heritage. Another perspective reflects an assimilation of Euro-American culture. The third and most dominant perspective reflects a culture representing varying degrees and mixtures of both African and Euro-American cultural frames of reference. The final perspective represents a state of alienation and disaffiliation from any viable and sustaining cultural perspective. This perspective represents those who have no buttress against the forces of racism and poverty.

These perspectives are represented in the diverse life styles and cultural perspectives of individual African Americans. From these diverse perspectives, a rich and diverse community with a unique history and heritage has emerged. Correspondingly, a set of institutions and organizations that identify with this heritage have developed. These organizations and institutions form the sustaining and nurturing infrastructure of the African American community. Such institutions and organizations include African American churches, mutual aid societies, fraternal orders, women's clubs, unions, orphanages, senior citizen homes, hospitals, educational institutions, protest movements, and race consciousness organizations (Martin & Martin, 1985).

Grounded in the historical, social and economic experiences of African Americans, these institutions shape the communal experiences of African Americans. They form the nucleus for the tradition of self help within the African American community (Martin & Martin, 1985). As community-based institutions, they provide for the experience of collectivity, in that they are the repositories of the communal narratives. These community-based institutions provide the format for communal celebration; and hence they provide succor and care during individual and/or communal tragedies.

The African American Helping Tradition

One domain in which the African American sense of community is evident is in the traditional forms of helping and mutual aid, self-help and informal social support. Informal social support can be defined as "an interwoven network" (Lubben & Becerra, 1987, p. 130) of family and friends who without training for the provision of care, undertake to provide a variety of services without compensation yet with a sense of obligation, loyalty or love (Barker, Morrow, & Mitteness, 1998). Martin and Martin (1985, pp. 4-5) describe the key concepts that recur throughout this communal sense of self-help.

- The African American helping tradition refers to the largely independent struggle of African Americans for their survival and advancement from generation to generation.
- The African American extended family consists of a multigenerational interdependent kinship system held together basically by a sense of obligation to the welfare of members of the kin network.
- Mutual aid, a dominant element in extended family life, involves a reciprocal effort of family members to pool the resources necessary for survival and growth.
- Social-class (status-group) cooperation is the endeavor of family members of different incomes, educational and social class levels to downplay class distinctions in giving and receiving aid.
- Prosocial behavior involves the attitudes and practices of cooperation, sharing, and caring that black adults consciously strive to in-

still in African American children so the tradition of black self-help will be passed on to future generations.

- Fictive kinship is the care giving and mutual-aid relationship among non-related African Americans that exist because of their common ancestry, history and social plight.
- Racial consciousness is the keen awareness by many African Americans of their history and condition as a people and their overwhelming desire to uplift their race to a state of dignity and pride.
- Religious consciousness refers to deliberated attempts of African Americans to live accordingly to those religious beliefs that call for acts of charity and brotherliness and neighborliness toward one another as a means of coming closer to God and carrying out God's will.

In various African traditions as well as among African Americans, there is clear veneration of the elders. With age comes wisdom and respect. Among the Ashanti, elderly men and women were the ones who had accurate knowledge (Rattray, 1923; Holmes & Holmes, 1995). In West Africa, elderly men and women were give respect by kin and non-kin alike and were referred to as "grandfather" and "grandmother" (Wylie, 1971). Notwithstanding their close affinity to the ancestors by virtue of their age, the elders as grandparents served as importance agents of socialization. Within traditional African American culture, and especially in rural culture, the elderly African Americans, especially grandmothers (Barer, 2001), maintain the role of matriarch, kinkeeper, perpetuators, models and finally benefactors of this helping tradition.

The African American Church: An Institutional Expression of the Helping Tradition

The African American church is one of the primary structures in the African American community. No other institution claims the loyalty and attention of African Americans including elderly African Americans as does the Black church (Boyd-Franklin, 1989; Taylor, 1985; Taylor & Chatters, 1986). The African American church can be described as an ontological community or a community of meaning in that it provides the spiritual, emotional, and existential meaning and supports for a vast group of African Americans (Brueggemann, 1996). For many, the African American church symbolizes the heart and soul of the community.

The church as a community institution serves multiple functions as it addresses the needs of African Americans. The church is a source of psychosocial support and can have an impact on every aspect of life. In addition to providing African American families with social services such as senior citizen activities, child care, educational groups, parenting groups, and housing development, the church also provides latent functions such as helping to maintain family solidarity, conferring of social status, leadership development, release of emotional tensions, social/political activity, and recreation (Staples, 1991).

Because the African American church has been ever present in the provision of human services, it has become an alternative social service delivery system for many African American families, and in this sense an institutional expression of the African American helping tradition. This is especially true for older African Americans in the rural areas. For example, elderly African Americans turn to their church for assistance more than elderly whites when community-based services are not available (Cantor & Mayer, 1978). Further, elderly African Americans rely on informal assistance from the church second only to support provided by their families (Dancy, 1977; Taylor & Chatters, 1986; McGadney, 1997). Given the extensive use of informal care support among rural African American elders, a question could be posed regarding the role of formal care services for older African Americans in rural communities. The next section will examine that concern.

FORMAL CARE SYSTEMS FOR RURAL AFRICAN AMERICAN OLDER ADULTS: IMPLICATIONS FOR SOCIAL WORK INTERVENTION

Some of the key problems in the developing and implementing services to older adults in rural communities are summarized by Krout (1992, p. 4) when he states that:

- Compared to urban elders, rural older persons generally have access to a smaller number of and more narrow range of community-based services, especially services for the severely impaired.
- Clear gaps exist in the continuum of care in rural communities, with few alternatives for those who cannot live independently but do not require institutionalization.

- Too little attention has been given to designing service delivery models and strategies specifically for rural areas and populations.

For Wood and Wan (1993) the gaps in continuum of care and poor access to services can create a greater reliance on informal care as the primary mode of services for rural elders. The use of informal care as the primary mode of service provision to rural African American elders is particularly evident due to an array of sociocultural and economic factors. There are many challenges in developing formal services. One challenge is found in the characteristics of many rural communities. These characteristics include low population density and size, which in turn can impact service access due to lack of transportation, and a lack of available information about existing though limited services.

Another challenge for rural communities is inadequate state and federal funding for elder services and restrictive and culturally insensitive elder services. Krout (1994) points out that in planning, implementing, and evaluating elder services in rural communities, they must be examined in terms of their availability, accessibility, appropriateness, acceptability, awareness, affordability, and adequacy.

We might add the factor of cultural competence as a challenge, especially as it relates to services for African American elders. Culturally competent services should involve the recognition and utilization of health protective behaviors and the health belief systems that are part of the cultural fabric of rural African American culture. These culturally competent services should also acknowledge and incorporate the African American helping traditions as a part of the service delivery design. A provider must bear in mind that due to the minority status of African American elders and their experiences with discrimination and racism, they are sensitive to the lack of respectful treatment by white service providers (such as the use of first name, etc.). Thus they would rather rely on the informal care system than to experience or re-experience discrimination.

SOCIAL WORK INTERVENTIONS WITH THE RURAL AFRICAN AMERICAN OLDER ADULTS

The goals for social work with this population are three fold: (1) to support and enhance those informal community-based levels of care for rural elderly African Americans that will allow them to function independently in their own homes, or homes of family utilizing the strength of the extended informal support network that exists in rural areas;

(2) to facilitate and expand the helping network to solve the psychosocial problems of African American rural older adults; and (3) to strive to create sound formal care organizations that can provide culturally competent services to rural African American elders. The latter goal is significant in that not all the physical and mental health issues of African American elders can be addressed through community-based informal support and caregiving. Community-based human service programs or long-term care facilities are necessary for a significant number of these individuals.

Social workers who work with older African Americans in rural communities should: (1) design strategies of intervention and support services within the sphere of religion or embedding these interventions and support services within the rural African American church; (2) advocate for increased financial support and governmental funding for those caretakers "recruited" by the older adult from their helping network; and (3) involve the elders in the service planning, implementation, and delivery of rural and community-based elder care systems. Such interventions would create avenues for participation, belonging, and mutual aid and support for elderly rural African Americans.

REFERENCES

Bane, S.D. (1991). Rural minority population. In. E.P. Stanford, & F.M. Torres-Gill (Eds.) Diversity: New approaches to ethnic minority aging [Special issue]. *Generations*, *15*(4), 63-65.

Barker, J.C., Morrow, J., & Mitteness, L.S. (1998). Gender, informal social support network, and elderly urban African Americans. *Journal of Aging Studies*, *12*(2), 192-222.

Barer, B.M. (2001, March). The 'grands and greats' of very old Black grandmothers. *Journal of Aging Studies*, *15*:1. Retrieved November 1, 2002, from *http://weblinks2.epnet.com/citation.asp?tb=1&_ug=dbs+0+In+en%2Dus+sid67.*

Barresi, C.M., & Menon, G. (1990). Diversity in black family caregiving. In Z. Harel, E.A. Mckinney, & M. Williams (Eds.), *Black aged: Understanding diversity and service needs*, (pp. 221-235). Newbury: Sage.

Billingsley, A. (1992). *Climbing Jacob's ladder*. New York: Simon and Schuster.

Blackwell, J.E. (1975). *The black community: Diversity and unity*. New York: Harper and Row.

Boyd-Franklin, N. (1989). *Black families in therapy: A multisystems approach*. New York: Guilford.

Brueggemann, W.G. (1996). *The practice of maco social work*. Chicago: Nelson-Hall.

Cantor, M., & Mayer, M. (1978). Factors in different utilization of services by urban elderly. *Journal of Gerontological Social Work*, *1*(1), 47-62.

Carlton-LaNey, I. (1992, November). Elderly black farm women: A population at risk. *Social Work, 37*: 6. Retrieved November 1, 2002, from *http://weblinks2.epnet.com/citation.asp?tb=1&_ug=dbs+0+In+en%2Dus+sid+3.*

Chatters, L.M., Taylor, R.T., & Jackson, J.S. (1986). Aged blacks' choices for an informal helper network. *Journal of Gerontology, 41*, 94-100.

Chatters, L.M., Taylor, R.T., & Jackson, J.S. (1985). Size and composition of the informal helper networks of elderly. *Journal of Gerontology, 40*, 605-614.

Cowgill, D.O. (1988). Aging in crosscultural perspectives: Africa and the Americas. In E. Grot (Ed.), *Aging in crosscultural perspective*. New York: Phelps Stokes Fund.

Dancy, J. (1977). *The black elderly: A guide for practitioners*. Ann Arbor: University of Michigan Press.

Day, J.C. (1993). *Population projection of the United States by age, race, and Hispanic origin: 1993 to 2050.* U.S. Bureau of the Census, Current Population Reports (pp. 25-1104). Washington, DC: U.S. Government Printing Office.

Ford, M.E., & Hatchett, B. (2001). Gerontological social work with older African American Adults. In E.O. Cox, E.S. Kelchner, & R. Chapin (Ed.), *Gerontological social work* (pp. 141-155). Binghamton, NY: The Haworth Social Work Practice Press.

George, L.K. (1988). Social participation in late life: Black-white differences. In J.S. Jackson (ED.). *The black American elderly*. New York: Springer.

Greene, R.L., & Seigler, I.C. (1984). Blacks. In E. Palmore (Ed.), *Handbook on the aged in the United States.* Westport, CT: Greenwood Press.

Harper, M., & Alexander, C. (1990). Profile of the black elderly. *U.S. Department of health and human services minority aging*. Washington, D.C: U.S. Public Health Service.

Harris, D.M., & Guten, S. (1979). Health-protective behavior: An exploratory study. *Journal of Health and Social Behavior, 20*, 17-29.

Holmes, E.D., & Holmes, L.D. (1995). *Other cultures, elder years*. Thousand Oaks: Sage.

Hooyman, N., & Kiyak, H. (2002). *Social gerontology*. Boston, MA: Allyn and Bacon.

Jackson, J.J. (1971). Age Blacks: A potpourri in the direction of the reduction in inequities. *Phylon, 32*, 260-380.

Jackson, J.J. (1972). Comparative life styles and family and friend relationship among older black women. *Family Coordinator, 21*, 477-484.

Krout, J.A. (1994). An overview of older rural populations and community-based services. In J.A. Krout. (Ed.), *Providing community-based services to the rural elderly*. (pp. 3-18). Thousand Oaks: Sage.

Krout, J.A. (1992). *Rural aging community-based services*. Paper prepared for heath and aging in rural America: A National Symposium. San Diego, CA.

Lubben, J.E., & Becerra, R.M. (1987). Social support among black, Mexican and Chinese elderly. In D. Gelfand, & D. Barresi (Ed.), *Research and ethnic dimensions of aging*. (pp. 130-144). New York: Springer Publishing Company.

Martin, J.M., & Martin, E.P. (1985). *Helping tradition in the black family and community*. Silver Spring, MD: National Association of Social Workers.

McGadney, B.F. (1997, February). Correlates of informal supportive church services for Black American and White family caregivers of frail elders. Paper presented at the Annual Scientific Meeting of the Michigan Academy. Retrieved March 28, 2003, from *http://www.imgip.siu.edu/journal/caregiver.html.*

Rattray, R.S. (1923). *The Ashanti*. Oxford: Clarendon.

Rosen, A.L., & Zlotnik, J.L. (2001). Demographics and reality: The "disconnect" in social work education. In E.O. Cox, E.S. Kelchner, & R. Chapin (Ed.), *Gerontological Social Work* (pp. 81-97). Binghamton, NY: The Haworth Social Work Practice Press.

Solomon, B.B. (1976). *Black empowerment*. New York: Columbia University Press.

Spence, S.A., Yogtiba, J.A., Perry, T.E., & Black, S.R. (1998). Older Rural African Americans: A study of the relationship between socio-demographic characteristics and informal caregiving. *The Research Association of Minority Professors Journal*, *2*(2), 67-83.

Staples, R. (1991). *The black family: Essays and studies*. Belmont, CA: Wadsworth.

Taylor, R. (1985). The extended family as a source of support to elderly blacks. *The Gerontologist, 25, 488-95.*

Taylor, R.J., & Chatters, L.M. (1986). Church-based informal support among elderly blacks. *The Gerontologist*, *26*, 637-642.

Torres-Gill, F., & Moga, K.B. (2001). Multiculturalism, social policy, and the new aging. In E.O. Cox, E.S. Kelchner, & R. Chapin (Ed.), *Gerontological social work* (pp. 13-32). Binghamton, NY: The Haworth Social Work Practice Press.

U.S. Bureau of the Census. (1996). *65+ in the United States*. Current Population Reports, Special Studies, pp. 23-190. Washington, DC: U.S. Government Printing Office. Retrieved November 8, 2002 from *http://www.census.gov/pro/1/pop/p23-190/p23-190.html.*

U.S. Bureau of the Census. (2000). Census 2000. Table DP-1 Profile of General Demographic Characteristics for the United States. Retrieved November 8, 2002 from *http://www.census.gov/Press-relaeas/www/2001/tables/dp_us_2000PDF.*

Wan, T.H. (1977). The differential use of health services. A minority perspective. *Urban Health*, *16*, 47-49.

Williams, S., Padgett, R., Blank, M., Guarini, J., Morton, S., Wilson, S., & Simmons, W. (2002). Comparison of specific illness beliefs of rural and urban blacks and whites. *Southern online journal of nursing research*, *7*:2. Retrieved January 24, 2003 from http:*//www.snors.org/members/SOJNR_articles/iss07vol102.htm.*

Wilson-Ford, V. (1992). Health-protective behaviors of rural black elderly women. *Health and Social Work*, *17*:1. Retrieved November 1, 2002 from *http://weblinks2.epnet.com/citation.asp?tb=1&_ug=dbs+0+In+en%2Dus+sid+F2.*

Wood, J. B., & Parham, I.A. (1990). Coping with perceived burden: Ethnic and cultural issues in Alzheimer's family caregiving. *Journal of Applied Gerontology*, *9*, 325-339.

Wood, J.B., & Wan, T.H. (1993). Ethnicity and minority issues in family caregiving to rural black elders. In C. Barresi, & D. Stull (Eds.), *Ethnic elderly and long-term care*. (pp. 39-56). New York: Springer.

Wylie, F.M. (1971). Attitudes toward aging and the aged among black Americans: Some historical perceptions. *International Journal of Aging and Human Development*, *2*, 66-69.

Chapter 9

Rural Latino Elders

Steven Lozano Applewhite, PhD
Cruz Torres, PhD

SUMMARY. This chapter presents relevant theories, demographic data and introduces guidelines for culturally relevant practice with rural Latino elders. Demographic characteristics of rural Latinos focus on age distribution, economic conditions, living arrangements, and language and service utilization issues. Cultural competence is discussed as a viable approach to cross-cultural practice based on a knowledge base, culturally relevant skills and a value orientation that embraces diversity. *[Article copies available for a fee from The Haworth Document Delivery Service: 1-800-HAWORTH. E-mail address: <docdelivery@haworthpress.com> Website: <http://www.HaworthPress.com> © 2003 by The Haworth Press, Inc. All rights reserved.]*

KEYWORDS. Rural Latinos, Latino elders, cross-cultural practice

INTRODUCTION

Diversity in rural America is a significant and growing area of interest in the field of gerontology. Emerging demographic trends and social indi-

[Haworth co-indexing entry note]: "Rural Latino Elders." Applewhite, Steven Lozano, and Cruz Torres. Co-published simultaneously in *Journal of Gerontological Social Work* (The Haworth Social Work Practice Press, an imprint of The Haworth Press, Inc.) Vol. 41, No. 1/2, 2003, pp. 151-174; and: *Gerontological Social Work in Small Towns and Rural Communities* (ed: Sandra S. Butler, and Lenard W. Kaye) The Haworth Social Work Practice Press, an imprint of The Haworth Press, Inc., 2003, pp. 151-174. Single or multiple copies of this article are available for a fee from The Haworth Document Delivery Service [1-800-HAWORTH, 9:00 a.m. - 5:00 p.m. (EST). E-mail address: docdelivery@haworthpress.com].

http://www.haworthpress.com/web/JGSW
© 2003 by The Haworth Press, Inc. All rights reserved.
Digital Object Identifier: 10.1300/J083v41n01_09

cators forecast a growing elderly population unparalleled in U.S. history. One group embedded within the rural population is the elderly Latino.[1] This population, comprised primarily of rural Mexican Americans and new immigrants from Mexico and Latin America, is estimated to be about 2.5 million in size and living primarily in agriculturally based areas of the rural Southwest and the borderlands (Glasgow & Brown, 1998; Torres, 2000). Growth patterns in the 1980s indicated that among the new rural residents, one in four was Hispanic (Cromartie, 1993), and in 1996, foreign-born persons made up two percent of the nonmetropolitan population (ERS, 1997; Ricketts, Johnson-Webb, & Randolph, 1999). Assuming that Latino immigrant settlement patterns increase as projected, the population of foreign-born Hispanics will grow in size, and these individuals will settle in nonmetropolitan areas of the country (Ricketts et al., 1999) and face a myriad of problems and challenges in years to come. Among these are widespread poverty, higher rates of chronic diseases, racial and ethnic disparities in health status, limited access to services, housing and transportation problems, social and geographical isolation, as well as cultural and linguistic problems. Equally problematic will be the difficult task of providing services to a greater number of elderly Latinos in nonmetropolitan settings. For many elders the cultural context of life in rural settings may act as a buffer against social, cultural, and economic affronts. Many others will seek help from families, church, friends, and community in situations where health and social needs are high, and access to services severely limited. However, the vast majority may ultimately seek help from agencies and service providers to meet their basic needs. The challenge therefore is to develop culturally proficient systems of care and culturally competent service providers that demonstrate the capacity to deliver services in a sensitive, relevant and appropriate manner congruent with the needs and expectations of elderly clients.

This chapter explores the nature and quality of life for elderly Latinos in rural America. It begins with a set of critical theories and perspectives in gerontology and social work that provide conceptual insight for understanding the aging experience in a cultural context. Secondly, a profile of elderly Latinos focuses on demographics, language, living arrangements, and economic status. The third area focuses on defining features of the Latino culture and familism that sustain and strengthen elderly Latinos in the face of adversity. Finally, a practice approach is discussed focusing on knowledge, skills, and values essential for culturally competent practice with rural elderly Latinos.

THEORETICAL PERSPECTIVES

Theories and perspectives provide a contextual framework for understanding the nature of old age and the interaction of culture, ethnicity and human development. Several theories are particularly significant and relevant for cross-cultural practice with rural elderly Latinos. The following discussion introduces the life course perspective, general systems theory, ecological perspective and the integrated ecological/systems perspectives with its emphasis on person-environment interaction. It highlights concepts that have cultural relevance for practice with elderly rural Latinos and serves as a starting point for further discussion on theory and practice integration.

The life course perspective views aging as a process that occurs from birth to old age involving biological, psychological, social, and cultural processes and life patterns shaped by cohorts-historical factors (Passuth & Bengson, 1988, in Cavanaugh & Whitbourne, 1999). Timing of life events, duration, sequencing and order of events, social structures and historical changes that affect these events are central to the life course. Building on this perspective, Gibson (1988), Devore and Schlesinger (1999), and Green (1995) developed a critical theme of significance in understanding the life course of ethnic minorities. Gibson (1988) states that the study of elders of color is more appropriately served by focusing on the life course perspective and "the interrelatedness of changing social structures, social-historical periods, personal biographies, life cycle stages, personal adaptive resources, life events and well being as integral to the study of minorities as they age" (p. 559). Devore and Schlesinger expanded the notion of life course to include race, gender, social class and ethnicity termed *ethnic reality* (p. 64). Quadagno (2002) further notes that life course research also incorporates the Theory of Cumulative Disadvantage to explain why inequality increases with old age, particularly for racial and gender groups. Inequality is viewed as a cumulative process with patterned differences in opportunities across the life course. Advantages early in life, such as greater resources, lead to greater opportunities to acquire additional resources. Conversely, disadvantages early in life with few opportunities and resources result in a steady state or decline in the social ladder. Historical analysis is significant in understanding patterned differences in opportunities across the life course. Thus, for many rural elderly Latinos, growing old is an *ethnic reality* based largely on social inequality, discrimination, and injustice experienced early in life, persisting over the life course, culminating in disadvantages in old age. Taken as a whole, the life course perspective provides a view of aging in an integrated fashion with culture, ethnicity, history and social inequality as pivotal concepts.

The second school of thought, general systems theory, focuses on structures (e.g., social, economic, etc.) and the systems with which people interact. Greene (1999) notes that systems theory is a unifying perspective or conceptual bridge that emphasizes multiple systems within which people interact, and places a person viewed as a biopsychosocial system within a multi-system context. Greene (1999) and Norton (1979) note that systems theory is useful in understanding cultural differences and interactions occurring across cultures. Greene adds that *culture, ethnicity, biculturalism*, the concept of *ethnosystems*, and the *dual perspective* are particularly relevant for understanding the worldview and way of life of diverse populations (pp. 234-236). Culture therefore is a critical concept interwoven into systems theory that recognizes distinct cultures, shared histories, values and belief systems, and patterns of social organization and social interaction.

The third school of thought, the ecological perspective, retains a systems view but focuses on the relationship of the person and the environment, and the ecological levels or subsystems within which individuals act (Bronfenbrenner, 1979). The first level is the microsystems which includes any person or environment in which the person has direct day-to-day contacts with influential others (e.g., extended family). Mesosystems involve the linkages of multiple settings involving the person in interpersonal face-to-face interactions (e.g., elderly person-church). Ecosystems involve larger systems and linkages between two or more settings, one of which may not typically involve the individual (e.g., decision making bodies, social service agency). The macrosystem represents the overarching social context or pattern of a given culture comprised of beliefs, societal attitudes and values that influence how individuals in different settings interact with one another (e.g., ethnic group system) (Greene, 1999; Hefferman, Shuttlesworth, & Ambrosino, 1988). The ecological perspective views people as connected and interacting within several systems simultaneously, and places importance on such concepts as *life course* (emphasis added), goodness of fit, relatedness, competence, role, habitat and niche, and adaptiveness. Other critical concepts are *cultural time*, defined as cultural beliefs and attitudes about the timing of life events; *bicultural environments* or the clients' own ethnic community and environment; *institutional racism*, defined as the combination of networks that reinforce discrimination; and *social and economic justice* which focuses on the interventions needed to address inequities across different levels from individual to political arenas (Greene, 1999, pp. 277-278).

The integration of the previous schools of thought resulted in the widely adopted systems/ecological framework proposed by Compton and Galaway (1989) based on the earlier work of Bronfenbrenner (1979), Garbarino (1982), Germain (1979), and Meyer (1973). This framework conceptualizes interactions between people and their physical and social environments across different levels or subsystems, while simultaneously considering the impact of social systems and structures on individual and group functioning. The value of this integrated approach lies in its special attention to *individual and structural factors* to explain human behavior (Hefferman et al., 1992, p. 55). Thus *individual factors* such as competence, adaptiveness, and coping may combine with *structural factors* such as poverty, discrimination, classism and racism to reveal individual functioning, relationships and human behavior in the context of rural social environments. To further apply the person-environment perspective, Lawton and Nahemow (1973), Lawton (1989), and Parmelee and Lawton (1990) proposed a *competence model* focusing on the interaction occurring between the person's physical and psychological characteristics and their social and physical environment. According to this model, *environmental press* places social and physical demands on an elderly person to adapt, respond or change. *Individual competence* refers to an individual's ability to adapt to his or her environmental press based on his or her level of functioning in terms of cognitive, behavioral and health status. Thus the higher the level of individual competence exhibited by the elderly person in such areas as optimal health, problem solving, and management of activities of daily living, the greater will be the level of tolerance for the environmental press (Hooyman & Kiyak, 2002). For rural elderly Latinos, knowledge about their rural environment; the interaction that occurs between the elderly, family and community systems; their functional capacity and personal attributes; and the cultural context of aging across the life course must be fully understood and considered essential in working with and planning for this population.

THE RURAL ELDERLY POPULATION

In recent years the socio-demographic emergence of Latinos nationally termed Latinoization, and the aging of the population has been at the forefront of demographic news. Notwithstanding the demographic shifts, the Latino elderly remain invisible to two arenas, the growing and youthful Latino population and the growing and white elderly population. Currently few national surveys on the elderly adequately sized samples to conduct comparative analyses of the Latino elderly population. National sampling techniques produce inappropriately small Latino samples; consequently these studies give little if any specific data on Hispanic elderly. What we do know is that Latinos, like the rest of the U.S. population, will continue to enjoy longer and healthier lives. Population projections indicate that the number of Latino elderly will dramatically increase in the next decades, and it is expected to grow faster than that of any other group by 2005. Without adequate data we risk introducing policies based on stereotypes rather than on real needs and problems (Torres, 1992). Researchers and policy makers still do not have the type of data that will allow us to inform policymakers on the long-term needs of the rural Hispanic elderly. What we do know is that we still have to proceed with caution when explaining service use by Latino elderly. Lack of data should neither imply lack of need or lack of use. Neither should social and environmental factors be confused with cultural factors.

In 2000 there were 35 million persons age 65 or older in the United States, accounting for over 12% of the population. Hispanics, with almost 1.9 million Latinos ages 65 and older, represent 5.7% of the elderly population (U.S. Census Bureau, 2001b). As evidenced by the 2000 Census, Latinos and people ages 65 and over are two of the fastest growing populations. Latino elders represent an equally small proportion of the youthful Latino population and of the mostly non-Hispanic white aging population. Under normal circumstances, it is the absolute population size that drives service demands, not the proportion of the population; however, given the unprecedented growth of the Latino and aging populations, the relatively small proportion of elderly Latinos within these two special populations makes Latino elderly invisible in both groups. Consequently, issues and policies relevant to Latino elderly receive very little attention (Torres, 2001). Table 1 provides the age numerical distribution of Latinos according to age categories and residence status. In Table 2 we provide the data according to percent of population and percent of the population ages 60 and over.

The population age 85 and older is currently the fastest growing segment of the older population. Among all populations and all age categories, women comprise a larger share of the older population, especially the oldest old. In 2000, women accounted for 58.7% of the Latino population age 65 and older and 67.1% of the population age 85 and older.

TABLE 1. Age Distribution of Older Latino Population by Metro-NonMetro Residence, 2000

Age Group	Residence	Total	Total Male	Total Female
Total Latinos		35,305,818	18,161,795	17,144,023
60 years and over	Total	2,483,998	1,074,283	1,409,715
	Metro	2,249,086	966,246	1,284,840
	NonMetro	234,912	110,037	124,875
60-64 years old	Total	750,409	266,504	402,998
	Metro	682,113	313,563	368,550
	NonMetro	68,294	33,846	34,448
65-74 years old	Total	1,076,619	473,875	602,744
	Metro	974,783	425,031	549,752
	NonMetro	101,836	48,844	52,992
75-84 years old	Total	506,264	203,382	302,882
	Metro	456,725	181,709	275,016
	NonMetro	49,539	21,673	27,866
85 years and over	Total	150,708	49,617	101,091
	Metro	135,465	43,943	91,522
	NonMetro	15,243	5,674	9,569

Source: U.S. Census Bureau, Census 2000 Summary File1, advanced national machine-readable data files, 2002.

Figure 1 illustrates the male/female ratio within each age category. Clearly, the female to male ratio is greater in the metropolitan than in the nonmetropolitan older Latino populations.

In 2000, 8.7% of the older Latino population was age 85 and older. Figure 2 illustrates the widening gap in the nonmetro male/female ratio with increased age. While nationally women represented slightly over 71% of the 85 and over 2000 population, among Latinos, women were only 63% of the population 85 and over. The male/female ratio approaches parity only in the young-old cohort, ages 60-64. Although the

TABLE 2. Age Distribution of Older Latino Population by Metro-NonMetro Residence, 2000

	60 years and older		85 years and older	
	Number	Share of total population	Number	Share of 60 and older population
Metro Total	2249086	90.5	135465	5.5
Male	966246	43.0	43943	4.6
Female	1284840	57.1	91522	7.2
NonMetro Total	234912	9.5	15243	6.5
Male	110037	46.8	5674	5.2
Female	124875	53.2	9569	7.7

Source: U.S. Census Bureau, Census 2000 Summary File1, advanced national machine-readable data files, 2002.

FIGURE 1. Metro-NonMetro Age Distribution by Sex

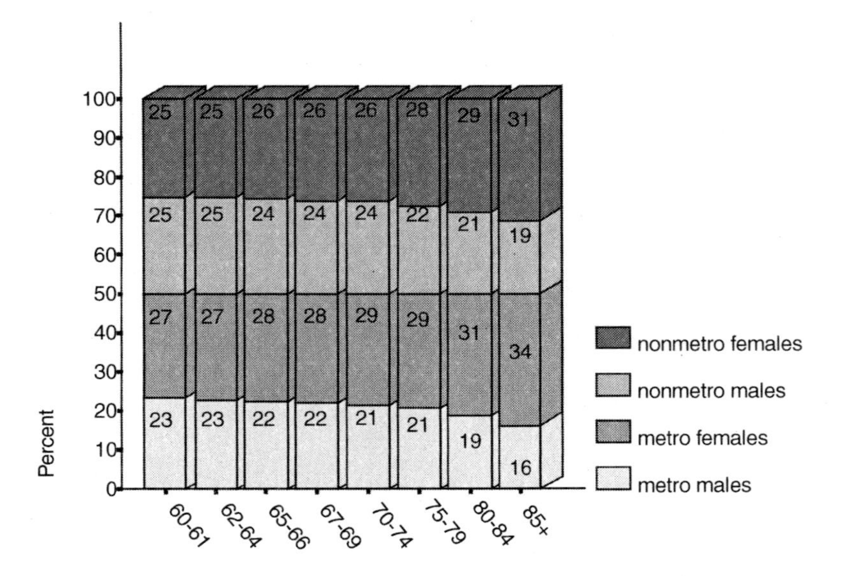

Note: Hispanics may be of any race.
Reference population: Civilian uninstitutionalized population.
Source: U.S. Census Bureau, Census 2000 Summary File1, advanced national machine-readable data files, 2002.

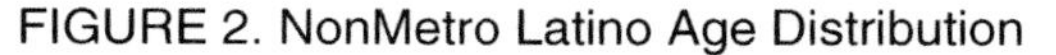

FIGURE 2. NonMetro Latino Age Distribution

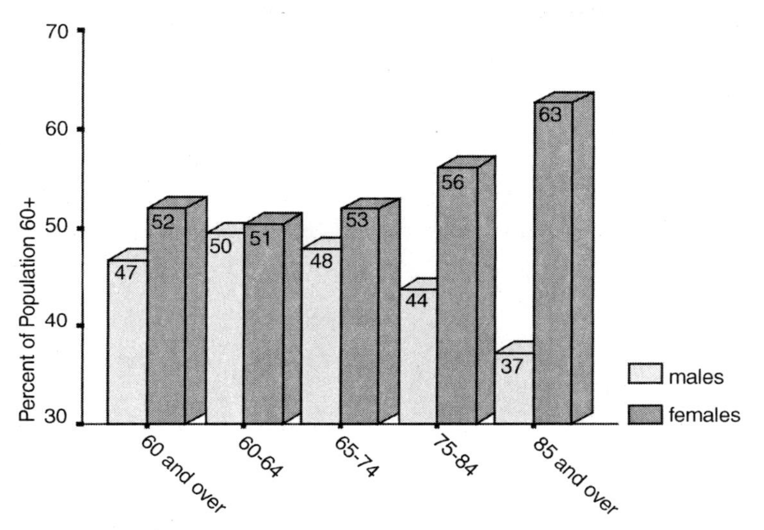

Note: Latinos may be of any race.
Reference population: Civilian uninstitutionalized.
Source: U.S. Census Bureau, Census 2000 Summary File1, advanced national machine readable data files, 2002.

older populations will increase among all ethno-racial groups, the Latino older population is projected to grow the fastest. By 2050, Hispanics are projected to account for 16% of the older population.

LANGUAGE

In the United States an estimated 27 million persons speak Spanish at home and more than 12 million cannot speak English very well or at all (U.S. Census Bureau, 2001d). Latino migration and settlement patterns shifted between the 1980s and the turn of the 21st century and dispersed Latinos away from the traditional Southwest; as a result, Latinos are no longer exclusively a borderlands population. This demographic shift promises to be one of the most serious challenges facing the service provider community. Especially challenging for locales without any previous experience with linguistically different populations will be the language barrier. Unequivocally, English is a social asset; not being able to speak English places Latinos at a disadvantage in negotiating complex bureaucracies, i.e., social and health services. Distinct languages, dialects and language use represent the most significant cultural difference and barrier that non English-speaking Latinos and host communities must bridge. As the provider/client social realities diverge, communication problems are magnified. Consequently, service planners must negotiate both the social reality and cultural reality that shape both the help seeking and care giving behaviors of client and practitioner (Torres, 2002). In a previous study (Torres, Salazar, Villas, & Garza, 1999), 31% of elderly Latino respondents who required translation reported service dissatisfaction and believed that some of the message was lost in the translation. Language discordance provides fertile ground for misinterpreting clients' concerns, promotes poor client compliance, inappropriate follow-up, and poor client satisfaction. In institutional settings, limited availability of bilingual, culturally competent professionals make it more difficult to bridge the language barrier and insure full access to institutional services. Moreover, the language barrier is more pronounced for the older Latino population, consequently meeting the needs of a linguistically isolated aging Latino population can be a monumental challenge (Torres, 2000) and can only aggravate existing service underutilization by the Latino community.

LIVING ARRANGEMENTS

Living arrangements and marital status can strongly impact economic and overall well-being. Those living alone are more likely to lack social and caregiving networks and experience greater poverty. As individuals age, their social networks tend to shrink. Network downsizing occurs at a time when the availability of instrumental and expressive aid is critical to the well-being of the older person. There is an erroneous assumption that Hispanic elderly do not live alone. The cultural myth of *familism* portrays a culturally insulated *viejito*, especially older women, and thus negates the need for formal institutional services. Is this image of the insulated elder a cultural characteristic or an adaptive technique borne of economic necessity, or is it a traditional norm that will give way to population mobility and urbanization? Of the non-institutionalized civilian Latino population age 65 and older, most live with a family member. Older Latinos head 11% of all rural households. Six percent of these households have a non-family member. Seventy-seven percent of Latino family rural households headed by a person 65 and over represents married couples. Elderly men are most likely to be married; elderly women are not. In 2000, 63.7% of Latino males ages 65 and over lived with their spouse in family households, compared with 32.2% of women in the same age group. Over 31% of households run by a person 65 and older are persons living alone. Older women are more likely to live alone than older men; only 14% of Hispanic males over the age of 65 live alone, compared with 27% of older Latinas. Approximately 15% of older Hispanics live with other relatives, and 4.3% live with non-relatives (U.S. Census 2001d) (see Figure 3).

ECONOMIC PROFILE

Traditionally, rural populations are more likely to be employed in agriculture, in unskilled labor or service sectors. These are jobs that frequently have low wages; offer no health insurance, pension plans or survivor benefits; and evidence higher health hazards. These characteristics are similar, if not identical, to the employment characteristics associated with Latinos. As a subpopulation, the economic profile of Latinos reflects the lowest levels of education, low-skill, low-wage

FIGURE 3. Latino Elderly Living Alone

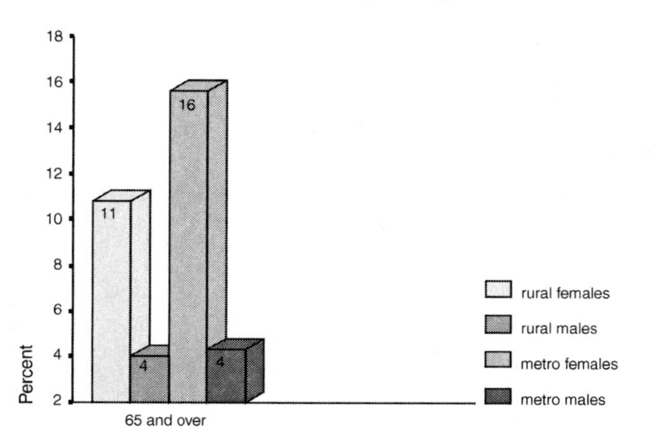

Note: Hispanics may be of any race.
Reference population: Civilian uninstitutionalized population.
Source: U.S. Census Bureau, Census 2000 Summary File1, advanced national machine readable data files, 2002.

jobs, and high levels of unemployment, resulting in the lowest per capita income. This education and workforce experience for older rural Latinos predicts an inadequate retirement income and lack of health insurance in their advancing years. For the past five decades a major public policy has been to reduce the level of poverty among the elderly population. The continued economic support from Social Security and the introduction of Medicaid in 1965 (Bok, 1996) have contributed significantly to the economic well-being of today's elderly. Additionally, Supplemental Security Income (SSI), a means-tested support program that assists older individuals who did not contribute enough to the system to qualify for regular earnings-based benefits, has been a particularly important source of income for older individuals without assets or private retirement income. Notwithstanding these major improvements, there is still extensive evidence that rural and minority populations are more likely to be at-risk of poverty. Thus, rurality and minority status combine to strongly influence the economic conditions of rural elderly Latinos. In addition, poverty increases with age, and older women and older persons living alone are more likely to be poor than married couples. In 2000, income per family member for Latinos living in married-couple households was $13,773 for individuals age 65 to 69, $12,907 for individuals age 70 to 74, and for those aged 75 and over the amount is $10,139. In contrast, income per family member for Latina households (husband absent) age 65 to 69 was $12,789, $9,592 for those ages 70 to 74, and $9,728 for those ages 85 and over (U.S. Census 2001c).

Poverty

Poverty is linked to inadequate nutrition, substandard housing, exposure to environmental hazards, unhealthy lifestyles and decreased access and use of health care facilities. Nationally poverty rates are highest in rural areas and rural minorities can be separated out as having the highest poverty rates. Latinos age 65 and over are more likely to be poor or near poor than any ethnic group. At age 65 and over, 18.8% of Latinos are poor and another 36.8% are near poor, compared to 8.3% and 26.0% for non-Hispanic whites in the same age category (U.S. Census Bureau, 2001c).

Much like all other older Americans, poverty rates are highest among the older Latinos. Figure 4 illustrates the poverty rates for older Latinos. In 2000, 18.4% of all Latinos ages 65 to 74 were below the poverty level; the poverty rate for rural Latinos in this age category was 19%. In

FIGURE 4. Percent Below Poverty

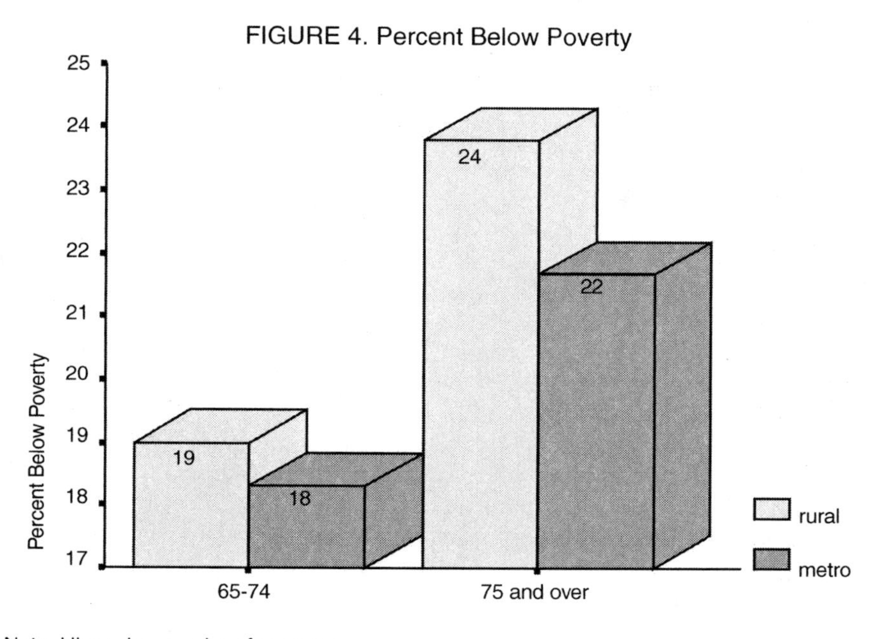

Note: Hispanics may be of any race.
Reference population: Civilian uninstitutionalized population.
Source: U.S. Census Bureau, Census 2000 Summary File1, advanced national machine readable data files, 2002.

comparison, the percent of persons below poverty level for rural Latinos 75 and older was 23.8%.

The oldest-old are the most economically vulnerable population and at the same time present the greatest need for health, medical and other services. This heightened level of need becomes especially troublesome in rural areas where the availability of these services is more limited. Moreover, in nonmetro communities the proportion of oldest-old (85 and older) is greater than in the metropolitan areas. Serving the needs of this special population is an urgent issue for rural service providers.

Insurance

According to the Institute of Medicine (2001), more than any other demographic or economic barrier, the availability of health insurance is the most important determinant of timeliness and quality of care. Nevertheless, access to private health insurance is a direct outcome of economic conditions, more specifically employment history. For persons age 65 and over, access to adequate health insurance is more likely linked to previous economic/employment conditions. We have already identified an employment history for rural and Hispanic populations that preclude optimal access to employment-based insurance in later life; similarly several conditions may also preclude older Latinos from Medicare eligibility, such as an employment history in industries not originally covered by Social Security legislation or legal residency. In 2000, only 17.5% of Latinos age 65 years and over reported employment based insurance coverage. Medicare covers 91% of this population; Medicaid supplements 26.3% of this population's health insurance. Approximately 95% of all Latinos age 65 and over have some type of health insurance; nevertheless, almost five percent of this very vulnerable population has no coverage at all. Nativity also impacts the level of insurance coverage for older Latinos. The level of coverage drastically declines as residency status decreases. Native born residents have much higher coverage than foreign-born, and naturalized citizens have greater coverage than non-citizens. In 2000, only three percent of non-citizen Latinos over age 65 were covered by Medicare (U.S. Census Bureau, 2001a).

Besides insufficient economic resources, transportation provides another barrier to access to services. Public transportation is either inadequate or nonexistent in rural communities. With uneven geographical distribution of service/health care facilities and providers, access to these services becomes especially problematic to rural Latino elders (Angel, Angel, McClellan, & Markides, 1996; Torres et al., 1999). Older Latinos are the most seriously impacted, since they are the ones least likely to either own a car or drive. Most often older Latinas rely on their close social network of family, friends and neighbors for transportation.

Disabilities

Old age is accompanied by certain diseases and disorders that affect physical functioning. The level of disability can become a significant burden and hamper the individual's capacity to live alone. Over 41% of U.S. Hispanics ages 65 to 74 report some physical disability (40% and 42% for males and females respectively). Rural Latinos report lower rates of disabilities (39.5%). Among rural elderly, a slightly higher percent of men than women report a physical disability (40.9% and 38.1% respectively). Among the older (75 years and over) the rate of disability increases significantly to 61.5%. At this life stage a higher percent of women (63%) report physical disabilities compared to men (60%) (see Figure 5).

FIGURE 5. Latino Elderly with Disabilities

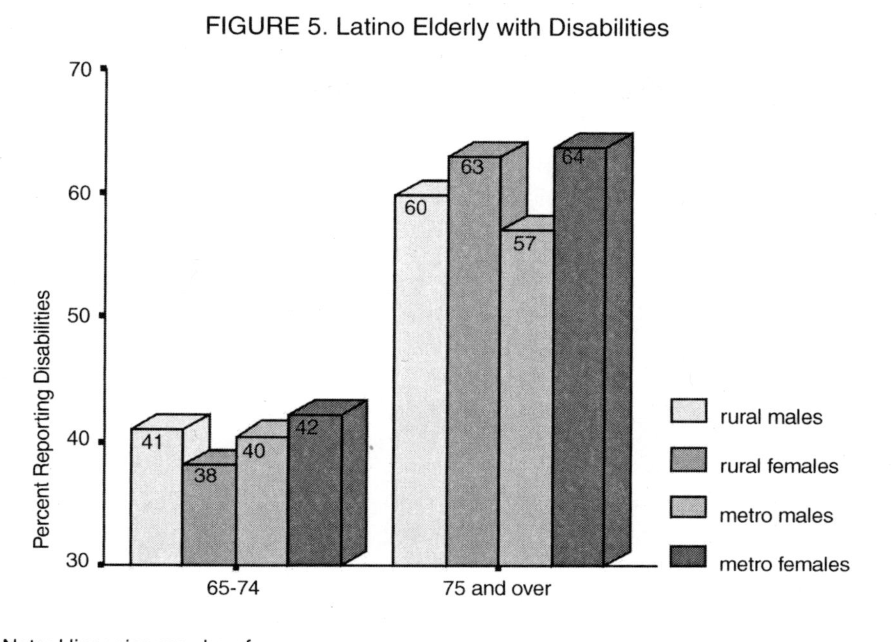

Note: Hispanics may be of any race.
Reference population: Civilian uninstitutionalized population.
Source: U.S. Census Bureau, Census 2000 Summary File1, advanced national machine readable data files, 2002.

Resource Access

Access to resources has long been a focus of concern for rural America and also holds true for rural Latinos. However, older Latinos' life experiences are vastly different from their non-Latino age cohort. Hence, we cannot assume that the aging experience is similar across all ethnic groups or that they share the same needs and face the same problems as their non-Hispanic counterparts in rural areas. Hispanic life cycle characteristics, e.g., high levels of unemployment and underemployment, disproportionate participation in occupations characterized by higher health risks such as agricultural work, and inadequate retirement and health plans, set them apart from their non-Hispanic aging cohort. In later life, these earlier life experiences may have more serious implications for health and social well-being, and limit their ability to access available resources (Saenz & Torres, in press). In addition to the general lack of services, geography plays an important role in accessibility of resources by rural residents. Because public transportation is very limited in rural areas and elderly Latinos are more likely to lack reliable private transportation, fewer provider options are open to them. Long distances aggravate service accessibility for older rural Latinos who may be unable or unwilling to travel long distances in order to access available services.

CULTURAL CONTEXT

Much of the literature documents that Hispanic elderly are more traditional in their help seeking behavior (Markides & Coreil, 1988) and tend to underutilize formal services (Wolinsky & Tierney, 1998; Angel & Angel, 1997a). Suggested reasons for underutilization include economics, language and education barriers, lack of transportation, uneven distribution of service providers, use of alternative services, and most importantly, culture. Specifically cited are the cultural distance between service provider and the Latino client (Angel & Angel, 1997b) and the persistent belief that the Hispanic culture dictates that Latinos provide for and take care of their own elders (Wong, Capoferro, & Soldo, 1999). Irrespective of the reason, the reality is that historically, access to services has been more problematic for Latinos than for whites. Yet, little specific attention has been given to the needs and the care-seeking behaviors of older Hispanics. Without specific knowledge of care/help seeking behaviors within this rapidly growing population, it will be difficult to plan for its future needs. We lack a basic understanding of the complex interaction between language, culture and social class, how these variables impact the biopsychosocial aspects of aging and the cognitive process of perceiving, interpreting and reporting health/well-being status among older rural Latinos.

The culture of rural America, like the Hispanic culture, plays both positive and negative roles in the social and economic well-being of its population. Rural communities are known for the strong social networks that bind small communities together. The strong familiarity that permeates small close-knit rural communities can deter the implementation and use of formal services. Social networks based on familiarity provide empathy and support but may result in over reliance on informal rather than formal institutions. Besides deterring the use of formal services, this reliance on informal networks places undue onus on an already resource poor Latino community.

Extended family living arrangements are more likely to be an adaptive response to socioeconomic inequality (Angel & Tienda, 1982). Familism is characterized by the hierarchical structure and roles assumed by members of the extended family. The two components within the concept of *familism*, family unity and expected mutual aid, directly speak to socioeconomic issues. The additional income realized from extra wage earners in a household provides valuable economic resources that mitigate poverty. As such, *familism* is perceived as a characteristic of family strength and vitality. Viewed as such, economic uncertainty and life course position, more than cultural preference, are the most important predictors of coresidence among elderly Latinos.

Growing old, poor and isolated in rural communities will continue to have serious implications for elderly Latinos. With projected population increases and limited accessibility to institutional resources, elderly Latinos may be at-risk for health and mental health problems with greater and more costly needs than their non-Hispanic white counterparts. And since most rural elderly Latinos have a history of agricultural work as well as underemployment, most may expect to enter old age with limited assets, pensions or other financial resources. However, several cultural factors are in place to significantly ameliorate the negative geographic and socio-demographic barriers. First, the large social networks that are characteristic of both rural and Hispanic communities will serve to significantly neutralize some of the negative consequences of social, economic and geographical isolation. Most elders have access to the English speaking community by proxy, e.g., family and friends. Second, cultural practices, such as dietary patterns and health behaviors (lower rates of drinking and smoking), buffer rural Latinos against potentially negative health outcomes in later life. Third, the extended family continues to serve as a viable cultural support and identity source. Elderly Latinos assume a pivotal role in the extended family structure, filling key roles and functions such as caretaking; advice giving; folkhealing; religious and spiritual advising; and transmitting cultural knowledge, history and traditions to younger generations.

Culture is clearly a crucial concept and a tool for understanding and working with rural elderly Latinos. It can bridge the gap between service providers and the elderly interacting across different cultures. Providers should embrace diversity and a desire to gain greater understanding, sensitivity, and awareness. Ultimately, culturally competent practice with rural elderly Latinos is essential and indeed warranted as rural populations continue to grow in size and diversity.

CULTURALLY COMPETENT RURAL PRACTICE

Cultural competence has emerged as the most critical aspect of service provision today facing social workers, counselors, physicians, nurses and related professions in the health and human services. Cross, Bazron, Dennis, and Issacs (March, 1989) describe cultural competence as a goal and developmental process that agencies, providers and systems pursue along a cultural continuum that extends from cultural destructiveness to cultural proficiency. Cultural competence acknowledges and incorporates differences in behaviors, beliefs and values and includes the use, when appropriate, of family and other natural support networks (church, minority community, etc.) in a more culturally responsive environment. A culturally competent system of care requires systems, agencies, and practitioners to value diversity, conduct cultural self-assessments, recognize the dynamics of difference, institutionalize cultural knowledge, and adapt services to address diverse cultural needs (Cross et al., pp. 19-21).

Cross-cultural competent practice with elderly Latinos calls attention to knowledge, values, skills and attributes that differ across cultures and provide a basis for cultural interventions. The current literature on cultural competence provides guidelines and principles for culturally competent intervention at the individual, provider, agency, and policy levels (see Applewhite, 1998; Cross et al., 1989; Devore & Schlesinger, 1999; Green, 1995; Leigh, 1998; Lum, 2003; Romero, 1996; Winkelman, 1999). The following guidelines, while not exhaustive, recognize the value-added dimension that diversity brings. They illustrate that the application of cultural knowledge for rural practice should include:

1. Knowledge about Latino and rural cultures and the intersection of these cultural systems.
2. Knowledge about acculturation and the impact that modernity and conflicting intergenerational values have on older rural Latinos.
3. Knowledge about social stressors and cultural coping mechanisms that affect elderly well-being in rural environments.
4. Knowledge about scarcity of personal and community resources that affect accessibility and utilization of existing resources.
5. Knowledge about the changing role and relative position of *ancianos* in the family hierarchy due to rural outmigration and shifting family patterns.
6. Knowledge about the acculturation continuum, the behaviors associated with the different stages, and how this impacts the inter-

actions of elderly Latinos with their family, community, and social environment.

7. Knowledge of *familismo* (familism), *jeraquismo* (family hierarchy), *curanderismo* (folk healing), and *presentismo* (present-time oriented) as key concepts to be understood and operationalized according to the elderly's ethnic reality.
8. Knowledge about individual and structural factors and the interaction between rural elderly Latinos, their families, communities, and society in the cultural context.
9. Knowledge about human behavior including individual and family life course considerations of elderly Latinos, and the effect that biopsychosocial, cultural, and spiritual systems have on their behavior.

In addition to new knowledge, providers are expected to acquire new skills for cross-cultural practice. Among the skills needed are the:

1. Ability to adapt formal acquired skills to function in less than optimal rural environments and impoverished communities lacking needed resources.
2. Ability to develop new approaches or adapt existing ones to assure cultural relevance and congruence with the needs, expectations and characteristics of rural elderly Latinos.
3. Ability to communicate effectively by incorporating preferred language, dialects, values, and traditions of the local community.
4. Ability to recognize temporal and spatial dimensions unique to rural communities (e.g., landmarks, cultural time, etc.).
5. Ability to recognize natural support networks as viable caregiving systems and to integrate these with formal delivery systems.
6. Ability to make culturally competent assessments that incorporate personal and cultural strengths, cultural coping mechanisms, natural support systems, care-seeking behaviors, and cultural beliefs and practices unique to rural elderly Latinos.
7. Ability to recognize family structures, especially extended family and fictive kin, elderly roles and expectations, family integration, and decision-making based on cultural tradition and level of acculturation.
8. Ability to apply ethnocultural factors (e.g., cultural beliefs and attitudes, cultural nuances, communication patterns) in client-provider interactions.

In cross-cultural encounters, values will differ between the provider and elderly Latinos. It is important therefore to value diversity by considering the following values:

1. Embrace cultural values that reflect *personalismo* (personalism) with its emphasis on *confianza* (mutual trust), *confianza en confianza* (trusting mutual trust), *respeto* (respect), *orgullo* (pride), and *dignidad* (dignity).
2. Value the elders' language and/or their preference for the mother tongue in situations where the individual demonstrates a traditional orientation.
3. Value the sense of place and belonging that rural elders acquire with longevity in a rural community.
4. Value their socio-historical experiences, their personal biographies, and their critical life-events that reflect their life course and rural ethnic realities.
5. Value the sense of spirituality and faith that serves as a buffer against social, economic, and cultural affronts and sustains them in profound ways.

The knowledge, values and skill essential for culturally competent practice must also be framed as a "cultural desire" or motivation to learn, to engage in a self-assessment across different levels including the practitioner, policymaking, and administrative levels. Finally cultural competence must be operationalized with benchmarks or standards for practice such as those established by the National Association for Social Work that serve as clear measures of accountability in practice.

CONCLUDING REMARKS

It is relatively certain that the population of elderly Latinos in rural areas will continue to grow in size and diversity based on shifts in rural to urban residence patterns. In addition a growing influx of new immigrant populations moving into rural areas will result in new challenges and issues related to health and social services, employment, and resource availability. A timely and appropriate response to the growing needs in rural communities will necessitate the development of a more comprehensive system of policies and programs aimed at addressing the needs and gaps in service delivery to rural elderly populations. Chief among these will be increased community service and resources, greater coordination of existing services, creative and alternative programming, accessible, affordable and available services, accurate representative data, and culturally competent workers in social work, nursing, public health, and related professions prepared to work in rural areas. Achieving these goals will be difficult indeed and must be tempered with the understanding that aging, ethnicity, culture and rurality are interwoven inextricably. Continued attention to the needs and aspirations of this elderly population is likely to improve the quality of life and subjective well being of rural elderly Latinos.

NOTE

1. Latino and Hispanic are used interchangeably in referring to individuals of Spanish-speaking origin.

REFERENCES

Angel, J.L., Angel, R.J., McClellan, J.L., & Markides, K.S. (1996). Nativity, declining health, and preferences in living arrangements among elderly Mexican Americans: Implications for long-term care. *The Gerontologist, 36*(4): 464-473.

Angel, R.J., & Angel, J.L. (1997a.) *Who will care for us? Aging and long-term care in multicultural America*. New York: New York University Press.

Angel, R.J., & Angel, J.L. (1997b). Health service use and long-term care among Hispanics. In K.S. Markides, & M.R. Miranda (Eds.) *Minorities, aging and health*. (pp. 343-366). Thousand Oaks, CA: Sage Publications.

Angel, R.J., & Tienda, M. (1982). Determinants of extended household structure: Cultural pattern or economic need? *American Journal of Sociology, 87*: 1360-83.

Applewhite, S. (1998). Culturally competent practice with elderly Latinos. *Journal of Gerontological Social Work, 30*(1/2): 1-15.

Applewhite, S.R., & J.M. Daley. (1988). Cross-cultural understanding for social work practice with the Hispanic elderly. In S. Applewhite (Ed.) *Hispanic elderly in transition: Theory, research, policy and practice* (pp. 3-16). New York: Greenwood Press.

Bok, D. (1996). *The state of the nation: Government and the quest for a better society*. Cambridge, MA: Harvard University Press.

Bronfenbrenner, U. (1979). *The ecology of human development*. Cambridge, MA: Harvard University Press.

Cavanaugh, J.C., & Whitbourne, S.K. (Eds.). (1999). *Gerontology: An interdisciplinary perspective*. New York: Oxford University Press.

Compton, B., & Galaway, B. (1989). *Social work processes*. Homewood, IL: Dorsey Press.

Cross, T.L., Bazron, B.J., Dennis, K.W., & Issacs, M.R. (March, 1989). *Towards a culturally competent system of care. Volume I.* Washington, DC: Child and Adolescent Service System Technical Assistance Center, Georgetown University Child Development Center.

Cromartie, J. (1993). Blacks maintain small nonmetro growth: One in four new nonmetro residents is Hispanic. *Rural Conditions and Trends, 4*, 16-19.

deAnda, D. (Ed.). (1997). *Controversial issues in multiculturalism.* Needham Heights, MA: Allyn and Bacon.

Devore, W., & Schlesinger, E.F. (1999). *Ethnic-sensitive social work practice.* (5th Ed.). Boston: Allyn and Bacon.

Economic Research Service (ERS). U.S. Department of Agriculture. (1997). Fewer immigrants settle in nonmetro areas and most fare less well than metro immigrants. *Rural Conditions and Trends, 8*(2): 60-65.

Garbarino, J. (1982). *Children and families in the social environment.* New York: Aldine.

Germain, C. (1973). An ecological perspective in casework practice. *Social Casework, 54*(6): 323-331.

Germain, C. (1979). *Social work practice: People and environments.* New York: Columbia University Press.

Germain, C., & Gitteman, A. (1980). *The life model of social work practice.* New York: Columbia University Press.

Gibson, R.C. (1991). Minority aging research: Opportunity and challenge. *The Gerontologist, 28*(4): 559-61.

Glasgow, N. & Brown, D.L. (1998). Older, rural and poor. In Coward, R.T., & Krout, J.A. (Eds.). *Aging in rural settings* (pp. 187-207). New York: Springer Publishing.

Green, J. (1995). *Cultural awareness in the human services.* Boston, MA: Allyn and Bacon.

Greene, R.R. (1999). *Human behavior theory and social work practice* (2nd ed). New York: Aldine De Gruyter.

Hefferman, J., Shuttlesworth, G., & Ambrosino, R. (1992). *Social work and social welfare* (2nd ed). New York: West Publishing.

Hooyman, N.R., & Kiyak, H.A. (2002). *Social gerontology* (6th ed.). Boston: Allyn and Bacon.

Institute of Medicine. (2001). *Health and Behavior: The interplay of biological, behavioral, and societal Influences.* Washington, DC: National Academy Press.

Lawton, J.A. (1989). *Behavior-relevant ecological factors.* In K.W. Schaie, & C. Scholars (Eds.). *Social structure and aging: Psychological processes.* Hillsdale, NJ: Erlbaum.

Lawton, M.P., & Nahemow, L. (1973). Ecology and the aging process. In C. Eisdorer, & M.P. Lawton (Eds.), *Psychology of adult development and aging.* Washington, DC: American Psychological Association (pp. 619-674).

Leigh, J.W. (1998). *Communicating for cultural differences.* Needham Heights, MA: Allyn and Bacon.

Lum, D. (2003). *Culturally competent practice* (2nd ed.). Pacific Grove, CA: Brooks/Cole.

Marin G., & Marin B.V. (1991). *Research with Hispanic populations*. Newbury Park, CA: Sage Publications.

Markides, K., & Coreil, J. (1988). The health status of Hispanic elderly in the Southwest. In S. Applewhite (Ed.) *Hispanic elderly in transition: Theory, research, policy and practice* (pp. 36-59). New York: Greenwood Press.

Meyer, C.H. (1973). *Social work practice* (2nd Ed.). New York: Free Press.

McLaughlin, D.K., & Jensen, L. (Eds.). (1998). *The rural elderly: A demographic report*. New York: Springer Publishing.

Norton, D.G. (1976). *The dual perspective*. New York: Council on Social Work Education.

Passuth, P.M., & Bengson, V.L. (1988). Sociological theories of aging: Current perspectives and future directions. In J.E. Birren, & V.L. Bengtson (Eds.) *Emergent theories of aging* (pp. 333-355). New York: Springer.

Parmelee, P.A., & Lawton, M.J. (1990). The design of special environments for the aged. In J.E. Birren, & K.W. Schaie (Eds.), *Handbook of the psychology of aging* (3rd ed). San Diego: Academic Press.

Perez-Stable, E.J., Napoles-Springer, A., & Miramontes J.M. (1997). The effects of ethnicity and language on medical outcomes of patients with hypertension and diabetes. *Med Care, 35*, 1212-9.

Quadagno, J. (2002). *Aging and the life course*. New York: McGraw-Hill.

Ricketts III, T.C., Johnson-Webb, K.D., & Randolph, R.K. (1999). *Rural health in the United States*. New York: Oxford University Press.

Romero, J.T. (1996). *Managed care and its implication for services to the Latino community*. Santa Jose, CA: Santa Clara County Mental Health Department.

Saenz, R., & Torres, C.C. (in press). Latinos in rural America. In D. Brown, & L. Swanson (Eds.) *Challenges for rural America in the 21st century*. Penn State University Press.

Torres, C.C. (1992). *Hispanic elderly: Lack of need or lack of data*? Paper presented at the American Sociological Association Meetings.

Torres, C.C. (2000). *Emerging Latino communities: A new challenge for the rural South. The rural South: Preparing for the challenges of the 21st century*. Southern Rural Development Center, Policy Brief no. 12. Mississippi State, MS: Southern Rural Development Center.

Torres, C.C. (2001). Elderly Latinos along the Texas-Mexico border: A health care challenge for the 21st century. *Journal of Border Health*, *7*(2): 28-37.

Torres, C.C. (2002). *Critical issues in Latino health*. Paper presented at the Rural Sociological Society, August 2002, Washington, DC.

Torres, C.C., Salazar, D., Villas, P., & Garza, D. (1999). *Factors influencing health seeking behaviors: Data from a pilot study of elderly Mexican Americans in the Lower Rio Grande Valley*. Paper presented at the Healthy Aging in the Next Millennium Conference. October, 1999.

U.S. Census Bureau. (2001a). *Housing and household economic statistics*. Table H109A. Retrieved December 11, 2001, from: *http://ferret.bls.census.gov/macro/032001/health/h09a_001.htm.*

U.S. Census Bureau. (2001b). Census supplementary survey. Table 2. Retrieved September 24, 2001 from the World Wide Web: *http://www.census.gov/c2ss/www/Products/Profiles/2000/index.htm.*

U.S. Census Bureau. (2001c). Poverty in the United States: 2000. Current population reports, Series P-60 no. 214. Washington, DC: U.S. Government Printing Office, 2001; Table 2. Age, Sex, Household Relationship, Race and Hispanic Origin by Ratio of Income to Poverty Level: 2000. Retrieved September 24, 2002 from: *http://ferret.bls.census.gov/macro/032001/pov/new02_004.*

U.S. Census Bureau. (2001d). Census 2000 Summary File 1, machine-readable data files. Washington: U.S. Census Bureau.

Winkelman, M. (1999). *Ethnic sensitivity in social work.* Dubuque, IA: Eddie Bower Publishing, Inc.

Wolinsky, F.D., & Tierney, W.M. (1998). Self-rated health and adverse health outcomes: An exploration and refinement of the trajectory hypothesis. *Journal of Gerontology, Social Sciences, 53B*(6): S336-S340.

Wong, R., Capoferro, C., & Soldo, B.J. (1999). Financial assistance from middle-aged couples and children: Racial-ethnic differences. *Journal of Gerontology, 54B*(3) S145-S153.

Chapter 10

Rural Disabled Elders

Elizabeth DePoy, PhD
Stephen French Gilson, PhD

SUMMARY. In this chapter we focus on social work practice with rural disabled elders. After discussing the tension between nomothetic and idiographic thinking about populations, we advance a definition which embodies both. Rural disabled elders are therefore a diverse set of members who both share some commonalities and are rich in their diversity and difference. To belong to this group, members must live outside of urban areas, be advanced in age and experience, and exhibit at least one atypical characteristic that carries an explanation which fits legitimate disability determination by a formal source. We then advance an approach to social work practice guided by the synthesis of two ideologies, self determination and legitimacy, and informed by systematic examination and analysis of social problems that affect individuals and groups. We conclude by advancing positive and negative principles for practice. *[Article copies available for a fee from The Haworth Document Delivery Service: 1-800-HAWORTH. E-mail address: <docdelivery@haworthpress.com> Website: <http://www.HaworthPress.com> © 2003 by The Haworth Press, Inc. All rights reserved.]*

KEYWORDS. Disabled elders, rural elders, self-determination

[Haworth co-indexing entry note]: "Rural Disabled Elders." DePoy, Elizabeth, and Stephen French Gilson. Co-published simultaneously in *Journal of Gerontological Social Work* (The Haworth Social Work Practice Press, an imprint of The Haworth Press, Inc.) Vol. 41, No. 1/2, 2003, pp. 175-190; and: *Gerontological Social Work in Small Towns and Rural Communities* (ed: Sandra S. Butler, and Lenard W. Kaye) The Haworth Social Work Practice Press, an imprint of The Haworth Press, Inc., 2003, pp. 175-190. Single or multiple copies of this article are available for a fee from The Haworth Document Delivery Service [1-800-HAWORTH, 9:00 a.m. - 5:00 p.m. (EST). E-mail address: docdelivery@haworthpress.com].

http://www.haworthpress.com/web/JGSW
© 2003 by The Haworth Press, Inc. All rights reserved.
Digital Object Identifier: 10.1300/J083v41n01_10

INTRODUCTION

Although we initially thought that this would be a straightforward chapter to write, we soon found that we struggled with how to delimit the boundaries and members of this group, and the issues of importance to social workers. The complexity of who fits into the category of disability, the slippery and differential meaning of elderly, the vast differences among geographic areas that are considered to be rural, and the diversity of individual, family, small group, and cultural experience in each and all three contexts can be confounding. Yet, we also recognize the critical importance of being able to address the nature, social issues, and related needs of groups, since no policy, program or community response could possibly take into account the vast range of individual diversity. We therefore approached our task from the perspective of tension and balance. That is to say, we present the tension between nomothetic (general principles about groups) and idiographic (individualistic) understandings of and responses to humans, and advance an analysis and exemplars for balance between the two poles which we believe can guide social workers towards thinking and action that help communities become socially just and respectful environments for the range of human diversity. We begin with the task of defining our terms and then move to a discussion of social work with rural, disabled elders. We conclude with positive (what should be) and negative (what should not be) principles for practice with rural disabled elders.

DEFINING OUR TERMS–WHO ARE RURAL DISABLED ELDERS?

While it is purposive and important to develop a generalized impression of what we might mean by the category rural disabled elders, it is obligatory to avoid a simplistic at best and potentially harmful homogenization of the diverse range of members in this group (Hudson, 1997). Many taxonomies describing and explaining human experience have been and continue to be posited. Thus, categorization is a dynamic thinking process (DePoy & Gilson, 2003) in which discourse and debate give rise to diverse conceptual frameworks which differ in their delineation of categorical boundaries, contexts, epistemological foundations, axiological dimensions, and ontology (Hutchison, 1999). Because of this complexity and the presence of three variables in our domain of concern, we begin our discussion by exploring each variable (rural, disability, and elder) individually. We then synthesize the lexical definitions to delimit our scope and to provide an understanding of the tension between the commonalities that comprise the conceptual category and the diversity of its individual members.

RURAL

As a beginning point, we examine just what we mean by rurality. The United States Census Bureau (2002) defines rural by what it is not. According to the Census Bureau, rural is classified as "all territory, population, and housing units located outside of UAs [urbanized areas] and UCs [urbanized clusters]. The rural component contains both place and nonplace territory" (p. 1). Roughly, urbanized areas are defined as densely settled areas that have census a population of at least 50,000 people, commonly with 1,000 people per square mile, and with adjacent block areas with at least 500 people per square mile. Urban clusters are settled geographic areas that have a density of 2,500 to 49,999 people, consisting of blocks or block groups of at least 1,000 people per square mile and adjacent blocks and block groups of at least 500 people per square mile.

Consulting the census definition provides us with a point, but only a starting point for our consideration of the scope of the concept of rurality. Unfortunately, while numerically clear, this approach to setting definitional boundaries and identifying essential elements of the concept of rurality does not take into account the factors that are relevant and necessary to understanding rural experience and needs, including but certainly not limited to economic activities, land values, political power, as well as primary language, educational opportunity, race, ethnicity, and cultural diversity. We all are aware that geographic areas that meet the Census 2000's definitional criteria for rurality exhibit tremendous contrasts in culture, climate, regional median income, occupational or career opportunities, and land use patterns. It therefore follows that we might expect vast differences in life opportunities, daily tasks, and availability and accessibility of health and social service offerings among locations such as a winter snow ski resort in Maine, a coal mining town in West Virginia, a farm in Iowa, a cattle ranch in Wyoming, or an American Indian reservation in Arizona. Each of these geographic settings provides both extraordinary opportunities for as well as unique challenges to daily life and experience.

Although diverse, there are some commonalities among rural areas that are relevant to social work and can be aggregated to produce a general definition that is useful for our discussion. Following the definitional approach of the Census Bureau, we also define rurality by what is not. That is to say, rural denotes a geographic area that, in comparison to urban areas, is less populated and has a limited array of formal resources, including those relevant to social work, such as health and social services. Although we highlight rural areas for what they are not for the purposes of this paper, we do not mean to imply that rurality is not rich with natural and human resources and opportunity. Rather, definition by comparison allows us to see what part of the literature on urban areas does not fit the nature of rural geographies.

DISABILITY

Similar to the difficulty in identifying a single but useful definition of rurality, defining disability provides confounding dilemmas that have been the source of debate and discourse for centuries (Longmore & Umansky, 2001). Looking back as far as ancient Greece, historical accounts reveal a nonlinear and multidirectional movement of the meaning of disability, spanning a continuum from the diagnostic-medical approach to an interactive complex person-in-environment perspective (Stiker, 1999).

The diagnostic approach to disability is based on medical explanations of individual human conditions. Accordingly, disability is defined as a long term to permanent diagnosed impediment that positions individuals with disabilities as less able than those who can recover from illness or who are non-disabled (Mackelprang & Salsgiver, 1997). As a form of biological determinism, the focus of disability in this definition is on physical, behavioral, psychological, cognitive, and sensory inadequacy, and thus disability is portrayed as a human characteristic situated within the disabled individual (Shakespeare, 1996). In large part, the diagnostic approach is based on the historic notion of illness advanced by Parsons in the early 1950s in which an individual who was deviant and deficient as a result of a diagnostic condition relinquished responsibility in exchange for professional care (Goffman, 1963).

The constructed approach to disability is the set of models in response to the medically deviant view that locates disability in the environment external to the individual. While a condition is acknowledged, it is not necessarily undesirable, in need of remediation (Quinn, 1988) or even relevant to understanding the circumstance of disabled people. Moreover, the notion that all individuals have diverse conditions is central to this approach. Why some conditions can be constructed as disabilities (i.e., mobility impairments in which individuals cannot walk) and others are not (mild nearsightedness), despite being correctable with adaptive equipment, is a fundamental question raised by this framework.

Simply put, the diagnostic-medical explanation of disability places the locus of disability within the individual who has experienced illness, insult, or anomaly. This internal focus results in an interpretation of the disabled individual as defective with reference to normative physical being. The constructed lens, on the other hand, looks at factors external to an individual that interact with diverse human conditions to create a disabling experience. Between these two views, numerous other explanations and understandings of disability exist, including ideas as extreme as disability being caused by spiritual demonization of individuals (Gilson & DePoy, 2000).

An analysis of the multiple definitions of disability reveals definitional vagueness, in that no distinction is made among definitions that approach the construct of disability from the perspective of description, explanation, and value. Synthesizing the approaches allows an overarching definition to be formulated. We therefore define disability as a value judgment regarding the degree to which the explanation for atypical human experience meets the legitimate criteria for a determination of disability. This definition does not take a single stance on disability as internal characteristic or external barrier. Rather, the disabling factor is the judgment regarding the fit of the label and relevant responses to explanations for why an individual or group lies outside of what is considered to be typical (DePoy, 2002; DePoy & Gilson, in press).

ELDERLY

In defining the term elderly, we encountered many words or phrases that seemingly are used interchangeably but may not have equivalent meanings. Here we distinguish *elderly* as a human attribute, *elder* as a noun for an individual who is elderly, and *aging* as a process. We agree with Harrigan and Farmer (2000) that aging "begins at birth, continues throughout life, and marks the passage of years" (p. 26). However, what chronological marker denotes the beginning of elderly is not as clear. As evidenced by even a cursory examination of agency, organization, and legislative policy, regulations, and program eligibility guidelines, what qualifies as the "legitimate age" beyond which one is an elder or elderly is both highly variable and determined by value. For example, the age for eligible membership in the AARP is 50; Medicare eligibility begins at age 65; individuals are eligible to begin receiving their Retirement Social Security benefits as early as age 62; and the determination of an individual's eligibility to retire from many white collar professional positions is often based upon a mathematical formula that factors in both the chronological age of the individual and the number of years that the individual has been employed at the designated setting.

If we use chronology alone as the determinant of elderly status, we quickly realize the universe of confounding variables. Consider gender for example. The issues, experiences, and potential needs of elderly women may be significantly different from those of men in the same age range (Beckett, Schneider, Vansburger, & Stevens, 2000). Variations and differences also exist when we consider characteristics of race, ethnicity, primary language, immigration status or land of origin, sexual orientation, faith and/or religions, educational attainment, economic status, or other individual or group characteristics, just to name a few. Further, because aging is intimately associated with the psychological, social, spiritual, economic, and political dimensions of an individual's and community's life, when one becomes elderly is influenced by all of these variables as well (Minkler & Fadem, 2002).

Synthesized from the vast literature, we propose a generalized definition of elderly as the chronological time of life which is advanced in years and life experience. Furthermore, consistent with Minkler and Fadem (2002), elderly individuals have experienced aging as a process of loss and gain over the lifespan and have a significant personal history on which to reflect.

SYNTHESIS

From the three definitions above, we now have a basis for delimiting rural, disabled elders as individuals who live outside of urban areas, who are advanced in age and experience, and whose explanations for an atypical nature are determined by at least one formal source to fit legitimate eligibility criteria for disability. Thus, the distinction between rural elders and rural elders who are disabled is the absence or presence respectfully of an atypical phenomenon that is explained with a legitimately disabling rationale. Although the likelihood of need for support for an individual with a disability is higher than for a non-disabled counterpart, we wish to clarify that the presence of a disability does not automatically necessitate services, supports, or caregivers. We return to this point later in the chapter.

Just to estimate the scope of individuals who may be members of the broad category of rural disabled elders, 23% of those who attained or passed the age of 65 now live in non-metropolitan areas, and of those, we can extrapolate from national data that approximately 55% (extrapolated from 1997 report, Profile of Older Americans, Administration on Aging, 2001) have at least one disability, with the higher age ranges reporting increasingly higher rates of disability. Moreover, as aging proceeds, the numbers reporting disability increase disproportionately (Administration on Aging, 2001).

As we noted above, not all disabled individuals need assistance and thus, the numbers of individuals who are both disabled and report needing assistance is of relevance to our continuing discussion. The numbers of those reporting both expand exponentially from 8.1% of the total population at the age range of 65-69 to 34.9% of individuals aged 80 and over, clearly highlighting the association between advancing age and need for assistance (Administration on Aging, 2001).

And while a disproportionately high number of elders, regardless of disability status, indicate the need for help, distinguishing who is defined as disabled because of the aging process from who enters the elder time of life already being disabled is important to consider in the current climate of categorical legitimacy for services. There are several reasons why. First, social workers can assist disabled elders to access the existing resources that address their category membership. But second, because current eligibility criteria for formal disability resources are anchored in nomothetically derived assertions of categorical needs, social workers looking to the future are in a crucial position to question the efficacy of the current service structures. These too frequently miss the important idiographic range of diversity and individuality within the membership of rural disabled elders. The challenge for social workers is therefore to seek a balance between the nomothetic and idiographic approaches to need of this population, among others. To accomplish this task, the thinking process of problem identification, embedded within the ideologies of self determination and legitimacy, provide important guidelines for identifying issues and related needs for rural, disabled elders, and for determining needed responses on the part of social workers. We turn to these now, beginning with ideology.

SELF DETERMINATION AND LEGITIMACY IDEOLOGY

Self-determination is a phrase that has come to be used by professionals to describe elements of progressive social, human, and health service work and by individuals to define a preferred approach to services, programs, organizations, policies, legislation, and research agendas (Tower, 1994). The ideology illustrates the balance of nomothetic and idiographic concerns, in that it recognizes the importance of choice within the constraints of social, economic and political contexts.

Within the field of disability studies, the ideology of self-determination places the disabled person at the "center of decision making and control" (Tower, 1994, p. 101). We have modified this ideology for social work practice with rural, disabled elders by suggesting that practice based in self determination ideology is at least a two layered approach. To address immediate need expressed by rural, elder, disabled individuals, social workers can identify and assist in the selection and organization of currently available resources. The second layer, focused on the future, is the obligation to systematically study and identify what social work and other community supports do not exist but are needed to resolve social problems. And on the flip side, it is incumbent on social workers to study what does exist and eliminate the services that do not meet the community needs, or perpetuate the growth of professional practice programs on the basis of the assumption that they are needed. Thus, social work practice guided by self-determination ideology is both immediate and future directed since it moves selection into choice. Choice involves developing desired positive (expansion of what is present) and negative (elimination or absenting what is currently present) options that reshape a list from which existing options can be selected. The distinction between choice and selection is a critical one in this model, in that selection, while more advanced on the thinking continuum than nomothetically based solutions to normative problems, actualizes thinking as a shared responsibility where the only step conducted by providers alone is the initial delimitation of service and support options. Choice is a thinking process in which existing options do not limit possibilities, but rather provide the grounding upon which to ascertain what else may be needed, decreased and/or eliminated to resolve identified social problems. Choice is idiographic in that it not only places an individual in control of his or her selection of options, but provides the forum to envision service and support options that are not available. This point is critical for social work with rural disabled elders.

Within the service system, self-determination requires that providers adjust their relationships with rural disabled elders and recognize that agency policies and procedures based on traditional paradigms of professional expertise commonly serve to diminish selection and choice necessary for self-determination (Freedberg, 1989). Fundamental to self determined human services is the recognition that rural elders with disabilities are the experts on their own lives and provide the idiographic understanding of their own needs. Within this conceptualization, the rural, elder, disabled person moves out of the role of client, patient, or recipient of services (Tower, 1994), to occupy the position of an educated, thoughtful, and informed user of services. This redefinition serves to place the elder in control of and directing his/her services (Brooke, Wehman, Inge, & Parent, 1995) as well as defining the range of "non-service" needs, desires, and interests.

A major consideration for social workers is that ideology of self-determination acknowledges that individual decisions are a civil right, but that the capacity to set one's own goals; decide what one needs and wants; and control how goals, needs, and wants are to be actualized may be shared. We mention capacity at this point, not to suggest or open the door for the denial of capacity, which is too frequently the experience of members of marginalized and oppressed groups, and particularly so with elderly and disabled persons, but rather to acknowledge that a critical role of social work is to uphold the practice of self-determination.

Third, self-determination must engender recognition from other groups regarding entitlement of the self-determining group not only to civil rights but also to equal opportunity and support in achieving both. This dimension is a critical factor in our assertion of the fundamental right of rural, elderly, disabled persons to choose their living environments, which may include a full range of options from their own homes to assisted living and nursing facilities.

Legitimacy is a concept that we have mentioned above in several instances. By legitimacy, we mean the values and parameters that bestow a label, category or power on an individual or group (Jost & Major, 2001). Legitimacy is a value-based process whereby determinations are made by different groups about the membership and worth of the groups or individuals of concern. Applied to disability and elders, legitimate disability and elder status may be promulgated by legislation, health care providers, or even disabled individuals themselves. Legitimacy involves not only a determination of membership, but also guides how members will be treated. Although we do not see people clamoring to join the ranks of the disabled elderly because of their devalued position in mainstream culture (Charlton, 1998), legitimacy as disabled, elder or disabled elder does have its benefits in our current categorically based health and social service systems (Hudson, 1997; Stone, 1986). What is exchanged for those benefits in terms of seeking a legitimate label of disabled elder may for some be an unwanted compromise. This point brings us to the integration of self determination and legitimacy as the ideological basis for social work practice with rural disabled elders. Attention to legitimacy is critical to understand the current systems, the values that shape them, why they are structured categorically, and how they may need to be changed to meet the self determined needs of rural disabled elders. Embedded within this ideology, systematic, logical, and shared thinking processes are necessary to derive an accurate explanation for problems and points of need which provide a balanced idiographic and nomothetic social work response. Although there are many thinking structures to meet this challenge, we have been successful with a technique called problem mapping (DePoy & Gilson, 2003). Let us look at this now.

PROBLEM MAPPING

Problem mapping is a systematic technique for analyzing and expanding our understanding of problem statements and their contexts. Further, this technique makes a clear distinction between problem and need, in which a problem is a legitimacy statement about what is undesirable, and a need is an empirically supported claim of what steps are necessary to resolve problems (DePoy & Gilson, 2003). Through the thinking process of problem mapping, the multidimensionality of problems, including their explanations, causes, and consequences, can be hypothesized, verified with credible evidence and linked to strategies that are needed to resolve all or part of the problem.

Current theory and research conducted through both nomothetic and idiographic approaches to inquiry have identified several broad problem areas experienced by rural disabled elders. First, many disabled elders have health problems which require specialized health care services. In rural areas, in which resources are less available and accessible than in urban areas, it is highly feasible to expect that specialists will not be available. Second, the limited population density of rural areas frequently means that individuals are not available for employment as providers of specialized or assistant services. Third, transportation is most frequently private, rendering travel even to local areas difficult for those who are unable to drive. Fourth, housing and recreation opportunities are less prevalent for rural disabled elders than for rural elders and for urban dwellers. Although not a definite factor in all rural areas, limited resources often mean underemployment and poverty. Given this variety of life issues that are quite often faced by rural disabled elders, we have selected the problem statement that follows to illustrate problem mapping anchored on our ideological framework:

Rural disabled elders are forced to live in nursing homes against their will.

Using problem mapping, we would conceptualize this initial problem statement as only one part of a larger phenomenon, with the metaphor of a single rock in a river. Mapping upstream, we name the explanatory causes for the originally articulated problem statement. Mapping downstream, we identify the consequences of the problem if it continues. Although these maps can be extremely complex, because we are limited in space, we present a truncated problem map for illustration purposes.

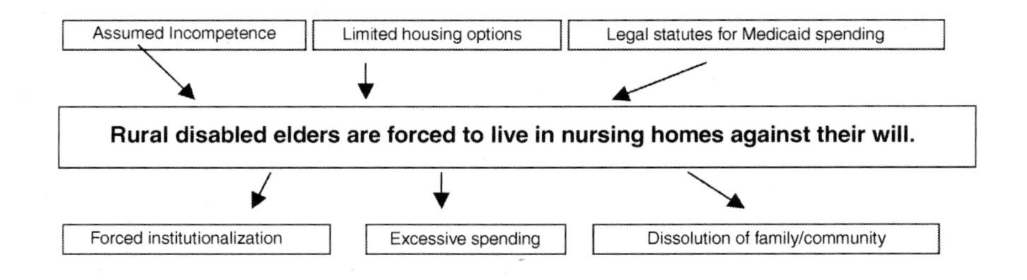

This problem map identifies three causal statements: (1) assumed incompetence of the rural disabled elder to make decisions about need; (2) limited housing options in rural areas for disabled elders; and (3) the legal statutes that direct payment for attendant care services to institutional settings.

The consequences of the problem as initially stated are: (1) forced institutionalization, (2) unnecessary expenditure of Medicaid funds for costly and unwanted institutionalization, and (3) the ultimate dissolution of families and communities who do not have the resources for community-based assistant services for disabled elders.

As you can see, as the initial problem statement is expanded by mapping, so understanding of needed interventions. Using thinking strategies to expand problems to nomothetic and idiographic causes and consequences provides the basis for balanced interventions within the ideology of self determination. Moreover, the areas where legitimacy criteria need to be changed are clearly highlighted.

From the idiographic perspective a social worker would focus on individual need. For example, in collaboration with the individual, a social worker might determine the desire for alternative living options. Thus idiographically driven social work practice might involve procuring the financial support, home health care, and assistance with activities of daily living resources that are commonly considered to be elements and experiences that define "living in the community." Concurrent with identifying and securing the needed and necessary community services, resources, and supports for the individual, the informed social worker would expand his or her scope to an examination of the degree to which the occurrence of being forced to live in a nursing home is a shared actual or potential experience for others. Along with community action, the social work response to uphold self-determination would seek to change public policy that currently principally supports reimbursement for institutional health care services to in-home and community based health care services.

Consider the example of The Medicaid Community-based Attendant Services And Supports Act (MiCASSA), originally introduced in 1995 and reintroduced most recently in 2001 (Liberty Resources, 2001). Crafted to address the balance of nomothetic and idiographic concerns of all disabled people, this bill would be of particular value to resolving the problem identified above through addressing the causative factor of institutionally-focused Medicaid spending patterns. Although the bill has many provisions which we cannot address here, its primary aim is the return of control over services to the user. The bill revises Medicaid spending patterns away from nomothetically based prescription of standard, institutionalized attendant services towards meeting the assistant care needs of the disabled individual in the location and manner in which he/she specifies. Moreover, assistance is based on function, not diagnosis, providing that one initially qualifies as legitimately disabled according to Medicaid eligibility criteria. For those who do not have the capacity, the bill guides shared decision making among professionals, service users and families, as well as shared selection and supervision of those providing attendant services.

Social work actions of advocacy and support for MiCASSA would be examples of an informed, balanced macro social work practice response to support self determination while acknowledging the issues raised by legitimacy. The heterogeneity of the population group is not lost within categorical legitimacy, but rather would be advanced by the social worker who advocates for socially just responses within the nomothetic constraints of Medicaid eligibility.

PRINCIPLES FOR SOCIAL WORK PRACTICE WITH RURAL DISABLED ELDERS

As we noted above, the principles which we suggest are both positive, that is what should be, and negative, what should not be. Positive principles include the basic guiding ethics, values, knowledge and practice principles of social work with all populations and locations.

- Begin with problem analysis.
- Select the part of the problem that is within the scope of social work practice.
- Empirically determine what is needed to resolve the problem.
- Set goals and objectives to meet the need through social work intervention.
- Thoughtfully conduct the intervention while systematically monitoring the degree to which process and preliminary outcomes are meeting objectives.
- Make necessary changes in response to monitoring.
- Assess the degree to which the desired outcomes met the need to resolve the problem or part of the problem for which social work services were initiated. (DePoy & Gilson, 2003)

Negative principles are based on legitimacy concerns.

- Do not assume that your problem definitions are in line with the problem definitions of others.
- Do not assume homogeneity among rural disabled elders.
- Do not attribute nomothetically derived characteristics to individuals based on a characteristic of age, disability or rural residence.

- Do not assume that people want or need services on the basis of age or disability.
- Do not assume that more formal services are necessary for rural communities.
- When an empirically determined need for services is asserted, identify who is making the assertion, for what purpose, who defines the desired outcome, and who is affected by the services.
- Based on empirical support, determine if social work ethics, values, skills, and knowledge will benefit the disabled rural elders in a manner that is meaningful to and desired by them.

CONCLUSIONS

In summary:

1. We have defined the category of rural, disabled elders as a broad swath of membership, sharing some commonalities but displaying the rich diversity that is present in all categorical descriptions of humans.
2. We identified the ideologies of self determination and legitimacy as foundations in which this population could be viewed through nomothetic and idiographic lenses.
3. We provided a structured thinking tool, problem mapping, for organizing the complexity of problems facing the group and its members.
4. Using the tool, we illustrated how an initial problem could be mapped to provide points at which needed and balanced interventions could be crafted and enacted.
5. We presented two levels of intervention as a sound and balanced social work response to a problem statement.
6. We offered positive and negative principles for practice.

In conclusion, we suggest that a major role of social work is the multi-level and collaborative effort to develop and continually improve all communities, including those that are considered to be rural. In order to actualize this role within the ethical mandates of the social work profession, concern with social justice, and respect for the full range of human diversity, including elders and individuals with disabilities, are essential.

Drawing on current trends in research (Bickman & Rog, 1997; DePoy & Gitlin, 1998; Schutt, 1999), contemporary philosophy (Silvers,

Wasserman, & Mahowald, 1998), new political theory (Kymlica, 2001), and even math and computer science (Gleick, 1988; Wolfram, 2002), we have based our work and exemplars on multiple epistemologies that illuminate central tendencies along with the context embedded uniqueness and have integrated this scholarship into our discussion of social work practice with rural, disabled elders. We urge social workers to guide their practices by developing and applying systematic knowledge of groups and individuals, analyzing and articulating the legitimacy criteria that shape knowledge and action, using thinking and action processes to identify and address the complexity of social problems and needs, and collaborating to promote communities in which a balance is maintained between social equilibrium and individual experience.

REFERENCES

Administration on Aging. (2001). *A profile of older Americans: 2001. Health, health care, and disability*. Retrieved September 16, 2002 online http://www.aoa.gov/aoa/STATS/profile/2001/12.html.

Babbie, E. (2001). *The practice of social research* (9th ed.). Belmont, CA: Wadsworth.

Beckett, J.O., Schneider, R.L., Vansburger, E., & Stevens, E. (2000). In R.L. Schneider, N.P. Kropf, & A. Kisor (Eds.), *Aging women. Gerontological Social Work: Knowledge, Service Settings, And Special Populations* (2nd ed.) (pp. 302-342). Pacific Grove, CA: Wadsworth.

Bickman, L., & Rog, D.J. (Eds.). (1997). *Handbook of applied social research methods*. Thousand Oaks, CA: Sage.

Brooke, V., Wehman, P., Inge, K., & Parent, W. (1995). Toward a customer-driven approach to supported employment. *Education and Training in Mental Retardation and Developmental Disabilities*, *30*, 308-320.

Charlton, J.I. (1998). *Nothing about us without us: Disability oppression and empowerment*. Berkeley, CA: University of California Press.

DePoy, E., (2002). Will the real definition of disability please stand up. *Psychosocial Process*, Spring, 2002, 50-54.

DePoy, E., & Gilson, S.F. (in press). *Disability: Towards a critical theory of disability and community*. Pacific Grove, CA: Wadsworth.

DePoy, E., & Gilson, S.F. (2003). *Practice evaluation: Thinking & action*. Pacific Grove, CA: Wadsworth.

DePoy, E., & Gitlin, L. (1998). *Introduction to research* (2nd edition). St Louis, MO: Mosby.

Freedberg, S. (1989). Self-determination: Historical perspectives and effects on current practice. *Social Work*, *34*, 33-38.

Gilson, S.F., & DePoy, E. (2000). Multiculturalism and disability: A critical perspective. *Disability & Society*, *15*(2), 207-218.

Gleick, J. (1988). *Chaos: Making a new science*. New York, NY: Penguin.

Goffman, E. (1963). *Stigma: Notes on the management of spoiled identity*. New York, NY: Simon & Schuster.

Harrigan, M.P., & Farmer, R.L. (2000). In R.L. Schneider, N.P. Kropf, & A. Kisor (Eds.), The myths and facts of aging. *Gerontological Social Work: Knowledge, Service Settings, and Special Populations* (2nd ed.) (pp. 26-64). Pacific Grove, CA: Wadsworth.

Hudson, R.B. (Ed.). (1997). *The future of age-based public policy*. Baltimore, MD: Johns Hopkins Press.

Hutchison, E.D. (1999). *Dimensions of human behavior*. Thousand Oaks, CA: Pine Forge Press.

Jost, J.T., & Major, B. (Eds.). (2001). *The psychology of legitimacy: Emerging perspectives on ideology, justice, and intergroup relations*. Cambridge, United Kingdom: Cambridge University Press.

Kymlica, W. (2001). *Contemporary political philosophy: An introduction*. London, England: Oxford University Press.

Liberty Resources. (2001). *MiCASSA*. Retrieved on January 28, 2003 from http://www.libertyresources.org/mc/ca-index.html.

Longmore, P.K., & Umansky, L. (Eds.). (2001). *The new disability history: American perspectives (History of disability)*. New York, NY: New York University Press.

Mackelprang, R., & Salsgiver, R. (1999). *Disability: A diversity model approach in human service practice*. Pacific Grove, CA: Brooks/Cole.

Minkler, M., & Fadem, P. (2002). "Successful aging": A disability perspective. *Journal of Disability Policy Studies, 12*(4), 229-235.

Moody, H.R. (1998). *Aging: Concepts & Controversies* (2nd.). Thousand Oaks, CA: Pine Forge Press.

Quinn, P. (1998). *Understanding disability: A lifespan approach*. Thousand Oaks, CA: Sage.

Schutt, R. (1999). *Investigating the social world: The process and practice of research*. Thousand Oaks, CA: Pine Forge.

Shakespeare, T. (1996). Disability, identity and difference. In G. Barnes, & G. Mercer (Eds.), *Exploring the divide: Illness and disability* (pp. 94-113). Leeds, United Kingdom: The Disability Press.

Silvers, A., Wasserman, D., & Mahowald, M.B. (1998). *Disability, difference, discrimination: Perspectives on justice in bioethics and public policy*. Lanham, MD: Rowman & Littlefield.

Smith, D., & Tillipman, H. (2000). *The older population in the United States: Population characteristics* (P20-532). Washington, DC: U.S. Census Bureau, U.S. Department of Commerce, Economics and Statistics Administration. Retrieved September 12, 2002 online http://www.census.gov/prod/2000pubs/p20-532.pdf.

Stiker, H.J. (2000). *A history of disability (Corporealities)*. Ann Arbor, MI: University of Michigan Press.

Stoller, E.P., & Gibson, R.C. (2000). *Worlds of difference: Inequality in the aging experience* (3rd ed.). Thousands Oaks, CA: Pine Forge Press.

Stone, D.A. (1986). *The disabled state*. Philadelphia, PA: Temple University Press.

Tower, K.D. (1994). Consumer-centered social work practice: Restoring client self-determination. *Social Work, 39*, 101-106.

United States Census Bureau. (2002). Census *2000 urban and rural classification*. Retrieved September 7, 2002 from http://www.census.gov/geo/www/ua/ua_2k.html.

Wolfram, S. (2002). *A new kind of science*. Champagne, IL: Wolfram Media Inc.

PART II

SECTION IV
SPECIAL ISSUES AND PROGRAMS

Chapter 11

Older Adult Health Promotion in Rural Settings

Stephanie J. FallCreek, DSW

SUMMARY. Social workers bring powerful tools to health promotion program design and delivery with rural older persons. Social work values and core clinical and organizational competencies are aligned closely with health promotion models that depend upon comprehensive strength-based assessment, self-care, self-efficacy, and empowerment strategies. There are many possible roles, including, for example, work with individuals, groups and organizations as a direct service provider, serving as a trainer or leader of volunteers, or practicing as a member of an interdisciplinary team. Social workers may wish to consider incorporating health promotion as part of a generalist practice or as a primary practice focus.

[Haworth co-indexing entry note]: "Older Adult Health Promotion in Rural Settings." FallCreek, Stephanie J. Co-published simultaneously in *Journal of Gerontological Social Work* (The Haworth Social Work Practice Press, an imprint of The Haworth Press, Inc.) Vol. 41, No. 3/4, 2003, pp. 193-211; and: *Gerontological Social Work in Small Towns and Rural Communities* (ed: Sandra S. Butler, and Lenard W. Kaye) The Haworth Social Work Practice Press, an imprint of The Haworth Press, Inc., 2003, pp. 193-211. Single or multiple copies of this article are available for a fee from The Haworth Document Delivery Service [1-800-HAWORTH, 9:00 a.m. - 5:00 p.m. (EST). E-mail address: docdelivery@haworthpress.com].

http://www.haworthpress.com/web/JGSW
© 2003 by The Haworth Press, Inc. All rights reserved.
Digital Object Identifier: 10.1300/J083v41n03_01

[Article copies available for a fee from The Haworth Document Delivery Service: 1-800-HAWORTH. E-mail address: <docdelivery@haworthpress.com> Website: <http://www.HaworthPress.com> © 2003 by The Haworth Press, Inc. All rights reserved.]

KEYWORDS. Health promotion, rural gerontology, empowerment practice

INTRODUCTION

The intersection or common ground of social work practice, health promotion, and aging in rural America is rich in opportunity and challenge. This presentation will touch upon multiple aspects of the topic. Some definitions will be reviewed and principles identified to establish a common language and context for the discussion that follows. The limited recent literature on gerontological social work practice for health promotion in rural settings will be illustrated. Selected characteristics of rural settings and a rural older adult constituency will be shared, in terms of the implications these might have for health promotion efforts by gerontological social workers. Given the dearth of published, peer-reviewed research in this specific practice area, the discussion will focus on emerging possibilities that respond to the fit between social work values and practice competencies and rural older adult health promotion.

THE LANGUAGE OF HEALTH PROMOTION

The "language of health promotion" crosses multiple disciplinary boundaries. As there are various definitions of "health," so there are multiple definitions of health promotion. Several are presented to frame the concept.

Health promotion has been defined several ways over the past few decades, varying primarily in terms of how broad a scope of intervention and outcome is incorporated. Four definitions, one tailored to older adults, are offered to illustrate the range, each definition recognized by different audiences.

More than two decades ago, Green and Anderson (1982) provided the following definition of health promotion: "any combination of health education and related organizational, political, and economic interventions designed to facilitate behavioral and environmental changes conducive to health" (p. 16).

The World Health Organization (1986) characterized health promotion simply as "the process of enabling people to increase control over, and to improve, their health" (p. 1). Imbedded in that definition is the assumption that this improvement in health results in a valued outcome. This definition also encompasses both individual level interventions and broader socio-economic and environmental level approaches.

A definition, adapted from Green and Anderson that has been tailored particularly to older adults, also has been offered (FallCreek, 1992):

> Health promotion for older adults is planned action to maintain or improve physical, mental, or spiritual health. It can be accomplished through personal or collective, behavioral, and environmental change. The best methods are those that promote dignity and independence and build knowledge and skills to help older adults make informed decisions about health issues, for themselves and as members of the community. (p. 2)

Most recently (2002), at the Second United Nations World Assembly on Aging, the World Health Organization slightly revised their earlier definition to suggest that health promotion is "the process of enabling people to take control over and to improve their health" (p. 22). In the same document, WHO described disease prevention (for older adults) as "the prevention and management of the conditions that are particularly common as individuals age: non-communicable diseases and injuries, referring to primary and secondary prevention" (p. 22).

HEALTH PROMOTION AND AGING

Since older people increasingly experience chronic disease and/or functional impairment as they age, tertiary prevention interventions (i.e., those which focus on preventing disability, delaying functional decline and loss of independence) are an integral component of comprehensive older adult health promotion. Secondary prevention, e.g., screening for early detection of chronic disease, before symptoms develop, also plays an important role throughout the life course. Still, even among the very old, primary prevention activities, such as immunization against influenza and maintaining an appropriate level of physical activity remain important–with the potential to maintain or improve function in daily life, save dollars, prevent or delay disability, and minimize personal discomfort and distress.

The outcomes of health-promoting actions or programs are diverse, including: changes in personal habits (e.g., regular exercise, smoking cessation); related health measurements (e.g., blood pressure, cholesterol) and skill development (e.g., assertive, effective communication with health care providers, low-fat food preparation); social norms and actions (e.g., familial sensitivity to potential impact of secondhand smoke on elders with compromised respiratory function); and/or organizational practices (using wellness days as an alternative to sickness days) and public policies (installation of accessible restrooms for persons with limited mobility).

If optimal health or "wellness" is the desired outcome of best practice health promotion with older adults, what are the underlying components of high-level wellness? Six frequently recognized dimensions of wellness include: physical, emotional, intellectual, spiritual, social, and vocational (Armbruster & Gladwin, 2001). A recent task force on healthy and successful aging identified the core components of successful aging somewhat differently (Cleveland Foundation, 2002). The task force suggested that, as one ages, at least three elements comprise an overall sense of well-being (perhaps yet another, more person-centered definition of optimal "health" or wellness): dealing effectively with life's inevitable changes and challenges; sustaining positive, meaningful, dynamic relationships; and living with purpose and joy. These coping and interpersonal skills, and living with a sense of meaning and purpose supplement, and are entirely compatible with, the comprehensive, long-standing definition of health offered in the World Health Organization *Constitution* (1948): "A state of complete physical, social and mental well-being, and not merely the absence of disease or infirmity."

Within the context of health promotion, health is considered not so much an abstract state of being, but rather as a means to an end that may be expressed in functional terms. It is a resource that permits people to lead an individually, socially, and economically productive life. Health is a resource for everyday life, not the object of living. It is a positive concept emphasizing social and personal resources, as well as physical capabilities.

Further, the World Health Organization's (2002, p. 12-13) adoption of the concept "Active Ageing" calls for an interdisciplinary, proactive approach–potentially offering gerontological social workers the opportunity to perform key roles. Planning, policy development and advocacy, program development, and clinical practice is shifted away from the traditional "needs-based" approach (which runs the risk of "fixing" older people in a recipient role) towards one which is oriented toward empowerment and participation–foundations upon which the social work code of ethics and strength-based practice is built. This model positions social workers to assist older people to claim and exercise equality of opportunity and self-determination in all aspects of their lives.

To the extent that necessary resources (information, education, skills development, and services) are available, it further holds individuals of all ages appropriately accountable for shaping their lifespan course of learning, growth, and development. A holistic approach to health promotion with older adults examines each of these definitions and principles when developing a needs assessment, prioritizing among change goals, identifying an appropriate intervention or approach, implementing the selected intervention(s), and evaluating the results.

HEALTH PROMOTION AND SOCIAL WORK PRACTICE

The *Occupational Outlook Handbook* (U.S. Department of Labor, 2001) describes two social work specializations that seem particularly relevant to older adult and rural health promotion: healthcare social workers and gerontological social workers. "Healthcare social workers help patients and families cope with chronic, acute or terminal illnesses and handle problems that may stand in the way of recovery or rehabilitation . . . They may organize support groups . . . advise family caregivers . . . plan for patient needs" (p. 161). "Gerontological social workers specialize in services for senior citizens. They run support groups . . . advise elderly people or family members about . . . choices . . . and . . . coordinate and monitor services" (p. 161). In their overall discussion of the profession of social work, the handbook says: "Social workers help people function the best way they can in their environment, deal with relationships, and solve personal and family problems" (p. 160). When this assistance is focused on helping people to "take control over and to improve their health" (WHO, 2002, p. 22), social workers, whether generalist or specialists, are practicing at the core of health promotion. Both the Ottawa Charter (WHO, 1986) and the Jakarta Declaration (WHO, 1997) incorporate advocacy, skill development and mediation between differing interests in society as fundamental strategies for achieving the goals of health promotion.

There are several educational models that identify desirable practice competencies for professional social workers. The John A. Hartford Foundation funded CSWE/SAGE-SW project (Council on Social Work Education, 2003) recently identified a very large set of social work competencies for working with aging populations, differentiating between those needed by all social workers and a subset specifically for gerontological social workers. Another recent model, developed in Cleveland, Ohio at the Mandel School of Applied Social Sciences (MSASS) at Case Western Reserve University, identified core abilities for all master's level social workers (2001, pp. 5-18) in all concentrations, including aging. A few examples of blended (both generic and aging specific) model competencies illustrate their applicability to health promotion with older rural adults:

- *Awareness of personal values as they relate to aging/Integrating social work values and ethics.* Consider how elders' attitudes affect accepting help, and how various interventions present ethical dilemmas around self-determination, mutual decision-making, and degree of risk for the older adult. For example, should participating in a smoking cessation program be voluntary for an elder kinship caregiver with compromised respiratory function living in a multi-generational household, including young children with asthma?
- *Diversity and populations at risk as it applies to variations in aging/Valuing a diverse world and advocating for social justice.* Consider the inter-relationship of culture and personal identity, with respect to gender, race, ability, ethnicity, economic status, sexual orientation, and religion. For example, what program design and delivery elements could be put in place to facilitate access to participation of a relocated elder gay or lesbian couple in a group education intervention in a closely knit, conservative small town? Could participation in a carefully designed and delivered program not only promote personal health, but also reduce discrimination or oppression?
- *Human behavior as it applies to lifespan person-environment dynamics.* This includes the biological, sociological, cultural, psychological factors and lifespan spirituality. For example, in a health promotion program designed for American Indian/Native American family caregivers, how can awareness of family and

tribal expectations and local herbalist health assessment practices be used to shape a curriculum that will be culturally sensitive and at the same time facilitate access to choices that include technology-based disease screening services? Another example would be a program focused on Asian-Americans that strengthened intergenerational bonding between youths and elders, considering the many peer/environmental influences outside of the home, while emphasizing autonomy of lifestyle choices for both.

- *Social work methods.* Examples include: bio-psychosocial spiritual assessment of functional ability, advocacy to create responsive systematic change(s), case management to integrate services, and resources to maximize independence. For example, what are the implications of the assessment findings for selecting proposed approaches to better controlling diabetes among kinship caregivers (and preventing it in the children they are raising) whose tradition includes regular preparation and consumption of desserts after each Sunday's church service?
- *Policy (and the regulations which guide its implementation), particularly as it relates to the Social Security Act, Medicare, Medicaid, and the Older Americans Act.* For example, operating within all the regulatory guidelines, in a rural area with extremely limited organizational, financial and human resources, how does one design and deliver an ongoing health promotion program that integrates funding from multiple components of the Older Americans Act and the school district, that uses health professional, retired volunteers to deliver the program and yet is open to community members of all ages and affiliations?
- *Research and evaluation of one's own practice effectiveness on a regular basis/Critical thinking and professional use of self.* For example, knowing that home-based, telephone or Internet reinforced strategies may be as effective as community-based group education models to promote increased physical activity among older women, how can an existing program be adapted to test this concept, permitting professional time and travel expenses to be reallocated toward another health promotion intervention?

Advanced practice involves the capacity to engage, plan, intervene and evaluate in a social work environment and a community environment that is involved in ongoing dynamic change (Mandel, 2001). Such skill certainly describes the landscape of rural social work practice–challenged and inspired at every twist and turn of the community and the environment.

Each of the above competencies/abilities prepares social workers for aspects of generalist practice in health promotion with older adults in rural areas. Furthermore, each level of health promotion intervention–individual, system, and local or global policy–offers possibilities to social workers who are interested in or committed to different types of practice. Gerontological social workers can assist individuals and groups with: deciding what to tackle (needs assessment, community organizing, planning, and prioritization); identifying approaches to use (individual counseling, small group process, community resource assessment, and development, changes in the surrounding environment); implementing the agreed-upon approaches (education, training, group facilitation, policy development, advocacy) and evaluating and learning from each health promotion intervention experience to improve future results. Rural gerontological social workers who possess and use these competencies and abilities will be well positioned to have a positive impact on the health and well-being of both older individuals and the rural communities in which they live.

SOCIAL WORK, HEALTH PROMOTION, AND RURAL AGING: EXAMPLES FROM RESEARCH AND PRACTICE

There is little published literature in the last decade that notes the "intersection" of gerontological social work, health promotion, and older adults, much less how it might play out specifically in rural settings. A search of the AgeLine database (AARP, 2002), as well as other sources, for the most recent literature (2000, 2001 and 2002) that specifically addressed health promotion roles for social workers with older adults in rural settings yielded no peer reviewed publications. However, considering any two of the related topics–rural aging, health promotion, and social work–yields a body of literature to suggest that social work roles and opportunities in rural health promotion currently exist and can be further developed. This includes roles for individual/clinical social work practice, as well as community/organizational social work practice with and for older adults. This includes, for example, literature on social work and rural aging (Bull, 1993), rural aging and health promotion (FallCreek, Muchow, & Mockenhaupt, 1994; National Rural Health Association, 1992), and health promotion with older adults (Dychtwald,

1986; FallCreek & Mettler, 1984; Haber, 1999; Mettler & Kemper, 2000).

In the 1980s, several pioneering older adult health promotion demonstration projects featured social workers in administrative leadership, community organizing, advocacy, and clinical-educational roles (FallCreek & Mettler, 1984). Later, Bender, and Hart (1986) also described a community health project in Oklahoma using this experience to illustrate roles of social workers in promoting health. More recently, social workers were identified as recruiters and trainers of volunteers in a demonstration health promotion project with older adults (e.g., Lan, 1999), while Vest, Ronneau, Lopez, and Gonzalez (1997) explored a holistic approach to health promotion using collaboration between social workers and community health providers in rural health clinics. Academic social work programs have embraced health promotion with older adults, which includes offering field placements in health promotion for social workers (University of Omaha, 1998), as well as developing interdisciplinary curricula with social workers, both as students and educators (Western Maryland Area Health Education Center, 2003).

The modest documentation of work that incorporates health promotion, social workers, and rural aging does not indicate, necessarily, a dearth of practice in this area. Rather, it may reflect the reality that gerontological social workers in rural areas that are engaged in health promotion activities have not been "written up" for publication, nor have their efforts and outcomes been evaluated empirically. Also, in view of the overall scarcity of social workers in rural areas, many have a generalist practice and, therefore, health promotion activities may be undertaken and accomplished "at the margin," and therefore, not even recognized as a specific area of practice.

Social work, with its focus on ethics, empowerment, and self-determination (NASW, 2000), and in the context of integrated community values, seems ideally suited to organize and/or facilitate interdisciplinary and consumer-led approaches to health promotion. Lucchetti and Federica (2002), in an evaluation of a multi-site community-based health promotion intervention undertaken by trained volunteers, found excellent consumer satisfaction ratings, solid attendance, and positive impact on the participants' nutrition and social support networking. The greatest challenge to the success of the model lay in helping the volunteers with organizational skills and process issues. This type of training and facilitation is well within the purview of skilled social workers. Recognizing the continuing shortage of skilled health professionals and paraprofessionals in rural areas, the viability of training and empowering volunteer leadership for health promotion programs seems an obvious and appropriate role for gerontological social work.

CHALLENGES TO PROGRAM DESIGN IN RURAL SETTINGS

At least three characteristics of rural settings that impact other forms of rural social work also influence health promotion with older persons. Limited availability of health and human service professionals, especially specialists; the distance (proximity) between consumers and the resources upon which they need to draw; and low population density, all influence the possibilities for health promotion program design and delivery.

The restricted availability of professional service providers increases the probability of programs designed with greater personal reliance on self-care, longer waits for appointments of all kinds, and the development and use of generalist practitioners. Though distance between clients and providers and the overall scarcity of human services professionals pose many barriers to service delivery, both these factors encourage service providers to use models anchored in individual and community empowerment that rely heavily on self-care strategies. Low population density also works against service models that depend upon large group education and often make it difficult to capture any economies of scale in acquisition of materials and equipment. Low population density may also reduce available resources if a per capita funding formula is applied.

Lifestyle modification often depends on the individual to assess need, identify desired changes or services, and make a commitment to the change or participation, acquire the necessary information and skills, and, ultimately, adopt and maintain his or her progress. Mettler, a social worker and primary author of *Healthwise for Life* (2000), created a resource that has been used nationwide, by a variety of health and social services sponsors to benefit rural and urban elders alike, as an affordable self-care tool, as well as a "primer" for group educations programs.

Issues of proximity (or geographic isolation) between the consumer and needed resources are compounded by low-population density, and one result is limited availability of both public and private free, subsidized, or full fee for service transportation. This further restricts opportunity for consumers who already are limited in their ability to secure and keep appointments for the screening, education, counseling, or face-to-face support groups that are typical of health promotion interventions. This makes group activities and site-based programs more expensive, difficult to recruit for, and challenging to schedule. Distance also limits the ability of practitioners to make individual, small group home or community-based setting visits. Greater travel time required between appointments adds to the individual cost of services for personal visits in addition to the per mile cost of the transportation itself. Face-to-face access is more difficult to arrange and more expensive to support under these circumstances.

CREATING COLLABORATION AND SOCIAL CAPITAL FOR HEALTH PROMOTION

In more rural settings, where formal organizational resources are scarce and health and medical professionals are few and far between, Gillies' (1998) notion of using the power and prospect for alliances and partnerships to maximize the creation of social capital, the return on its investment, in health promotion outcomes at the individual and system level, is particularly intriguing. Social workers have long practiced advocacy, community organizing, collaboration, and cooperation across diverse disciplinary and organizational boundaries.

Gillies (1998) proposed two levels of alliance or partnership, each of which offers different opportunities for gerontological social work with rural older persons. First, at the micro level, alliances or partnerships between and among collaborators that seek to have a health promoting impact through individuals, groups or organizations could be developed. These would not be directed toward systematic or structural change. Second, alliances or partnerships would be developed to impact health promotion at the macro level. These could impact the structural determinants of health (p. 101).

Gillies' (1998) review of diverse international health promotion projects found that the greater the representation of many sectors of the community and, the greater the active engagement of the community–especially public representation–the greater the impact and more enduring the benefits which accrued. Although the projects reviewed are not focused specifically on elders or rural communities, two of the reviewed projects, "Health Promotion in Hungarian Gypsies" and the Canadian

"Healthy Start Project," specifically engaged and built upon the efforts of social workers to achieve the health promoting outcomes (pp. 108-109). Gillies identifies several features, common across successful projects, which appear to optimize the outcomes of organizing community resources for health promotion:

1. Creating durable structures for shared decision-making
2. Involving local people in planning, maintaining order and relevance
3. Providing for appropriate opportunities to dissent
4. Creating vehicles for direct engagement in practical activities of health promotion (p. 102).

In terms of advocating for system level changes and policy development that responds to a particular constituency, it may be important to refer to and draw upon the learning and critical knowledge developed through the interaction of the lay participants as well as the larger body of scientific, evidence-based knowledge. In an environment of mutual validation (drawing upon those critical social work communication skills), where scientific and professional experts work collaboratively with lay citizens, the prospects for planning and achieving meaningful health promotion goals are optimized.

The term social capital initially referred to the complex and varied social mechanisms that parents use to advance their children's success. Coleman (1988, p. 101) defined the function identified by the concept of social capital as "the value of these aspects of social structure to actors as resources that they can use to achieve their interests." Putnam (1993) adapted earlier work to develop his widely recognized definition of social capital as "features of social organization such as networks, norms, and social trust that facilitate coordination and cooperation for mutual benefit." Social workers can facilitate the development and maintenance of community networks, norms, and social trust to leverage personal and collective changes that promote health and wellness.

The creation of social capital needed to build and maintain alliances and partnerships for health promotion depends upon relationships between individuals, between individuals and organizations and between organizations and organizations. The participants, whose trust and energy create the needed social capital, must be able to freely cross boundaries and frontiers artificially drawn by inequities such as poverty and many forms of discrimination, including, for example, both ageism and sexism.

Despite low population density, there are many aspects of rural and small town living that offer opportunities to the gerontological social worker that is interested in promoting health through the development and reinvestment of social capital. In the "best" of small town North America, it has been suggested that there is a strong sense of community with an individual character, an awareness of place, and a sense of family and tradition. The fabric of community is comprised of close social and personal relationships coexisting with a low population base. One can readily envision the value that this might bring to creating self-help and mutual support groups for health promotion.

Of course, some of these same aspects of rural and small town living also pose challenges to gerontological practice. For example, how can confidentiality be best protected, where "everyone knows your name" (and your business!)? The need to balance the community's best interest with that of its individual citizens results in an ongoing requirement to analyze relationship issues very carefully. This is complicated by a tendency toward generalist practice in rural areas–the social worker who leads the older adult community health promotion class on stress management may also be the social worker who has shared responsibility with the public health nurse for investigating and reporting communicable diseases, in addition to counseling kinship caregivers about managing difficult intra-family relationships between custodial grandparents and birth parents whose parental rights have been terminated.

TECHNOLOGY OPTIONS FOR RURAL HEALTH PROMOTION

Considering the scarcity of health and human service professionals, and the low population density, using advanced technology for health promotion communication would seem promising. For example, in contrast to pervasive early skepticism about the acceptability and accessibility of computer and Internet-based programs with older persons, evidence has begun to suggest its potential. The tools of technology can strengthen the intervention and support and maintenance systems needed for rural social work practice in health promotion with elders. In a recent article, Kressig and Echt (2002) found that most of a community sample of older adults was willing and able to complete and understand a computer-based questionnaire and the recommendations it generated about their current levels of physical activity. Increased availability of both dial up and high-speed Internet connections in rural areas will substantially extend the potential of using technology in rural health promotion with older adults.

The older adult population in rural America is quite diverse, and the opportunities and challenges for social workers to engage in health promotion programs will be equally varied. The richness of the opportunity set is complicated, of course, by personal and organizational resource constraints. As Ginsburg (1998) suggests, many of those remaining in rural areas are older people whose health, economic, and social problems are, or have become, severe. Yet recent studies have suggested (Wallace & Wallace, 1998) that in terms of physical health, differences in health and illness rates may be modest between urban and rural elders. Instead, greater variation may exist between rural areas (e.g., access to care) and among specific demographic subgroups of elders, such as the oldest-old men (Krout & Coward, 1998) who may be disproportionately in poverty and poor health.

The behavior/lifestyle/environmental change "targets" chosen for rural health promotion programs may be similar to that of their more urbanized peers. It is, rather, the types of interventions and methods of delivering them that may need tailoring to be effective with rural older adults (e.g., using electronic communication instead of small group face-to-face education, focusing on home-based distance monitoring of clinical values rather that group screening and counseling appointments, creating chat rooms or telephone buddies for mutual support rather than gathering frequently at a senior center).

The evolution of information technology and increasing availability of Internet access in small towns and isolated rural areas also offers promise for social work practice. Although much distance learning has focused on professional education and development, there are multiple avenues to using technology to enhance education for health promotion among rural elders. Some of these include: audiotapes; videotapes; disk or CD-based computer instruction; and most recently, interactive, Internet-based diagnostic, education, support, and monitoring services.

Atienza (2001) reviewed research on home-based programs to promote physical activity among middle-aged and older women. Among the relevant findings were: home-based programs were often as effective as group-based and home-based programs with telephone-based counseling were particularly effective in facilitating participation among middle-aged and older adults.

As Dezendorf and Green (1999) suggested in a conference paper, *Electronic Social Work (ESW) and Rural Practice*, the greatest barrier to fulfilling the potential offered by contemporary technology to rural practice may be the resistance of the profession itself to incorporating technology in individual, community, and policy/advocacy practice. Although universal access to the Internet is far from assured, more and more older persons, regardless of socio-economic status or geographic residence, are gaining access to the information highway. It is important for rural social workers to be aware of and gain expertise in making the most of using electronic support groups, senior information gateways, and community advocacy opportunities.

Specifically, these electronic "tools" may help partially to overcome the scarcity of on-site specialized health professionals; the difficulties imposed by distance, physical isolation, lack of transportation; and even some of the self-image/privacy concerns of older consumers. The use of "high tech" should not be construed as completely replacing the need for personal presence in health promotion practice. Rather, it enables the social worker to provide a significant amount of information, facilitate the development of ongoing peer support and communication, and provide important feedback to community leaders and other decision-makers very cost-effectively while focusing limited face-to-face time on those issues and opportunities where the personal touch is most critical.

CULTIVATING THE CLIMATE FOR HEALTH PROMOTION WITH RURAL ELDERS

Despite a dearth of published, peer-reviewed literature relating to social work, health promotion with older adults and small town practice, the possibilities for social work practice are rich and varied. For those who are skeptical about the potential importance of social work's role in rural health promotion, consider the following as examples of some possible roles:

- To increase awareness of opportunities to promote personal, family, and community health through health promotion strategies.
- To assist individuals and communities to identify and prioritize opportunities to develop and implement health promotion strategies, considering individual, family, and community/system levels of intervention tailored to the special needs and resources of small towns and rural areas.
- To educate and assist consumers, service providers, and the public to discard ageist myths that limit older adults' access to health pro-

motion opportunities, and to adopt attitudes that empower older adults to undertake health promoting changes in their lives.
- To promote consumer and community appreciation of the powerful roles that people play in promoting their own health and well-being.
- To educate and assist social workers, other allied health professionals, leaders in the community, and the public to acquire the personal and professional knowledge and skills that are required for health promotion with older adults.
- To promote understanding of the interwoven social, cultural, economic and political factors that facilitate or limit access to health promotion for a community or its diverse older adult members.
- To advocate for policy and regulatory changes that increase the opportunities for health promotion with rural older persons.
- To educate others to advocate for policy changes that increase the opportunities for health promotion with rural older persons.

Social workers have the knowledge and skills to help cultivate a "climate" of health promotion in rural communities and to influence the health care system to redirect some of its resources. This redirection should support individuals and communities to make healthier choices.

Effective health promotion methods with rural elders promote dignity and day-to-day autonomy while strengthening knowledge and skills used to make informed personal and community health choices, including those which recognize the importance of, and positive nature of, interdependence among and between people and systems. A life course perspective also suggests that while autonomy for most people is a desired state, interdependence is not a "dirty" word, but rather a description of the ever changing reality of both the usual individual human condition and the community and global environment and context within which aging occurs.

Particularly as individuals age in place, accompanied by almost inevitable impairments in one or more functional domains, striving to achieve a healthy interdependence among individuals, families, friends, neighbors, and the communities in which they live may be a highly desired outcome. Social workers–specialists in weaving the fabric of collaboration and cooperation across relationships, disciplines, and environments–can be the change agents who facilitate this outcome. Some international studies have found that women are particularly adept at modeling and maintaining collaborative efforts for community health promotion (Gillies, 1998). It is important to consider this and make best use of effective gender-based resources. Yet, at the same time, social workers must maintain and deploy a perspective that offers opportunity to, and equally holds accountable, men and women as equal partners.

Clearly, individual and community health is influenced by genetics–inherited from parents and the personal and environmental history of the community and its citizens. It also is substantially created and lived by people as they accomplish their chosen daily activities, to learn, work, play, love, and worship throughout the lifespan. Assisting others to develop or acquire the ability to control, or at least influence, personal and corporate choices that affect one's health and well-being, and that of one's neighbors locally and fellow citizens globally, can be a "best practice" example of empowerment and self-determination.

CONCLUSION

Although it is somewhat disappointing that there has not been more emphasis given to the opportunities for rural gerontological social work in health promotion–in the published literature, in our educational curricula, and in our practice–it is not surprising. At least three barriers are apparent: the scarcity of funding for health promotion/disease prevention in the general population, and older adult health promotion in particular; turf and boundary issues related to inter and multidisciplinary practice; and a shortage of trained social workers serving in rural settings. While we wait and work for public policy that better addresses these barriers, social workers nonetheless have diverse opportunities to have an impact in this area.

Given the natural "fit" between the values held by social workers, the skills in the "toolkit" of professional social workers, and the approaches to intervention needed for older adult health promotion in rural settings, we might ask ourselves, who better to lead our small towns and rural areas toward wellness and wisdom? Or at least, who better to extend the hand of collaboration and spirit of interdisciplinary teamwork to allied health practitioners and community leaders? As our population ages, and as increasing emphasis (and even, perhaps, funding!) is given to disease prevention and health promotion interventions (e.g., the Robert Wood Johnson initiative to increase physical activities among older persons [Robert Wood Johnson, 2003]; the Centers for Disease Control Public Health and Aging Initiatives [The National Center for Disease Prevention and Health Promotion, 2003]) gerontological social workers should prepare themselves to embrace this promising arena of practice.

REFERENCES

Armbruster, B., & Gladwin, L. (2001). More than fitness for older adults: A "whole-istic" approach to wellness. *Health and Fitness Journal, 5*, 6-12.

Atienza, A. (2001). Home-based physical activity programs for middle-aged and older adults: Summary of empirical research. *Journal of Aging and Physical Activity, 9* Suppl. 2001. S38-S58.

Badger, L.W., Ackerson, B., Buttell, F., & Rand, E.H. (1997). The case for integration of social work psychosocial services into rural primary care practice. *Health and Social Work, 22*(1), 20-29.

Bender, C., & Hart, J.P. (1986). Rural health promotion: Bailiwick for social work. *Health and Social Work, 11*(1), 52-58.

Bryant, T. (2002). Role of knowledge in public health and health promotion policy change. *Health Promotion International, 17*(1), 89-98.

Bull, C.N. (Ed.). (1993). *Aging in rural America*. Newbury Park: Sage Publications.

Cleveland Foundation. (2002). *Successful aging initiative*. [Electronic version]. Accessed December 27, 2002, from www.successfulaging.org.

Coleman, James (1988). Social Capital in the Creation of Human Capital. *American Journal of Sociology, 94*: S95-S120.

Council on Social Work Education. (2003). *National Aging Competencies Survey Report*. Accessed February 15, 2003 from www.cswe.org/sage-sw/resrep/competencies rep.htm.

Dezendorf, P.K., & Green, R.K. (1999). *The impact of electronic social work on rural practice*. Presented at the Third Annual Technology Conference for Social Work Education and Practice, Charleston, SC, September 1-5, 1999.

Dychtwald, K. (1986). *Wellness and health promotion for the elderly*. Maryland: Aspen.

FallCreek, S., & Franks, P. (1984). *Health promotion and aging: Strategies for action*. (DHHS Publication No. (OHDS) 84-20818, pp. XX). Washington, DC: Government Printing Office.

FallCreek, S., & Mettler, M. (1984). *A healthy old age: A sourcebook for health promotion with older persons (Rev. ed.)*. New York: The Haworth Press, Inc.

FallCreek, S. (1992). *Health promotion and aging: An opportunity for advocacy*. Washington, DC: AARP.

FallCreek, S., Muchow, J., & Mockenhaupt, R. (1994) Health promotion with rural elders. In R. T. Coward, C. N. Bull, G. Kulkulka, & J. Galliher (Eds.) *Health services for rural elders* (pp. 182-203). New York: Springer Publishing Company.

Gillies, P. (1998). Effectiveness of alliances and partnerships for health promotion. *Health Promotion International, 13*(2), 99-120.

Ginsburg, L.H. (1998). "Introduction: An Overview of Rural Social Work." In Ginsburg, L.H. (Ed.) *Social work in rural communities* (pp. 3-23). (3rd Edition). New York: Council on Social Work Education.

Green, L., & Anderson, J. (1982). *Community health*. St. Louis: C.V. Mosby.

Haber, D. (1999). *Health promotion and aging: Implications for the health professions*. New York, NY: Springer Publishing Company, Inc.

Kressig, Reto, & Echt, K. (2002). Exercise prescribing: Computer application in older adults. *The Gerontologist, 42*(2), 273-277.

Krout, J., & Coward, R. Aging in rural environments. In R.T. Coward, & J.A. Krout (Eds.). *Aging in rural settings: Life circumstances and distinctive features.* New York: Springer Publishing Co.

Lan, J. (1999). Volunteer in health promotion for the elderly: An experimental project in fostering a healthy living to needy elderly by volunteer health promoters. *Journal of Gerontological Social Work, 32*(3), 81-107.

Lubben, J.P., Welier, I., Chi, I., & De Jong, F. (1988). Health promotion for the rural elderly. *The Journal of Rural Health, 4*(3), 85-96.

Luchetti, M., & Cerasa, F. (2002). Performance evaluation of health promotion in aging. *Educational Gerontology, 28*(1), 1-13.

Mandel School of Applied Social Sciences. (Rev. 2001). *Field Education Manual.* Cleveland: Case Western Reserve University, pp. 5-12.

Mettler, M., & Kemper, D. (2000). *Healthwise for life.* Boise, ID: Healthwise.

National Association of Social Workers. (2000). *Code of ethics.* Washington, DC: National Association of Social Workers.

National Center for Chronic Disease Prevention and Health Promotion. (2003). *Healthy Aging.* Accessed March 1, 2003 from http://www.cdc.gov/aging.

National Rural Health Association. (1992). *Health and aging in rural America.* Kansas City: National Rural Health Association.

Putnam, R. (1993). *Making democracy work: Civic traditions in modern Italy.* Princeton: Princeton University Press.

Robert Wood Johnson Foundation. (2003). *Active for Life Program.* Retrieved on February 28, 2003 from http://www.activeforlife.info/.

University of Omaha. (1998). *Practicum Agency Profile: Lifetime health at the Lincoln Area Agency on Aging.* Retrieved on December 14, 2002, from http://ww.unomaha.edu/~bhagen/Lifetimehealth/Lifetimehealth.html.

U. S. Department of Labor, Bureau of Labor Statistics. (2002). *Social Worker. Occupational Outlook Handbook 2002-2003.* Washington, DC: U.S. Government Printing Office.

Vest, G.W., Ronneau, J., Lopez, B., & Gonzalez, G. (1997). Alternative health practices in ethnically diverse rural areas: A collaborative research project. *Health and Social Work, 22*(2), 95-100.

Wallace, R.E., & Wallace, R.B. (1998) Rural-Urban contrasts in elder health status: Methodological issues and findings. In Coward, R.T., & J.A. Krout (Eds.) *Aging in rural settings: Life circumstances and distinctive features.* (pp. 67-83). New York: Springer Publishing Company.

Western Maryland Area Health Education Center. (2003). Retrieved on January 16, 2003, from http://www.allconet.org/ahec/rihp/ridcteam/stoc.html.

World Health Organization. (2002). *Active ageing: A policy framework.* A contribution of the World Health Organization to the Second United Nations World Assembly on Ageing. April 2002. Madrid, Spain: World Health Organization.

World Health Organization. (1997). *The Jakarta Declaration on leading health promotion into the 21st century.* Geneva: World Health Organization.

World Health Organization. (1986). *Ottawa charter: Health for all.* The First International Conference on Health Promotion. Geneva: World Health Organization.

World Health Organization. (1948). *Constitution.* Retrieved February 15, 2003 from http://poolicy.who.int/cgi-in/om_isapi.dll?hitsperheading+on&infobase=basicdoc&record={9D5}&softpage=Document42.

Chapter 12

Older Rural Workers and Retirement Preparation

Lorraine T. Dorfman, PhD

SUMMARY. This chapter first examines the impact of the rural environment on work and retirement by reviewing current socioeconomic conditions in rural areas, rural community infrastructure, and rural community change. It goes on to discuss the employment status and income of older rural workers, giving particular attention to gender and racial/ethnic differences in employment. Job training and job creation are also discussed. Next, the chapter turns to the retirement needs and retirement preparation of rural elders. It concludes with suggestions for gerontological social work practice in developing employment and retirement services and improving existing services and service delivery. *[Article copies available for a fee from The Haworth Document Delivery Service: 1-800-HAWORTH. E-mail address: <docdelivery@haworthpress.com> Website: <http://www.HaworthPress.com> © 2003 by The Haworth Press, Inc. All rights reserved.]*

KEYWORDS. Older workers, retirement, rural practice

[Haworth co-indexing entry note]: "Older Rural Workers and Retirement Preparation." Dorfman, Lorraine T. Co-published simultaneously in *Journal of Gerontological Social Work* (The Haworth Social Work Practice Press, an imprint of The Haworth Press, Inc.) Vol. 41, No. 3/4, 2003, pp. 213-228; and: *Gerontological Social Work in Small Towns and Rural Communities* (ed: Sandra S. Butler, and Lenard W. Kaye) The Haworth Social Work Practice Press, an imprint of The Haworth Press, Inc., 2003, pp. 213-228. Single or multiple copies of this article are available for a fee from The Haworth Document Delivery Service [1-800-HAWORTH, 9:00 a.m. - 5:00 p.m. (EST). E-mail address: docdelivery@haworthpress.com].

http://www.haworthpress.com/web/JGSW
© 2003 by The Haworth Press, Inc. All rights reserved.
Digital Object Identifier: 10.1300/J083v41n03_02

INTRODUCTION

Work and retirement among rural older persons take on particular significance for gerontological social workers because of labor market problems encountered by some older workers and the relative paucity of employment and retirement services in rural areas. Both work and retirement contribute importantly to the well-being and quality of life of older persons, not only in terms of their financial well-being, but also in terms of impacts on health, social participation, choice of housing environment, and sense of purpose in life (Bossé, Aldwin, Levenson, & Workman-Daniels, 1991; Dorfman, 1998). From a role theory/interactionist perspective, an individual's sense of self and identity are linked to the major roles that he or she plays, such as the occupational role (Burr, 1972; Cottrell, 1942; Kosloski, Ginsburg, & Backman, 1984). Therefore, knowledge about an individual's work life and preparation for leaving that work can provide valuable information in assessing the life situation of older persons and can serve as a useful guide for practice.

This chapter begins by examining the impact of rural environments on work and retirement and then reviews the current employment status of older rural persons. The chapter goes on to describe job training and employment opportunities that are being developed in rural settings. Next, retirement needs and retirement preparation of rural-dwelling elders are discussed. The chapter concludes with suggestions for gerontological social work practice in the areas of work and retirement.

THE IMPACT OF THE RURAL ENVIRONMENT ON WORK AND RETIREMENT

Socioeconomic Conditions and Infrastructure

Although there is considerable diversity in rural areas as to region, population density, farm or non-farm residence, ethnicity, and race, on average rural elders have lower incomes and less formal education, worse health, poorer housing, and less availability and access to services, including transportation, than do their urban counterparts (Bull, 1998; Dorfman, 1998; Krout & Coward, 1998). Several subpopulations of rural elders are at particular risk: racial and ethnic minorities, women, especially widows, and the very old (Bull, 1998). In a study conducted in Canada, Joseph and Martin-Matthews (1993) concluded that living conditions there are also worse in rural than in urban areas, so it appears that the situation of rural Canadian elders is similar to those in the United States.

One commonality of rural areas is that opportunities for earning income are often scarce, and sometimes non-existent, when compared to urban communities, particularly for older workers (Dorfman & Ballantyne, 1994; Joseph & Martin-Matthews, 1993; National Coalition on Rural Aging, 2001). There is some job loss in rural areas due to "depopulation" as the young migrate to metropolitan areas in search of higher-paying jobs, more educational opportunities, and a greater variety of cultural experiences. Other factors impacting rural economies and rural jobs include resource depletion, such as in the mining, forestry, and fishing industries; shifting markets and the competition of a global economy; a declining agricultural economy; new technology that is changing the face of agriculture; the appearance of large retailers that can force businesses in small towns to close; and the trend toward large-scale service industries, which do not usually locate in rural areas (Freshwater, 2000; Krout & Coward, 1998; National Coalition on Rural Aging, 2001). In such an economic environment, older workers may lack requisite job skills and have a difficult time finding and keeping employment.

Rural Community Change

Speaking to the need for rural economic development, David Freshwater, Professor in the Department of Agricultural Economics and the Martin School of Public Administration and Public Policy at the University of Kentucky, recently had this to say: "The future of rural America rests upon its ability–with governmental assistance–to define and develop competitive industries to replace the resource extraction and low-skill manufacturing industries upon which it has depended" (Freshwater, 2000, p. 6). There is some evidence that rural economies are showing resilience in nonfarm economic growth (Economic Research Service, 2000b). It is important to keep in mind, however, that some strategies for revitalizing the economic infrastructure of rural communities, including entrepreneurship and increasing tourism and recreational facilities, cannot be applied across all rural settings. For instance, rural communities located in areas that are not blessed with natural attractions like lakes, mountains or seashore may not be conducive to the development of tourism or recreational facilities and must therefore concentrate on developing other industries.

One of the positive developments contributing to rural community change is retirement migration. In-migrants to many rural areas, in search of a more relaxed life-style, lower cost of living, and respite from the pressures of urban life, are creating "mailbox economies" and demand for new services. Although such economic development can occur only with substantial in-migration to rural counties (Malroutu & Brandt, 1992), the in-migration of retirees can raise the tax base and create jobs in rural communities (Bennett, 1996; Stallman, Deller, & Shields, 1999). Using an econometric model, Stallman et al. estimated that five hundred new "young-old" (age 65-75) in-migrant households to rural areas would create 300 initial jobs, and that the same number of "old-old" (age 75+) in-migrant households would create one hundred initial jobs. However, population growth in rural areas has slowed in recent years, so that by 1999 it was only one-half that of the metropolitan growth rate (Economic Research Service, 2000a). This population slowing included a drop in in-migration to nonmetropolitan areas, and was particularly evident in the Western part of the United States and among college graduates.

RURAL EMPLOYMENT AND THE OLDER WORKER

Current Employment Status

In the late 1990s, unemployment continued to fall in nonmetropolitan areas, but more slowly than it had earlier in the decade (Economic Research Service, 2000a). Job growth slowed in the late 1990s; between 1995 and 1998, it slowed from 3.5% to 2% annually (Gale & McGranahan, 2001). Table 1 displays the employment status of the civilian noninstitutionalized population 45 years and older in both metropolitan and nonmetropolitan areas based on the 2000 Census. The table reveals that both the unemployment rate and the adjusted unemployment rate were higher in nonmetropolitan than in metropolitan areas for persons aged 45-54 and 55-64. However, this was not the case for persons 65 and older, where there was a higher rate of unemployment in metro than in nonmetro areas (3.2% vs. 2.7%, respectively, for unemployment; 6.2% vs. 5.8%, respectively, for adjusted unemployment) (Economic Research Service, 2000c). These figures indicate an interesting residential reversal in unemployment for people who are beyond the traditional retirement age. One possible factor contributing to this finding is that older rural men have historically tended to participate in

TABLE 1. Employment Status of the Civilian Noninstitutionalized Population 45 Years and Over in Metropolitan and Nonmetropolitan Areas by Age, 2000 Annual Averages (Numbers in Thousands)[a]

Age	Labor Force	Employed	Unemployed	Unemployment Rate	Adjusted Unemployment Rate[b]
Metro					
45-54	24,270	24,137	583	2.4	4.5
55-64	11,046	10,774	272	2.5	4.8
65+	3,328	3,134	104	3.2	6.2
Non-Metro					
45-54	5,747	5,580	166	2.9	5.5
55-64	2,928	2,853	75	2.6	5.6
65+	962	936	26	2.7	5.8

[a]Source: Economic Research Service, U.S. Department of Agriculture Briefing Room (2000c). *Rural labor and education: Employment and unemployment.* Adapted from Employment status of the civilian noninstitutionalized population 16 years and over in metropolitan and nonmetropolitan areas by age, sex, race, and Hispanic origin. *http://www.ers.usda.gov./Briefing/LaborandEducation/data/demographics00*

[b]The adjusted unemployment rate is defined as the total unemployed plus all marginally attached workers, plus total employed part-time for economic reasons, as a percent of the civilian labor force plus all marginally attached workers. Marginally attached workers are persons who currently are neither working nor looking for work but indicate they want or are available for work and have looked for work sometime in the recent past.

the labor force more than their urban counterparts. This may have been linked to the prevalence of farming, which allows one to work at one's own pace, and to higher rates of self-employment in rural areas (Moen, 1994).

Gender and Racial/Ethnic Differences in Employment

The 2000 Census also reveals gender differences in the unemployment rate among both metropolitan and nonmetropolitan dwellers: female unemployment across age was slightly higher than it was for males (4.0% vs. 3.8%, respectively, in metro areas and 4.4% vs. 4.3%, respectively, in nonmetro areas) (Economic Research Service, 2000c). Importantly, overall female unemployment in nonmetro areas exceeded that in metro areas (4.4% vs. 4.0%, respectively). Figures by age, gender, and metro/nonmetro residence were not yet available at the time of this writing.

With regard to minorities, Table 2 shows the overall unemployment figures for Whites, Blacks, and Hispanics by residential status from the 2000 Census (Economic Research Service, 2000c). Again, age break-

TABLE 2. Percent Unemployed of the Civilian Noninstitutionalized Population 16 Years and Over in Metropolitan Areas by Race and Hispanic Origin, 2000 Annual Averages (Numbers in Thousands)[a]

	Metro	Non-Metro
White	3.4	3.9
Black	7.4	9.4
Hispanic	5.6	6.3

[a]Source: Economic Research Service, U.S. Department of Agriculture Briefing Room (2000c). *Rural labor and education: Employment and unemployment.* Adapted from Employment status of the civilian noninstitutionalized population 16 years and over in metropolitan and nonmetropolitan areas by age, sex, race, and Hispanic origin. *http://www.ers.usda.gov/Briefing/LaborandEducation/data/demographics00*

downs are not yet available for these categories. The table reveals that there was a substantial difference among the three groups in both metropolitan and nonmetropolitan areas, with Blacks having the highest unemployment rate, followed by Hispanics. The highest unemployment rate (9.4%) was found among nonmetro Blacks, indicating double jeopardy when race and rural residence are considered. It is reasonable to expect that older minorities suffer "triple jeopardy" in employment when the effects of race, rural residence, and age are all considered.

Types of Employment

Recent data show that the greatest growth in employment in nonmetropolitan areas was in the services industries, followed by retail trade (Gale & McGranahan, 2001). Service industries employ over one-half of rural workers, with many of those industries related to recreation, retirement, and the natural environment, and also restaurants and retail shops (Economic Research Service, 1997). Telecommunications are also producing jobs in rural areas. Manufacturing is still relatively important in some nonmetropolitan areas, contributing 22.3% of earnings compared to 16% for metropolitan workers, but many of those jobs remain "old economy" low or medium skilled jobs (Gale & McGranahan, 2001). Although manufacturing industries had declined by the mid-1990s, they still employed nearly one-fifth of the rural workforce (Economic Research Service, 1997). Agricultural services related to forestry and fishing had substantial growth rates during the late 1990s, followed by finance, insurance, real estate, transportation, and public utilities (Economic Research Service, 2000b). There were regional differences in growth of employment, with gains particularly in the Rocky Mountain, South West, and Far West states.

It has been clear for some time that farming is no longer the main source of employment in rural areas. It remains the main source of jobs and income in relatively few areas, notably the sparsely populated areas of the heartland (Economic Research Service, 2000b). Farming employment dropped dramatically from about eight million to three million in the past forty years, with the number of farms dropping from nearly six million to a little more than two million (Economic Research Service, 1997). Only about five million people, comprising less than 10% of the rural population, live on farms, and most of those farms are classified as "small," with half having annual sales of less than $10,000 (Newton & Hoppe, 2001). Non-farm employment is very high among farm families and involves both farmers and their spouses. Even among persons living on large family farms, nearly two-fifths of farm spouses are employed off the farm (Newton & Hoppe, 2001).

Rural Employment and Income

Despite economic gains in rural areas during the 1990s, rural workers still earn only about four-fifths of what urban workers do (Huang, 1999). Employed women, Hispanics, and Blacks averaged real income gains in the 1990s, with income gains for both Hispanics and Blacks exceeding those of rural Whites (Huang, 1999). Although low wage jobs are still held disproportionately by women and minorities, the share of White men in low wage jobs has been growing in rural areas. An interesting shift also is that there is a smaller percentage of African-Americans in the low wage work force than previously; in contrast, the percentage of Hispanics in those low-wage jobs is increasing (Economic Research Service, 2000a).

Although poverty rates continued to drop during the late 1990s because of the then booming economy, poverty rates remained higher in rural than in urban areas, with a higher proportion of rural dwellers living just above the poverty line (Huang, 1999; Economic Research Service, 2000a). In 1999, over one-fourth of rural workers earned wages below the poverty threshold ($17,028 for a family of four) and Blacks and Hispanics remained disproportionately represented (Economic Research Service, 2000a).

Another disadvantaged group with regard to employment and income is older rural caregivers, who spend more time providing care than do urban caregivers (Dorfman, 2002; Horwitz & Rosenthal, 1994).

This burden falls particularly on rural women as they grow older because of the relative lack of health and human services in rural areas. Farm women experience the most demands and spend most time in caregiving activities, possibly because of the isolation of many farms and the inability of surrounding communities to provide needed services, but also possibly because of rural values of independence and self-reliance (Dorfman, 2002). This in turn affects women's ability to work and earn income.

JOB TRAINING AND EMPLOYMENT OPPORTUNITIES FOR OLDER WORKERS

Need for Older Workers in Rural Areas

As many rural areas depopulate because of the loss of jobs and migration of young people to metropolitan areas in search of better economic opportunities, older workers become an increasingly valuable source of human capital for many rural communities (Dorfman & Ballantyne, 1994). Older workers are more likely than younger workers to remain in their communities and can help build the rural community infrastructure (National Coalition on Rural Aging, 2001). It makes sense therefore to invest substantial resources in job training and retraining for middle-aged and older adults in order to fill existing jobs and jobs that may arise from rural community development efforts. Currently, however, few job skills training programs are available for older adults in rural communities. In 2000, in amendments to the Older Americans Act, Congress recognized that rural individuals face special challenges (National Coalition on Rural Aging, 2001). Among the policy recommendations of the National Coalition on Rural Aging was the importance of strengthening the economic infrastructure in rural areas by retraining older workers in job skills that are matched to community needs.

Job Training and Job Creation Programs

Private sector employment and training programs exist; however, government programs provide the bulk of training and employment programs, mainly for economically disadvantaged older persons. These programs are particularly important for rural-dwelling older workers because they generally have lower incomes than do their urban counterparts. Major government programs that provide job training, loans, and technical assistance include the following.

Title V of the Older Americans Act. A 1973 amendment to the Older Americans Act of 1965 funded the Senior Community Service Employment Program (SCSEP) which provides publicly subsidized minimum wage jobs in community service organizations for older persons aged 55 and older who have incomes no higher than 125% of the poverty level (Hale, 1990). The goal is to ultimately place those individuals in unsubsidized employment.

Job Training Partnership Act (JTPA). This act, passed by Congress in 1982, is a federal workforce development program. It provides educational and occupational skills training to economically disadvantaged older persons who have multiple employment barriers so as to prepare them for employment and self-sufficiency. Title IIA-3% is a special set-aside for persons aged 55 and older. Title IIA provides for assessment and testing, counseling, academic and occupational skills training, and job search training and placement assistance (Hale, 1990).

Department of Labor, Employment and Training Office–Job Training Partnership Act Microenterprise Grant Program. This program provides funding for community-based enterprise activities, with special emphasis on long-term unemployed and dislocated workers (Wallace, 2000). This technical assistance program may be particularly relevant for older rural workers who are negatively affected by the process of rural community change.

Green Thumb. A particularly useful source of employment for older persons in rural areas, Green Thumb is sponsored by the National Farmers Union with funds from the Department of Labor. It provides part-time employment for older persons in conservation, beautification, and community improvement projects (Dorfman & Ballantyne, 1994).

Department of Agriculture, Rural Business Service–Intermediary Relending Program (IRP). This program provides loans through an intermediary organization for businesses in rural areas with populations under 25,000. Funds, however, are not available for businesses involving tourism, recreation, or agricultural production (Wallace, 2000), which does restrict their applicability.

The Small Business Administration–Microloan Program. Loans are also provided through intermediary organizations in this program to fund local microenterprises. Some of the money can be used for technical assistance, such as marketing or management. A notable provision of the Microloan Program is that assistance is targeted to a number of at-risk groups including women, minorities, low-income people, and persons who have difficulty getting credit (Wallace, 2000).

One job creation strategy that seems to be taking hold in some rural communities is development of home-based businesses. The tradition of self-employment in rural areas may make "work at home" appealing, and modern technology and telecommunications may facilitate home-based businesses. Such business ventures eliminate the need to commute to often far-off metropolitan areas and can be a workable solution for older rural workers. Self-employment can also foster feelings of autonomy, control, and provide opportunities for social interaction (Kean, Van Zandt, & Miller, 1996).

RETIREMENT NEEDS AND RETIREMENT PREPARATION

The Context of Rural Retirement

There are many positive aspects of retiring in, or to, rural communities. These include a more leisurely life-style and less crowding than in urban areas, the reputed friendliness of rural people, open spaces, and clean air. On the other hand, negative aspects of retirement in rural communities may include lack of services, poor transportation, relatively few opportunities for part-time work in retirement, and the relative isolation of many rural communities.

There may be more flexibility in the retirement decision for some rural dwellers than for their nonrural counterparts because of the higher incidence of self-employment in rural areas. Rural workers may be able to choose when they retire and the rate at which they retire (Dorfman, 1989). The downside of self-employment, though, is that those workers are less likely to receive information about retirement and social security, or to be covered by company pension plans, than are nonrural workers. Consequently, rural workers may need to do more individual planning for retirement than do their nonrural counterparts, and rely more on informal sources of information about retirement and written or media information.

The Meaning of Retirement

Abrupt retirement from the labor force is far less common today than it was even a decade or two ago. Many older workers reduce their work to part-time or phase out their work lives, while others reenter the workforce after retiring (Knapp & Muller, 2000). Retirement, therefore, is no longer clear-cut or "crisp" for many older workers, but instead becomes more of a "blurred" and complex phenomenon (Henretta, 1997). Dorfman (1989) found that among Iowa retirees, almost one-half (48%) of rural men and nearly a third (29%) of rural women said they retired gradually, indicating a preference for phasing retirement. Similarly, Keating and Munro (1989) reported that 63% of farmers aged 60 and older had reduced their amount of work in the past five years.

Retirement Preparation of Rural Elders

Role theory suggests that adjustment to new social roles is associated with anticipatory socialization, or preparation, for those roles (Burr, 1972; Cottrell, 1942). It is therefore a useful theoretical perspective for examining the way individuals prepare for, and ultimately adapt to, loss of the work role. Among mechanisms that help individuals prepare for retirement are informal mechanisms, such as talking to people about retirement, reading books and articles about retirement, and listening to radio or watching television programs about retirement. More formal mechanisms include preretirement education or counseling, making specific plans for retirement, and retiring gradually. We know, however, that many people do little planning for retirement (Kosloski, Ekerdt, & DeViney, 2001). Ekerdt, DeViney, and Kosloski (1996), for example, report that about two-fifths of workers in their 50s have either made no plans whatsoever for retirement or have not given much thought to retirement.

Only a few studies have focused specifically on retirement preparation of rural-dwelling workers; those studies likewise suggest that there is relatively little planning for retirement. A prospective study of middle-aged (45-54) female members of the North Carolina Extension Homemakers Association and males of the same age revealed that 50% or more of respondents had made definite plans for retirement in only five of fifty-nine kinds of retirement planning behaviors investigated (Glass & Flynn, 2000). Three of those five types of planning involved financial planning, whereas other important aspects of retirement planning, such as how time would be spent in retirement or obtaining information about housing choices and where to live, were engaged in by only a minority of respondents.

The Iowa study of rural retirees (Dorfman, 1989) likewise revealed low rates of retirement planning. Only 13% of men and 15% of women in that sample said they had done either a "moderate" or "a great deal" of planning for retirement, and a majority said they had done no planning whatsoever before they retired. The most common type of preretirement planning was financial, but even in this area only about one-third of retirees had done any planning. A tiny percentage of retirees (3%) had attended preretirement classes, seminars, or counseling sessions, but this could have reflected lack of availability as much as lack of interest. More rural retirees, in contrast, had been involved in informal preparation for retirement, with 45% saying they had discussed retirement with other people before retiring and about one-third saying they had read articles or books about retirement. Additionally, more than one-fourth said they had listened to radio or watched television programs about retirement (Dorfman, 1989).

IMPLICATIONS FOR GERONTOLOGICAL SOCIAL WORK PRACTICE

This chapter has reviewed recent trends in employment, job training and job creation, and retirement preparation of older rural workers. The data suggest a number of implications for gerontological social work intervention in rural communities.

Develop and deliver services based on the needs and conditions of rural-dwelling elders. Employment and retirement services cannot rely on the dominant urban model, which is often inappropriate for rural populations (Dorfman & Ballantyne, 1994; Krout, 1998). The provision of services must be tailored to the cultural and demographic realities of rural life and to rural values of independence and self-reliance, and also recognize the diversity of rural communities with respect to region, gender, race, and ethnicity.

Inform older workers about their individual civil rights and the law. Age discrimination in employment remains a real issue, despite the Age Discrimination in Employment Act. Social workers can inform workers about their rights and also about unemployment benefits to which they are entitled. Likewise, social workers can help rural workers access those benefits by linking them with relevant services and programs.

Provide employment counseling services. Counseling can help older workers understand what skills they already have and might need to develop. Voluntary agencies around the country have done this kind of counseling for several decades and also offer help in developing self-assurance and occupational adjustment. One example is Senior

Action Services in Evanston, Illinois, which is locally funded and has placed workers in a variety of jobs (Gelfand, 1999).

Advocate for more job training and retraining for older workers. Practitioners can play an important "advocate" role (Compton & Galway, 1994) in helping to foster new employment opportunities for older workers. Likewise, they can strive to increase federal, state, and local funding for new and existing employment programs.

Increase access to employment and retirement services. Since access to these services is often a problem in rural areas, particularly in more isolated rural communities, social workers can help organize volunteer transportation to those services, which are sometimes located in regional centers. Local volunteers can be utilized, especially in off-peak hours. Practitioners can also play the "broker" role by coordinating job counseling and retirement services that may be available to far-flung communities, perhaps on an itinerant basis.

Encourage entrepreneurial activities. Social workers can assist older rural workers in accessing small business incubators and development centers, which are often associated with institutions of higher education (Dorfman & Ballantyne, 1994). Rural Initiatives at Cornell University, for example, has provided training and consultation for people who want to start entrepreneurial activities (Erikson, 1991). Such centers have been developed in other rural states such as Iowa.

Develop and deliver preretirement education and planning programs. Rural service providers may be able to develop these programs in conjunction with senior centers, churches, community colleges, and the Cooperative Extension Service. The Cooperative Extension Service has historically provided a great deal of education and outreach to rural elders. Retirement planning services should provide information that is particularly salient for rural-dwelling elders, such as the move from farm to town, and where to find health and human services. Several groups may be in particular need of such services: rural women, who may not have had much experience in handling money; older minorities, because of their relatively low incomes; and farmers, who may have wanted to continue working, but could not due to health or other reasons. One successful program that can be modeled by rural social workers is the AARP Women's Financial Counseling Program (AARP, 1991), a series of weekly classes to help empower midlife and older women to make financial decisions.

Train peer educators to inform rural adults about retirement. Here the "teacher" role is very important for social workers (Compton & Galway, 1994). Practitioners can help train peer educators to inform prospective retirees about retirement. Such peer educators, who are usually retired themselves, can help prepare preretirees for the coming transition and help them understand what to expect once they retire.

Assist in identifying and accessing volunteer, education, and recreational activities that can provide meaningful substitutes for the lost work role. This is a special challenge for rural social workers because there may be fewer organizational resources to offer such activities in rural than in urban settings. However, careful assessment of community resources and needs can identify meaningful and useful roles in retirement and can help maintain the social integration and productivity of retired rural elders.

Connect rural older workers to financial counselors and planners. As a help in planning for retirement, social workers can serve as a broker in connecting rural adults to financial advisors, who might visit rural areas on a rotating basis. This is important both before retirement and on a regular basis after retirement in order to help safeguard the financial status of rural elders.

Engage in thorough and rigorous program evaluation. Krout (1998) points out that there is a paucity of good program and evaluation data in rural areas. Employment and retirement services need to be carefully evaluated in cooperation with the agencies and programs that provide those services for older rural persons. It is very important, moreover, that such evaluation be conducted on an ongoing basis in order to assess how well programs and services are continuing to achieve their purpose.

CONCLUSION

Employment and retirement have often been seen as individual matters and not in need of practice intervention. The reality is that older workers, particularly in rural areas where incomes tend to be relatively low and services scattered or unavailable, are often in need of assistance when there is job loss or skill obsolescence and when opportunities to learn about and prepare for retirement are relatively few. Gerontological social workers can play a vital role in contributing to the well-being of rural elders by developing needed employment and retirement services and by improving existing services and service delivery to persons who live on farms, in open country, in small towns, and in other rural settings.

REFERENCES

American Association of Retired Persons. (1991). *Women's financial information program*. Washington, DC: Author.

Bennett, D. G. (1996). Implications of retirement development in high-amenity nonmetropolitan coastal areas. *Journal of Applied Gerontology*, *15*, 345-360.

Bossé, R., Aldwin, C., Levenson, M. R., & Workman-Daniels, K. (1991). How stressful is retirement? Findings from the normative aging study. *Journal of Gerontology: Psychological Sciences, 46*, P9-P14.

Bull, C. N. (1998). Aging in rural communities. *National Forum, 78*, 38-41.

Burr, W. (1972). Role transitions: A reformulation of theory. *Journal of Marriage and the Family, 34*, 407-416.

Compton, B. R., & Galway, B. (1994). *Social work processes* (5th ed.). Homewood, IL: Dorsey Press.

Cottrell, L. S. (1942). The adjustment of the individual to his age and sex roles. *American Sociological Review, 7*, 617-620.

Dorfman, L. T. (1989). Retirement preparation and retirement satisfaction in the rural elderly. *Journal of Applied Gerontology, 8*, 432-450.

Dorfman, L. T. (1998). Economic status, work, and retirement among the rural elderly. In R. T. Coward, & J. A. Krout (Eds.), *Aging in rural settings: Life circumstances and distinctive features* (pp. 47-66). New York: Springer.

Dorfman, L. T. (2002). Family networks and relationships among rural elders. *Geriatric Care Management Journal, 12*, 16-21.

Dorfman, L. T., & Ballantyne, R. L. (1994). Employment and retirement services for the rural elderly. In J. A. Krout (Ed.), *Providing community-based services to the rural elderly* (pp. 115-132). Thousand Oaks, CA: Sage.

Economic Research Service, U. S. Department of Agriculture. (1997). *Understanding rural America*. Retrieved November 29, 2001 from *http://www.ers.usda.gov/publications/aib710/aib710.C.*

Economic Research Service, U. S. Department of Agriculture. (2000a). Overview: Favorable rural socioeconomic conditions persist, but not in all areas. *Rural Conditions and Trends, 11*(2), pp. 4-7. Retrieved December 4, 2001 from *http://purl.access.gpo.gov/GPO/LPS1396.*

Economic Research Service, U. S. Department of Agriculture. (2000b). Overview: Nonfarm growth and structural change alter farming's role in the rural economy. *Rural Conditions and Trends, 10*(2), pp. 2-6. Retrieved December 4, 2001 from *http://purl.access.gpo.gov/GPO/LPS1396.*

Economic Research Service, U. S. Department of Agriculture Briefing Room. (2000c). *Rural labor and education: Employment and unemployment.* Retrieved February 22, 2002 from *http://www.ers.usda.gov/Briefing/LaborandEducation/data/demographics00.*

Ekerdt, D., DeViney, S., & Kosloski, K. (1996). Profiling plans for retirement. *Journal of Gerontology: Social Sciences, 51B*, S140-S149.

Erikson, L. (1991). Trends: Cultivating homegrown resources offers hope for rural America. *Inside Business, 9*, 51-53.

Freshwater, D. (2000). Rural America at the turn of the century: One analyst's perspective. *Rural America, 15*(3), 2-7.

Gale, F., & McGranahan, D. (2001). Nonmetro areas fall behind in the "new economy." *Rural America, 16*, pp. 44-52. Retrieved December 10, 2001 from *http://purl.access.gpo.gov/GPO/LP1396.*

Gelfand, D. E. (1999). *The aging network: Programs and services* (5th ed.). New York: Springer.

Glass, J. C., & Flynn, D. K. (2000). Retirement needs and preparation of rural middle-aged persons. *Educational Gerontology, 26*, 109-134.

Hale, N. (1990). *The older worker.* San Francisco: Jossey-Bass.

Henretta, J. (1997). Changing perspectives on retirement. *Journal of Gerontology: Social Sciences, 52B*, S1-S3.

Horwitz, M. E., & Rosenthal, T. C. (1994). The impact of informal caregiving on labor force participation by rural farming and nonfarming families. *The Journal of Rural Health, 10*, 266-272.

Huang, G. G. (January, 1999). *Sociodemographic Changes: Promises and problems for rural education.* Eric Clearinghouse on Rural Education and Small Schools, EDO-RC-98-7. Retrieved November 29, 2001 from *http://www.ael.org/eric/digests/edorc987.*

Joseph, E. J., & Martin-Matthews, A. (1993). Growing old in aging communities. *Journal of Canadian Studies, 28*, 15-29.

Kean, R. C., Van Zandt, S., & Miller, N. J. (1996). Exploring factors of perceived social performance, health and personal control among retired seniors and seniors owning home-based businesses in non-metropolitan counties. *International Journal of Aging and Human Development, 43*, 297-313.

Keating, N. C., & Munro, B. (1989). Transferring the family farm: Process and implications. *Family Relations, 38*, 215-218.

Knapp, K., & Muller, C. (2000). *Productive lives: Paid and unpaid activities of older Americans.* NY: International Longevity Center-USA, Ltd.

Kosloski, K., Ekerdt, D., & DeViney, S. (2001). The role of job-related rewards in retirement planning. *Journal of Gerontology: Psychological Sciences, 56B*, P160-P169.

Kosloski, K., Ginsburg, G., & Backman, C. W. (1984). Retirement as a process of active role transition: In V. L. Allen, & E. vande Vliert (Eds.), *Role Transitions* (pp. 331-341). New York: Plenum Press.

Krout, J. A. (1998). Services and service delivery in rural environments. In R. T. Coward, & J. A. Krout (Eds.), *Aging in rural settings: Life circumstances and distinctive features* (pp. 247-266). New York: Springer.

Krout, J. A., & Coward, R. T. (1998). Aging in rural environments. In R. T. Coward, & J. A. Krout (Eds.), *Aging in rural settings: Life circumstances and distinctive features* (pp. 3-14). New York: Springer.

Malroutu, Y. L., & Brandt, J. A. (1992). Nonmetropolitan retirement location: Preferred community characteristics. *Housing and Society, 19*, 31-41.

Moen, J. R. (1994). Rural nonfarm households: Leaving the farm and the retirement of rural men, 1860-1980. *Social Science History, 18*, 56-75.

National Coalition on Rural Aging. (2001). *Discussion of significant rural issues.* Retrieved November 29, 2001 from *http://www.ncoa.org/advocacy/issuebs/ ncra092701.*

Newton, D. J., & Hoppe, R. A. (2001). Financial well-being of small farm households depends on the health of rural economies. *Rural America, 16*(1), 2-11.

Stallman, J. I., Deller, S. C., & Shields, M. (1999). The economic and fiscal impact of aging retirees on a small rural region. *The Gerontologist, 39*, 599-610.

Wallace, G. (2000). Using microenterprise programs in the rural United States. *Rural America, 15*(1), 38-44.

Chapter 13

Rural Older Adults at Home

Whitney Cassity-Caywood, MSSW
Ruth Huber, PhD

SUMMARY. In this chapter, we discuss circumstances that affect rural seniors living in their own homes. The strengths perspective informs this discussion, allowing the reader to consider several alternatives to the deficit-focused mentality that often pervades those who work with elders who are, sometimes, and perhaps stereotypically, regarded as frail. Issues unique to rural areas are addressed, programs that serve rural seniors are reviewed, and suggestions are made for the service provider working with this population. *[Article copies available for a fee from The Haworth Document Delivery Service: 1-800-HAWORTH. E-mail address: <docdelivery@haworthpress.com> Website: <http://www.HaworthPress.com> © 2003 by The Haworth Press, Inc. All rights reserved.]*

KEYWORDS. Strengths perspective, rural elders, community servics

INTRODUCTION

This chapter is organized in four parts. First, the strengths perspective as a theoretical base is described and explained. Second is a discus-

[Haworth co-indexing entry note]: "Rural Older Adults at Home." Cassity-Caywood, Whitney, and Ruth Huber. Co-published simultaneously in *Journal of Gerontological Social Work* (The Haworth Social Work Practice Press, an imprint of The Haworth Press, Inc.) Vol. 41, No. 3/4, 2003, pp. 229-245; and: *Gerontological Social Work in Small Towns and Rural Communities* (ed: Sandra S. Butler, and Lenard W. Kaye) The Haworth Social Work Practice Press, an imprint of The Haworth Press, Inc., 2003, pp. 229-245. Single or multiple copies of this article are available for a fee from The Haworth Document Delivery Service [1-800-HAWORTH, 9:00 a.m. - 5:00 p.m. (EST). E-mail address: docdelivery@haworthpress.com].

http://www.haworthpress.com/web/JGSW
© 2003 by The Haworth Press, Inc. All rights reserved.
Digital Object Identifier: 10.1300/J083v41n03_03

sion of several factors that affect the ability of rural seniors to live independently, including home and dwelling needs, and the basic human needs of dignity and self-worth. The third section focuses on innovative programs or projects that were either developed for, or may be adapted to, the needs of rural elders in their own homes. The fourth and final section draws key concepts from the literature to inform strategies for social workers who serve the rural elderly.

THE STRENGTHS PERSPECTIVE

Working with elders who live in their own homes in rural areas will be explored from a strengths perspective. This approach is uniquely suited to work with this population as it allows the recognition of, and building upon, the distinct capabilities and resources of rural elders who, some believe, are the strongest among their peers. Perhaps best described as an evolving theory, the strengths perspective is an appropriate framework for considering the situations and needs of older adults living in rural areas who continue to live in their own homes. In contrast to traditional theories of interventions that focus on individuals' deficits and problems, the strengths perspective offers a core set of ideas that are perhaps more useful and certainly more aligned with social work philosophy. Saleebey (1992) discussed six key concepts in the strengths perspective: (a) empowerment, (b) membership, (c) regeneration and healing from within, (d) synergy, (e) dialogue and collaboration, and (f) suspension of disbelief.

Empowerment occurs while helping individuals locate and utilize the personal power and resources that are already within them, and these may be considerable in magnitude in the rural elderly who have managed to stay in their own homes–the desire of most elders (Kelley & MacLean, 1997). *Membership* refers to the development and maintenance of a sense of belonging. Humans have consistently demonstrated the need to belong–to one another, to families, churches, peer groups, and myriad organizations, teams, committees, and cohorts (Saleebey, 1992).

The strengths perspective assumes that individuals are capable of helping themselves cope with and recover from adversity, thus the concepts of *regeneration and healing* from within–drawing on inner resources, the favored philosophy of those from western/industrialized nations that were built on the bootstrap philosophy.[1] *Synergy* refers to the effects of individuals working in unison to develop new and perhaps unexpected outcomes, which relates both *back* to the membership notion, and *forward* to the next concept. *Dialogue and collaboration* require active participation with another person toward a common goal in an egalitarian manner–again in concert with membership, and regeneration and healing. And finally, *suspension of disbelief* refers to privileging clients' stories and personal perspectives. It is not our place, as social workers, to disbelieve that clients can achieve new or revisited goals, regardless of whether they seem worthy or possible to us (Saleebey, 1992).

Chapin (1995) noted that a social constructionist theoretical approach is the basic underpinning of the strengths perspective. This theory allows a reflexive and inquisitive approach to working with individuals that is the basis for respecting and accepting their individual realities. Additionally, a strengths perspective calls attention to the specific skills and coping mechanisms that individuals use to address the concerns of daily life, and how these skills and mechanisms may be elicited, supported, and expanded in times of need (Early & GlenMaye, 2000; Van Wormer, 1999). By regarding individuals and their environments as inherently possessing strengths, or key internal and external resources, this perspective privileges individuals' voices and perspectives, and uses them as the foundation on which respectful and empowering relationships can be built (Brun & Rapp, 2001; Cowger, 1994; Gowdy, Rapp, & Poertner, 1993).

Specific practice guidelines for working with individuals from a strengths orientation draw heavily upon the aforementioned ideology and might also include the following strategies: (a) privilege the client's understanding of the facts, including believing what the client says, (b) *with* the client, identify and promote the use of personal and environmental resources, (c) use language that the client understands, (d) offer assertive community involvement by case managers and other advocates, (e) emphasize the relationship between the client and social worker, (f) make assessment and service planning a joint activity between provider and client, (g) avoid focusing on blame as well as cause and effect thinking, and (h) think and work with the client toward an assessment rather than a diagnosis (Brun & Rapp, 2001; Cowger, 1994). In effect, the strengths perspective, while perhaps not a solidly developed theory, is a conceptual framework and emerging theory that can inform ethical and appropriate work with elders living in their own homes in rural environments.

FACTORS THAT AFFECT INDEPENDENT RURAL LIVING

This section addresses various factors that affect rural elders' abilities to continue living independently in their own homes. "Home," however, may mean many different things to rural elders, including a farm, house, apartment, mobile home, or even another town or city, or perhaps where they grew up. The notion of "home" could also have more individualistic meaning, i.e., states or countries of origin–perhaps Ireland or Iowa. For our purposes, we will consider home to mean some residence in which an elder lives that is not institutional (e.g., a nursing home), although home can also be defined as co-residence with a family member or friend. Our emphasis is more on those elders not requiring an institutional level of health care than on the actual physical location of home. However, we also include those whom others might deem to be in need of skilled nursing, but who, for various reasons, have chosen to remain in their own homes–perhaps as a result of being doggedly determined to do so, even in the face of familial and professional pressure to relinquish their most important, perhaps, token of independence–their own homes (Norris-Baker & Scheidt, 1994).

The main factors that affect elders' remaining in their own homes are (a) financial resources, (b) knowledge and utilization of community and environmental resources and supports, (c) interpersonal and relationship resources, and (d) intrinsic or personal resources. We discuss these factors individually but with specific attention to how they impact rural elders' attention to two specific categories of need: (a) home and dwelling needs, including social support, and (b) needs for dignity and self-worth (Cox, 1993; Dinkins, 1994; Gilderbloom, 1996; Glasgow, 1993; Heumann & Boldy, 1993; Krause, 1990; Lacayo, 1992; Pezzin, Kemper, & Reschovsky, 1995; Rathbone-McCuan, 1992).

Financial Resources

While money cannot buy everything, it can definitely put into place many of the resources in elders' lives that enable choices and independence. These include home renovations and repair, transportation, skilled and unskilled assistance, and adequate health care. Many rural elders lack such financial stability, which may severely limit their choices in accessing needed resources. Availability of financial resources is an important factor to explore when assessing the ability of older people to remain in their own homes (Cox, 1993; Dinkins, 1994; Gilderbloom, 1996; Heumann & Boldy, 1993; Lacayo, 1992).

Knowledge and Resource Utilization

For elders in need, even adequate funds may not ensure accessibility of services if the services are (a) not known about, or (b) not available near rural elders' homes (Chapleski & Dwyer, 1995; Cox, 1993; Glasgow, 1993; Krout, 1985; Krout, 1994; Mainous & Kohrs, 1995). Knowledge is a powerful tool that social workers should always, always, be able to give their clients.

Interpersonal and Relationship Resources

Having adequate social skills, friends, and adult children nearby are often seen as positives for rural elders. Many adult children, however, no longer live in the area, some small rural churches are no longer open, and many elders have survived most of their friends and family members of their generations. In such cases rural elders may feel quite alone and abandoned, even with adequate health and financial resources. It is important to be aware that rural elders do not universally experience strong social and kinship support networks, nor do they all experience dire isolation and hopelessness (Glasgow, 1993; Krout, 1988; Lockery, 1992).

Intrinsic and Personal Resources

Finally, the unseen and perhaps unexplainable inner resources may be the magic that is inherent in some–missing in others–that allows some elders to continue to grow intellectually, spiritually, and emotionally, while others seem unable to do so. One group of researchers headed by Drs. Nancy Hooyman and Naomi Gottlieb at the University of Washington studied "exceptional women" to learn what such women knew, or could draw upon or do, that enabled–even compelled–them to do exceptional things after age 50. Referred to as the Eleanor Roosevelt syndrome, they hoped to learn something about that inner magic that could be taught or passed along to others who seemed to be stuck in the more negative aspects of aging, regardless of where they lived. While this goal eluded them to some extent, it was clear that women who made significant contributions to art, music, education, business, and other arenas after age 50 did indeed have some inner magic, resources, curiosities, talents, questions, and interests that were uniquely theirs, as well as the inner resources to bring those gifts to fruition. When looking at intrinsic and personal resources, factors such as a sense of self, a sense of will, and awareness of personal capacity and potential must be considered (Rathbone-McCuan, 1992).

These four kinds of resources, financial, knowledge utilization, interpersonal and relationship, and intrinsic and personal, will be brought to bear more specifically on the next sections, (a) home and dwelling needs, including relevant social support, and (b) the dignity and worth of rural elders. The chapter will then close with key concepts for social workers whose privilege it is to serve the rural elderly.

Home and Dwelling Needs

Perhaps the most commonly cited concern about the home life of elders living in rural areas is their overall condition and the fit between their needs and the layout of their homes (Dinkins, 1994; George & Holden, 2001; Norris-Baker & Scheidt, 1994). Specifically, as homes age, they need general and sometimes extensive upkeep and repair, which may be a problem for older people if they do not have sufficient income to support such needs. Additionally, as people age, they may experience physical conditions which require (or could be handled better with) home modifications such as wheelchair ramps, widened doorways, grab bars in showers and bathrooms, and lowered kitchen and bathroom counters.

Home maintenance and modification are critical needs that may be addressed with both personal and environmental resources. Lack of resources and the inability to secure these services is linked to premature institutionalization for elders, and is generally tied to poverty (Cox, 1993; Dinkins, 1994; Gilderbloom, 1996; Heumann & Boldy, 1993; Tabbarah, Silverstein, & Seeman, 2000). This inability to meet housing rehabilitation and modification needs and subsequent premature institutionalization may be due not only to insufficient personal financial resources, but also to a lack of systemic programs that provide these services. Liebig (1995) studied the priorities of State Units on Aging (SUA), perhaps the major organizations providing services to elders, and found that, with few exceptions, SUAs devote "minuscule" amounts of their budgets to housing, and ranked housing a relatively low #6 in a list of 8 priority areas (Liebig, 1995, p. 80).

With only sparse and spotty availability of housing rehabilitation and modification resources, elders who are in need are left to either find ways to accommodate their needs themselves or go without the accommodations. Availability of personal financial resources for meeting these needs may be even less likely for elders in rural areas, as they are more likely to be impoverished than non-rural elders (Glasgow, 1993). Additionally, minority status may present not only increased need but also further barriers to housing rehabilitation and modification services for rural elders. Elderly African Americans historically (a) have poorer housing and are less likely to own their own homes, (b) experience discrimination in both their ability to earn and save money, and securing adequate housing, and (c) are less able to access home rehabilitation programs due to lack of awareness and cultural aversion to securing loans, and may, therefore, also be less able to modify their homes to meet emerging needs as they age (Lacayo, 1992; Martinez, 1979).

From a strengths perspective, Norris-Baker and Scheidt (1994) asserted that people in small towns where populations have dwindled may be the most resilient of all, as they have stayed and aged in place while others left. This may indicate that those elders who remain in rural areas with few financial and environmental resources have been the most effective in coping with stressors and maintaining their personal efficacy–perhaps through more reliance on intrinsic or personal resources. These researchers found rural elders living in residences that others considered barely habitable, but the elders still expressed overall satisfaction with their dwellings (Norris-Baker & Scheidt, 1994). This will be an important issue to consider in our later discussion of working with elder individuals in rural environments from a strengths orientation that privileges individuals' authority and perspectives.

Social Supports

Stereotypes of both rural and minority seniors as having access to large, informal support networks of family and friends to help with health and personal care needs, thereby enabling elders to remain in their own homes, have been challenged (Krout, 1988; Lockery, 1992). While these challenges do not propose that informal or relational support resources are not important and vital in helping elders remain in their own homes, they point out that over-reliance on such resources may not only overburden families but may also leave gaps in policies and practices aimed at addressing elders' needs.

Studies of formal and informal support have found that each seems to serve a distinct role in maintaining rural elders' capacities to remain in their homes. Krause (1990), and Pezzin, Kemper, and Reschovsky (1995) both found positive effects of formal support programs, and noted that using formal supports neither reduced or superseded use of informal care. Availability of community-based formal care has been found to be much more limited in rural areas, however, and seems to be a ripe subject for future research, policy, and programming endeavors to address the needs of rural elders (Krout, 1994).

Dignity and Self-Worth

The needs for dignity and self-worth receive perhaps the least attention in the literature, but are vitally important in considering service provision for rural elders. These needs are most closely tied to both relationship and intrinsic or personal resources and may be exemplified through feelings and perspectives of self-reliance, connectedness and reciprocal relationships with others, and personal generativity (Saleebey, 1992).

In a study of rural versus urban neighborhood preferences, Zimmer and Chappell (1997) found that when ranking desirable characteristics of a neighborhood, rural elders placed more emphasis on social interaction than life-enhancing amenities. This suggests that a sense of connection may be more important to rural seniors than the condition of their houses, and highlights our fear that seniors may be infrequently asked what they want when policy and program decisions are made, such as what type of housing services to provide.

Similarly, in a qualitative study of women 85+ in primarily rural areas, Van Zandt (1991) found that societal connectedness with family and friends was important to all of the women interviewed. Several of the hypotheses generated in this grounded theory approach also related to issues of relationships with others and personal feelings of dignity and worth. One was that there was a significant relationship between mental health in old age and the presence of multiple sources of inner strength and well-being, including feelings of self-worth as well as multiple supports and connections with others. This study further challenged myths that older adults, particularly those considered the "old old" (85+), are either uninterested or incapable of being active members of their communities. One of the participants in Van Zandt's study continued to run her own farm, including doing large amounts of manual labor around the house, garden, and yard, at age 88. Another woman, aged 90, operated a volunteer social service agency out of her home, which provided food, clothing, and other basic supplies to needy persons in her community. This woman may serve as a good example of how formal-resource-barren rural communities may meet the needs of their residents, while at the same time illustrating that elders should not automatically be seen as only the recipients of such services.

Related to the issue of social relationships and reciprocity, in a study of the informal support networks of older African Americans in a rural North Carolina community, Groger (1992) found that individuals who owned land had more consistent and dependable informal support networks than those who did not. Those owning land were seen as having power and connections that could result in assistance from those whom they had helped in the past. Such reciprocity in relationships and power may paint a very non-traditional picture of elders and is testament to both the standing of these individuals in their communities, as well as to their personal power and self-sufficiency.

A final issue related to dignity and self-worth is that of elders having different perspectives of themselves and their needs than those possibly held by social workers. One explanation identified by Krout (1985) for why seniors may indicate low levels of awareness about in-home services and referral programs is that they may not see themselves in need of services, simply are not interested, or see accepting services as being on the dole. Respondents in Van Zandt's study (1991) also reflected such a stand: Only 2 of 10 women aged 85+ reported subjective feelings of being "old," and one particular woman addressed the conflict between her wants and needs, and her daughter's perspective on the matter. This woman spoke at some length about feeling that her daughter was trying to impose her own ideas and values on her regarding the kind of lifestyle she should lead. It is clearly important for social workers to respect clients' self-perceptions and desires for services (or not), a value position that falls squarely in the strengths perspective camp.

INNOVATIVE PROGRAMS AND SERVICES

We now discuss some programs and services that have either been aimed at helping seniors remain in their homes or could be seen to benefit such efforts. In some cases, these programs took place in rural areas, and in others, the programs will be discussed in their potential applicability to rural settings. The three topics are (a) congregate housing, (b) empowerment and education, and (c) collaborative supportive services.

Congregate Housing

Hallman and Alun (1997) investigated housing rural elders in a congregate setting referred to as the Abbeyfield model. The study took place in Canada but the authors asserted that findings may generalize to rural areas in the United States. Major components of the model included a small residential setting with 5-10 residents, a full-time resident housekeeper, and private space for each resident including a bedroom/sitting room. The site facilities were funded through non-profit organizations and were financially self-sustaining. The residents in this study were basically self-sufficient, and this arrangement was considered non-institutional. Some major issues identified by Hallman and Alun (1997) were that (a) although the proportion of elders in rural areas is higher than in urban areas, the actual number of elders may be low, limiting congregate-type housing as an option, (b) the heterogeneity of elders in rural areas must not be overlooked–it should not be assumed that it will be easy or desirable for these individuals to adapt to congregate living, (c) relatively little is known about the use of housing alternatives such as this in rural communities, and (d) there was some disjunction between the perceptions of the elders in the study and those of municipal officials and service providers–the elders were less likely to see deficiencies in their pre-intervention housing arrangements and were considered by the professionals to be somewhat resistant to accepting the service model. This study raised these very important issues that may be generalized and will be discussed further in the section on the role of social workers.

Empowerment and Education

Cox and Parsons (1996) discussed the use of a small group model in developing personal and community strengths, and the efficacy of meeting the needs of a group of elderly women. The study referred to the use of an empowerment intervention in which a master's level social worker assisted elderly women in a low-income housing complex in developing a group that performed the following functions: (a) pursued educational information about Medicare and Medicaid, (b) researched and discussed local health care clinics and experiences with health care providers, (c) discussed and developed strategies for communication with health care professionals, other service providers and family members, (d) compared prices of medication from different sources, (e) explored resources for transportation, (f) developed mutual support relationships including accompaniment of others to doctors' appointments, and (g) discussed and pursued topics of political relevance to seniors. This group eventually became self-generated and continued after the research component and intervention of the professional social worker ceased. Although this model was not contextually described as taking place in an explicitly rural community, it could be based in a local senior center, church, or area ministry association.

Collaborative Supportive Services

George and Holden (2001) investigated the collaboration between governmental and local community supports in meeting the needs of rural seniors in four communities across the United States, and highlighted specific issues unique to each area. In the first site, Cateret County, North Carolina, two major issues with which the community dealt were (a) a prevalence of natural disasters (hurricanes) which led to frequent damage of elders' homes, and (b) an influx of elder immigrants who had higher incomes than long-time residents. This skewed economic data to give a false perception of the income base of the area and resulted in funding agencies' perceiving the area in less economic need for assistance, particularly following hurricane damage. This community responded to these needs through a very strong collaboration between the local community action agency and two non-profit organizations that had ties to religious organizations. One in particular was an agency connected with the local African Methodist Episcopal church. This agency (a) collaborated with a federally-funded job training program where trainees completed home rehabilitation projects for agency recipients, (b) made loans to individuals in need of housing repair and rehabilitation, (c) offered outreach seminars and counseling, and (d) assisted with grant and loan applications. Overall, the agencies in this rural county, both governmental and non-governmental, worked together effectively to provide a strong housing resource component. The authors highlighted the idea that the religious connections of two key organizations within this system may have increased accessibility of services by providing legitimacy and easing elders' fears of fraud and scams (George & Holden, 2001).

A second site was Chenago County, New York, where a major issue was the prevalence of elders residing in mobile homes–many of which had become substandard. George and Holden (2001) reported that (a) the collaboration of service providers in accessing funding reduced the competition for scarce resources, (b) close organizational collaboration facilitated more appropriate referrals, and (c) some of the rural homeowners were reluctant to apply for home repair loans, due to fear of having liens placed on their homes or inheritance consequences of re-mortgaging their homes (George & Holden, 2001).

Issues highlighted at a third site, Lake County, California, included the problem of older mobile homes being difficult to repair and less likely to meet housing regulations. Such conditions disqualified some homeowners from certain repair and modification loans. Some low-income seniors had poor credit that prevented them from securing loans or forced them to secure loans from sub-prime lenders who charge unreasonably high interest rates (up to 22%). This community did not have an active non-profit housing organization and therefore little collaboration, but did offer a legal aid service for seniors that gave them free legal and housing related advice and representation (George & Holden, 2001).

The fourth research site, Lowndes County, Alabama, was home to an active private, non-profit organization that also utilized a mutual self-help method for providing labor in rehabilitating older homes, as well as building new homes for elders and other community residents. Laborers worked on both their own and others' homes. This organization accessed a large grant from the W. K. Kellogg foundation for funding (George & Holden, 2001).

These three types of innovative programs represented (a) congregate housing, (b) education and empowerment, and (c) collaborative approaches to addressing the needs of elders living independently in rural communities (George & Holden, 2001). Issues identified in each of these areas will inform and provide useful questions for contemplation in the following section on social work roles and functions.

KEY CONCEPTS FOR SOCIAL WORKERS

We now focus on the roles and functions of the social workers serving rural elders living in their own homes. This discussion of service provision is grounded in the strengths perspective and suggests practice strategies that incorporate and exemplify strengths based practice.

Elders in rural communities who continue to live in their own homes may be seen in one or more of the following groups: the healthiest, most resilient, most supported, most supportive, most determined, and most at-risk. The very fact that they continue to live independently may inherently limit the role of the social worker, as these individuals may not be in need of services and/or may not perceive themselves to be in need of services. They might, however, need but not *want* services. Social workers who are privileged to work with these individuals may do so through a variety of avenues including the will of the individual, the will of the individual's family, the intervention of protective services, or referrals from other community contacts. We next discuss several key issues.

Congruent with the strengths-based philosophy of privileging the perspective of the client, a major theme throughout the literature is the need to recognize the heterogeneity of elders in rural communities. This issue may be particularly salient for elders who live in non-institutional settings as they maintain their places in the unique settings of their own homes and surroundings. Social workers who are truly able to recognize the heterogeneity of rural elders residing in their own homes will be more aware of personal and societal stereotypes and biases and will be less likely to make practice decisions based on such views. In addition to being sensitive to elders living in rural, non-institutional environments as a whole, social workers must be aware of the need for cultural sensitivity, including sensitivity to the needs and unique perspectives of individuals who are ethnic and racial minorities and those with life-long disabilities (Burton, Dilworth-Anderson, & Bengtson, 1992; Gilson & Netting, 1997; Rathbone-McCuan, 1992).

Related to sensitivity to heterogeneity and the strengths-based notion of privileging the individuals' perceptions is the need for social workers to respect individuals' conceptualizations of themselves. For example, social workers should make every effort to understand individuals' perspectives on themselves–their self-concepts and feelings of personal identity. Clients' self-perceived strengths must not be regarded by social workers as stubbornness that may be a barrier to effective service delivery, but as the foundation from which the social worker may assist clients in continuing to address their own needs. Rathbone-McCuan (1992) addressed the tendency of practitioners to conceptualize elders according to notions of emotional, physical, and resource *deficits*, which serves to justify and legitimize social work interventions in their lives. She suggested instead, that from a strengths-based perspective, we should focus on that which individuals can do to secure their own well-being. Rathbone-McCuan (1992) stated that

> We forget too easily that people with cognitive and physical changes have strengths. Even in the settings that offer the best rehabilitative and preventive services to older persons, the approach is to compensate for what people cannot do rather than [capitalize on] what they can do. (p. 104)

Related to building on strengths, social workers engaging with rural elders who live independently must acknowledge the elders' needs to be generative, and do everything possible to encourage that, including helping to remove any barriers that might pose threats to existing and desired activities.

In addition to privileging the individual's sense of self, social workers may be instrumental in helping clients maintain personal integrity, and/or negotiate with family members who have different opinions of the client's needs and capabilities. This may be particularly salient for rural elders who continue to live independently, as they generally do not receive comprehensive supportive services that might make an anxious family member feel like they were more "safe." Van Zandt (1991) illustrated the case of one woman whose daughter had very different ideas about how her mother should live her life. In the role of helper and advocate, social workers may mediate or advocate on behalf of clients with their families by (a) encouraging the family to support independence and reduce paternalism, (b) providing information about available community resources, and (c) helping clarify issues between the client and family members if tensions should arise. On the other hand, social workers as advocates may need to advocate for their client moving if that is their desire. For example, when the second author cautiously broached to her mother the idea of moving out of her home of 40 years, her mother said, "Don't worry about *me* moving out of that old house to a nicer one!" A part of serving in this role may also include being sensitive to the stress and needs of family caregivers and providing emotional and educational support to them, when doing so does not compromise the worker's allegiance to the client.

Another advocacy function may be to secure and keep current information about governmental housing and other resources that may not be readily available near the client's home. This may include various types of housing grants and loans available at state and national levels, including local or regional programs such as Habitat for Humanity. Also related to advocacy, social workers must stay engaged with community decision and policy-makers, stressing the need for services that allow individuals to remain in their homes (e.g., housing repairs and modifications, transportation services, and job programs for seniors). Too many policy and program decisions are made without the presence of either clients or their social workers; and social workers are remiss in their responsibilities if they are not also intervening at that level.

Finally, and perhaps blatantly obvious, service providers at all levels should ask elders what they want and what would best assist them in maintaining life in their own homes, if that is their desire. Kelley and MacLean (1997) found that the seniors in their study not only expressed the desire to continue to live in their own homes permanently, but also requested services that were not normally provided, e.g., assistance with home maintenance, prescription delivery, assistance with spring cleaning, and transportation. Social workers should place themselves in the role of speaking up when they recognize that policy and programmatic decisions affecting elders are being made without client input, or with minimal input. They should also encourage elders to seek public office, participate in political activities, or simply vote.

A summary of key concepts for social workers working with elders in rural settings who continue to live in their own homes includes:

- Recognize the heterogeneity of this population–don't make assumptions
- Respect individuals' self-concepts
- Encourage maintenance and development of self-efficacy if desired by the client
- When appropriate, interact with the clients' families on their behalves
- Be sensitive and supportive to the needs of family and other caregivers
- Stay current on local and regional resources
- Educate the community about clients' needs for self-sufficiency and support
- Ask clients what they want–privilege their voices and encourage their participation in decisions that affect them.

NOTE

1. As in "I pulled myself up by my own bootstraps."

REFERENCES

Brun, C., & Rapp, R. (2001). Strengths-based case management: Individual's perspectives on strengths and the case manager relationship. *Social Work, 46*(3), 278-288.

Burton, L., Dilworth-Anderson, P., & Bengtson, V. (1992). Creating culturally relevant ways of thinking about diversity and aging: Theoretical challenges for the Twenty-First century. In E. Stanford, & F. Torres-Gil (Eds.), *Diversity: New approaches to ethnic minority aging* (pp. 129-140). Amityville, NY: Baywood.

Chapin, R. (1995). Social policy development: The strengths perspective. *Social Work, 40*(4), 506-514.

Chapleski, E., & Dwyer, J. (1995). The effects of on- and off-reservation residence on in-home service use among Great Lakes American Indians. *The Journal of Rural Health, 11*(3), 204-216.

Cowger, C. D. (1994). Addressing client strengths: Clinical assessment for client empowerment. *Social Work, 39*(3), 262-267.

Cox, C. (1993). Housing needs and options. In C. Cox (Ed.), *The frail elderly: Problems, Needs, and Community Resources* (pp. 83-102). Westport, CT: Greenwood.

Cox, E., & Parsons, R. (1996). Empowerment-oriented social work practice: Impact on late life relationships of women. *Journal of Women and Aging, 8*(3/4), 129-143.

Dinkins, J. (1994). Rural Southern elderly: Housing characteristics. *Family Economics Review, 7*(2), 11-18.

Early, T., & GlenMaye, L. (2000). Valuing families: Social work practice with families from a strengths perspective. *Social Work, 45*(2), 118-131.

George, L., & Holden, C. (2001). Federal programs and local organizations: Meeting the housing needs of rural seniors. (Housing Assistance Council) on-line: 1/13/02 at *http://www.ruralhome.org/pubs/hsganalysis/elderly/index.htm.*

Gilderbloom, J. (1996). Housing modification needs of the disabled elderly: What really matters? *Environment and Behavior, 28*(4), 512-535.

Gilson, S., & Netting, E. (1997). When people with pre-existing disabilities age in place: Implications for social work practice. *Health and Social Work, 22*(4), 290-298.

Glasgow, N. (1993). Poverty among rural elders: Trends, context, and directions for policy. *The Journal of Applied Gerontology, 12*(3), 302-319.

Gowdy, E., Rapp, C., & Poertner, J. (1993). Management is performance: Strategies for client-centered practice in social service organizations. *Administration in Social Work, 17*(1), 3-22.

Groger, L. (1992). Tied to each other through ties to the land: Informal support of black elders in a southern U.S. community. *Journal of Cross-Cultural Gerontology, 7*, 205-220.

Hallman, B., & Alun, J. (1997). Housing the rural elderly: A place for Abbeyfield? In L. Pastalan (Ed.) *Shelter and service issues for aging populations: International perspectives.* New York: The Haworth Press, Inc.

Heumann, L., & Boldy, D. (Eds.). (1993). *Aging in place with dignity.* Westport, CT: Praeger.

Kelley, M., & MacLean, M. (1997). I want to live here for the rest of my life: The challenge of case management for rural seniors. *Journal of Case Management, 6*(4), 174-182.

Krause, N. (1990). Perceived health problems, formal/informal support, and life satisfaction among older adults. *Journals of Gerontology: Social Sciences, 45*(1), S193-S205.

Krout, J. (1985). Service awareness among the elderly. *Journal of Gerontological Social Work, 9*(1), 7-19.

Krout, J. (1988). Rural versus urban differences in elderly parents' contact with their children. *The Gerontologist, 28*(2), 198-203.

Krout, J. (1994). Rural aging community-based services. In R. Coward (Ed.), *Health services for rural elders* (pp. 84-107). New York: Springer.

Lacayo, C. (1992). Current trends in living arrangements and social environment among ethnic minority elderly. In E. Stanford, & F. Torres-Gil (Eds.) *Diversity: New approaches to ethnic minority aging.* Amityville, NY: Baywood.

Liebig, P. (1995). State units on aging and housing for the elderly: Current roles and future implications. *Journal of Housing for the Elderly, 11*(2), 67-84.

Lockery, S. (1992). Caregiving among racial and ethnic minority elders: Family and social supports. In *Diversity: New approaches to ethnic minority aging.* E. Stanford, & F. Torres-Gil., (Eds.). Amityville, NY: Baywood.

Mainous, A., & Kohrs, F. (1995). A comparison of health status between rural and urban adults. [Electronic version]. *Journal of Community Health, 20*(5). Retrieved November 9, 2001, from First Search.

Martinez, C. (1979). Policy and research strategies pertinent to the housing needs of minority aged. In E. Stanford (Ed.), *Minority aging research–old issues, new approaches* (pp. 181-199). San Diego, CA: San Diego State University Press.
Norris-Baker, C., & Scheidt, R. (1994). From 'Our Town' to 'Ghost Town': The changing context of home for rural elders. *International Journal of Aging and Human Development*, *38*(3), 181-202.
Pezzin, L., Kemper, P., & Reschovsky, J. (1995). Does publicly provided home care substitute for family care? *The Journal of Human Resources*, *31*(3), 650-676.
Rathbone-McCuan, E. (1992). Aged adult protective services clients: People of unrecognized potential. In D. Saleebey (Ed.), *The strengths perspective in social work practice*, pp. 98-110. New York: Longman.
Saleebey, D. (Ed.). (1992). *The strengths perspective in social work practice*. NY: Longman.
Tabbarah, M., Silverstein, M., & Seeman, T. (2000). A health and demographic profile of institutionalized older Americans residing in environments with home modifications [Electronic version]. *Journal of Aging and Health*, *12*(2), 204-228.
Van Wormer, K. (1999). The strengths perspective: A paradigm for correctional counseling. *Federal Probation*, *63*(1), 51-58.
Van Zandt, P. (1991). *The invisible woman: Women over age 85 in today's society*. New York: Garland.
Zimmer, Z., & Chappell, N. (1997). Rural-urban differences in seniors' neighborhood preferences. In L. Pastalan (Ed.), *Shelter and service issues for aging populations* (pp. 105-124). Binghamton, NY: The Haworth Press, Inc.

Chapter 14

Specialized Housing and Rural Elders

Sandra S. Butler, PhD
Donald W. Sharland, MSW

SUMMARY. This chapter begins with an examination of current living arrangements and housing conditions among the elderly in general and for rural elders in particular. The environmental press and empowerment-oriented practice models provide readers with a framework for understanding the underlying tension between autonomy and security faced by rural elders and the social workers who assist them. Drawing from in-depth interviews with nine geriatric social workers working with elders in rural housing settings, we explore practice challenges, particular issues related to rurality, and innovative techniques and programs. The chapter concludes with policy implications and practice guidelines. *[Article copies available for a fee from The Haworth Document Delivery Service: 1-800-HAWORTH. E-mail address: <docdelivery@haworth press.com> Website: <http://www.HaworthPress.com> © 2003 by The Haworth Press, Inc. All rights reserved.]*

KEYWORDS. Empowerment practice, rural elders, elder housing

[Haworth co-indexing entry note]: "Specialized Housing and Rural Elders." Butler, Sandra S., and Donald W. Sharland. Co-published simultaneously in *Journal of Gerontological Social Work* (The Haworth Social Work Practice Press, an imprint of The Haworth Press, Inc.) Vol. 41, No. 3/4, 2003, pp. 247-263; and: *Gerontological Social Work in Small Towns and Rural Communities* (ed: Sandra S. Butler, and Lenard W. Kaye) The Haworth Social Work Practice Press, an imprint of The Haworth Press, Inc., 2003, pp. 247-263. Single or multiple copies of this article are available for a fee from The Haworth Document Delivery Service [1-800-HAWORTH, 9:00 a.m. - 5:00 p.m. (EST). E-mail address: docdelivery@haworth press.com].

http://www.haworthpress.com/web/JGSW
© 2003 by The Haworth Press, Inc. All rights reserved.
Digital Object Identifier: 10.1300/J083v41n03_04

INTRODUCTION

In this chapter we will be examining housing needs of rural elders and the role social workers can play in assisting older adults to secure optimal housing and services. We will begin by reviewing current trends and preferences for various housing types among U.S. seniors. This will be followed by an exploration of some of the special housing issues and circumstances facing elders in rural areas, with a focus on supported housing, or housing with services. The competence model, first proposed by Lawton and Nahemow in 1973, will provide a framework for our discussion of the challenges social workers face as they try to balance their elder clients' need for autonomy with their need for security in making housing choices. Empowerment-oriented practice will be offered as an effective approach for managing these tensions. This will be followed by practice illustrations from a series of interviews with rural gerontological social workers regarding the challenges and opportunities of meeting the housing and services needs of their clients. We will conclude with policy implications and best practice guidelines pertaining to housing and rural elders.

CURRENT LIVING ARRANGEMENTS AND HOUSING CONDITIONS AMONG THE ELDERLY

Older adults live in a wide range of housing settings–from single family homes, to full-service retirement communities, to nursing facilities. In the United States, only one in ten older adults live in age-restricted communities–90% of people age 70 and older live in conventional housing (Schafer, 2000). In fact, older adults have the highest homeownership rates of any age group, comprising nearly one quarter of all owners (Schafer). However, as people age in their homes, they often require home modifications and/or support services. Only about half of disabled elders have the home modifications they believe they need, leaving hundreds of thousands of older disabled individuals without the structural modifications that would allow them to more easily function in their own homes (Pynoos & Golant, 1996; Schafer, 2000). Furthermore, approximately 3% of elderly householders occupy dwellings with severe physical problems, and an additional 4.8% have moderate physical problems. Elders living in rural areas are more at risk of occupying housing in poor condition than their urban counterparts (Golant & LaGreca, 1994; Pynoos & Golant). Moreover, about one quarter of elderly homeowners paid more than 30% of their income for housing, the federal government's threshold for excessive housing costs (Pynoos & Golant).

Special arrangements to receive care in regular housing are made by about 15% of older adults (Schafer, 2000). For some (about two thirds of this group), this means moving in with a non-elderly individual or having a non-elderly person move in with them for the purpose of receiving care. The remaining third of this group obtains support services in the home from an outside organization or non-relative. While only 5% of elders between the ages of 70 and 79 receive outside support services in their home, the percentage rises to 20% for those 90 and older (Schafer). Level of disability, proximity of children, and presence or absence of a spouse are all important factors in whether an older adult will choose shared or supported housing.

Some elders–about 10%–choose to live in age-restricted communities. Just over two thirds of this group (about 2 million seniors) live in communities that do not provide services and that are tailored for residents who are relatively healthy and who lead active lifestyles (Schafer, 2000). Assisted communities are home to only 3% of the nation's seniors, 70 and older, who do not live in nursing homes; for those 85 and older, the percentage rises to 7%. These assisted communities range from congregate housing, which provide meals and limited services, to settings, which provide on-site nursing care.

In all, about one million elders currently occupy unsubsidized supportive housing options (Pynoos & Golant, 1996). Assisted communities, which are not covered by Medicare at all, are costly:

> The out-of-pocket monthly costs of assisted communities without income restrictions average $1500. And even these relatively steep rents do not necessarily cover all costs of care received by residents. One-fifth of residents in assisted communities contract for outside help at an average cost of nearly $1300 per month. (Schafer, 2000, p. 3)

Though state Medicaid waivers may cover limited costs for some low-income residents in assisted communities, for the most part, poor seniors who need assistance with daily activities must choose lower-cost, and often undesirable, board and care facilities or nursing homes, which are Medicaid reimbursed (Pynoos & Golant). Furthermore, a larger group of poor and near poor elders needing in-home care lack government assistance in paying for these services (Schafer). The proportion of the elderly population residing in nursing homes has remained relatively stable during the past two decades, despite the growing number of persons over 75 years of age; it has ranged from about 4 to 5% of the population over 65 (Pynoos & Golant).

HOUSING FOR ELDERS IN RURAL AREAS

About one quarter of households headed by individuals over 65 in the U.S. exist in rural areas (Pynoos & Golant, 1996). Approximately 80% of these rural elders are homeowners, and 70% of these owners have paid off their mortgages (Prosper & Clark, 1994). Nonetheless, because of the high rate of poverty among rural elders (27%), nearly a third (31%) spent more than 30% of their income on housing (Prosper & Clark); among poor households, the proportion rises to 69% (Lazere, Leonard, & Kravitz, 1989). Given that many of these households have paid off their mortgages, high housing costs occur due to the rising cost of utilities, property taxes, insurance, maintenance, and repairs (Lazere et al.). Moreover, as stated earlier, rural elderly householders are more likely to live in substandard housing than are their metropolitan counterparts. Thus, while the rural elderly represent just over a quarter of all elderly households, they occupy 43% of elderly substandard households and 57% of severely substandard elderly households (Lazere et al.).

Rural elders seeking housing with services have fewer alternatives than do their urban counterparts.

> The lower population density and smaller proportion of high-income consumers found in rural areas generally make it difficult to develop housing with services facilities that are large enough to take advantage of economies of scale in construction and service delivery or to use rent-skewing approaches to subsidize low-income tenants with the rents of higher income tenants. (Bolda et al., 2000, p. i)

Those facilities that do exist in rural areas tend to be smaller than metropolitan facilities, typically servicing from five to 20 residents. A positive outcome of this smaller size is that facilities tend to be more home-like in appearance and more easily integrated into a residential area or town center (Bolda et al.). "Tenants in small facilities also tend to form close bonds with both staff members and other tenants, reducing social isolation and the risk of health problems or other needs going unnoticed" (Bolda et al., p. i).

According to Bolda and her co-authors (2000), the greatest challenge to financing rural housing with services projects lies in funding the services rather than the housing. States often rely heavily on Medicaid waiver programs, which have medical and financial eligibility requirements that create oversight and licensing burdens too costly for small facilities, exclude residents with moderate levels of impairment, and may discourage measures designed to prevent institutionalization (Bolda et al.). The goal of aging in place may be particularly important to rural elders who face moving to a distant city if long-term care options are unavailable near their homes. The 24-hour staffing necessary to allow people to age in place is especially expensive to provide in small rural facilities (Bolda et al.). In the final analysis, "[b]uilding and service regulations and licensing requirements often make current care models too expensive to build and operate on a scale small enough for rural communities to support" (Bolda et al., p. iii).

Krout (2001) concurs that rural elders have constrained housing choices due to lack of alternatives. He submits that the high rate of home ownership in rural areas may reflect a housing preference, but it may just as easily reflect the lack of alternatives such as service-enriched housing. Rural elders not wanting or unable to remain in their own homes have few local choices and often need to relocate. Unfortunately, the one service that is the exception to the rule of rural scarcity is nursing home beds, leading to the possible over institutionalization of elders in rural areas (Krout).

Given the inadequate supply of elder housing with services in rural areas, rural seniors in need of supportive housing are often confronted with difficult choices. Should they continue to live in inappropriate housing or accept premature institutionalization? Should they remain in a familiar community that lacks services or move to a more urban area that offers greater choice (Hallman & Joseph, 1997)? When one's home is no longer appropriate due to increased disability and service needs, and no alternatives are available, then housing becomes a source of stress, as leaving behind one's home and community may come at great psychological cost (Norris-Baker & Scheidt, 1994). Rural elders may forgo more suitable housing in order to remain in the home and neighborhood that is loved and familiar.

> If the neighborhood and service characteristics of the housing context are considered, very small towns are likely to offer major defi-

> cits when compared even with larger towns. Yet, even for physically substandard housing, elderly individuals tend to express satisfaction, that may in turn be related to *place* meaning. (Norris-Baker & Scheidt, p. 185, italics added)

The tension of balancing autonomy with security that arises for rural elders and their families as they face often difficult housing choices will be examined next using the environmental press and competence models developed by Lawton.

BALANCING AUTONOMY AND SECURITY

The environmental press model is based on theory proposed by psychologist Kurt Lewin and his associates in the first half of the 20th century (Hooyman & Kiyak, 2002). Lewin's field theory suggested that a person's "life space" includes not only the person and the interacting environment, but also the psychological space in which the person-environment interaction takes place.

> Lewin captured the relationships in his ecological equation [B = f(P,E)], where behavior (B) is a function (f) of the personal characteristics (P) and environmental characteristics (E), together comprising a "subjective reality" by which the individual perceives the life condition not only through the present situation but through future expectations as well as through past experience. (Cvitkovich & Wister, 2001, p. 3)

Lawton and Nahemow (1973) build on this theory in the development of their competence model, which emphasizes the interaction between personal and environmental characteristics (Cvitkovich & Wister). The competence model assumes that the impact of the environment is mediated by the individual's level of ability. "The ultimate goal of any modification should be to maximize the older person's ability to negotiate and control the situation, and to minimize the likelihood that the environment will overwhelm the person's competence" (Hooyman & Kiyak, p. 331). The environmental press in this model refers to the demands that physical and social environments make on an individual to adapt, respond and change (Hooyman & Kiyak).

An underlying theme when examining environmental press is the tension between autonomy and security (Parmelee & Lawton, 1990).

The balance between autonomy and security becomes particularly salient when discussing specialized housing. Parmelee and Lawton define autonomy as the ability (perceived or actual) to pursue life goals through one's own resources–"free of choice, action and self-regulation of one's life space" (p. 465). Security, on the other hand, suggests that life goals are "linked to, limited by, and aided by dependable physical, social, and interpersonal resources" (p. 465). Parmelee and Lawton further submit that in the normal aging process, there is an ongoing dynamic between autonomy and security. As an individual ages, physical security and psychological feelings of safety and stability are important concerns. Nonetheless, of equal importance, is the individual's need to maintain a sense of self-efficacy.

Finding the equilibrium between autonomy and security is an ongoing process. Gains in security may result in loss of autonomy, and vice versa. "Overly secure environments produce boredom, apathy, and withdrawal; too much autonomy (i.e., in the absence of security) leads to stress and its documented effects" (Parmelee & Lawton, 1990, p. 468). Social workers, working with rural elders in specialized housing, must be ever vigilant about their clients sometimes competing needs for autonomy and security.

EMPOWERMENT-ORIENTED PRACTICE

By necessity, most rural social workers are generalists; they assist their clients with a wide range of issues, having fewer specialists to call upon than do social workers in metropolitan areas (Ginsberg, 1998). Virtually every practitioner working with elders in rural areas will eventually be faced with the need to assist their clients with housing choices. As described above, these choices may be constrained due to a scarcity of alternatives and will undoubtedly involve attention to the balance between autonomy and safety. Empowerment-oriented practice provides a structure for assisting rural elders around housing issues in a manner that is strengths-based and client-centered.

> Empowerment-oriented social work practice is a model through which social workers can assist older people to utilize their strengths, abilities, and competencies in order to mobilize their resources toward problem solving and ultimately toward empowerment. Empowerment-oriented practice recognizes that elders

> frequently experience substantial loss of power for a variety of reasons. (Cox & Parsons, 1994, p. 19)

The relationship between the worker and client in empowerment-oriented practice is one of collaboration and mutual responsibility. It is important for the client to experience a sense of power within the relationship. "Empowerment is clearly not something that is done to another person, but a process that must be engaged in by mutual effort" (Cox & Parsons, 1994, p. 38). Principles and strategies identified by Cox and Parsons (p. 39) as being a part of an empowerment-oriented practice model include:

- Basing the helping relationship on collaboration, trust, and shared power;
- Accepting the client's definition of the problem;
- Identifying and building upon the client's strengths;
- Involving the client in the change process;
- Utilizing mutual support and self-help networks or groups; and
- Mobilizing resources or advocating for clients.

In order to illustrate how these principles can be integrated into practice, we turn now to findings from a series of interviews with social workers who had many years of experience working with elders in rural Maine.

ILLUSTRATIONS FROM THE FIELD

From December 2001 to April 2002, the second author conducted in-depth interviews with nine geriatric social workers, currently working with elders in rural housing settings. Since rural elder housing programs tend to be very small and do not include professional social workers, it was determined that geriatric social workers who provide clinical mental health services would have the widest practice experience from which to contribute. Nearly all participating social workers had more than 10 years clinical practice experience in community mental health agencies.

Informants reported that their services were reimbursed by a variety of funding programs including state and federal mental health grants, Medicaid and Medicare. They noted that the funding source determines the type and extent of services provided. Practitioners having the most latitude are funded by geriatric mental health service grant funds that allow a wide range of services from psychotherapy to consultation and education services. Medicaid and Medicare programs have reimbursement limitations that restrict eligibility for and extent of social work interventions.

Social workers reported working with clients residing in a range of rural housing settings including retirement communities, publicly subsidized independent elder housing projects, congregate services programs, assisted living facilities, residential care facilities and nursing homes. The semi-structured interviews addressed the following topics:

- Important issues for rural social workers with regard to rural elder housing programs;
- Roles social workers fulfill in serving elders residing in rural settings;
- Barriers encountered in their work with elders around rural housing issues;
- Impact of rurality on their practice;
- Impact of rurality on the quality of life for elders;
- Potential functions and roles for rural social workers in elder facilities; and
- Innovations in their practice related to working with elders and housing in rural areas.

Findings from these rich interviews are highlighted below.

Important issues for rural social workers with regard to rural elder housing programs. The nine rural social workers reported that the most common issues confronting their clients were lack of local housing options, lack of transportation to community services and social isolation.

Lack of housing options in small rural communities leaves many frail elders with no choice but to remain in their own homes. While remaining in one's home is the preference of many elders, as they become very frail, the care and support burden placed on families and neighbors can be burdensome and exhausting. At the point when it becomes impossible to remain at home, frail elders may be forced to move away from their hometown family and support systems to larger service center communities. In instances where local housing options are available in small towns, they tend to be at the extreme ends of the housing and services continuum, either independent apartments with part-time managers and no support services, or residential care and nursing home facilities.

Lack of readily available transportation and long travel distances to medical and other services is a major disadvantage for residents of rural elder housing programs. Social workers have found that in order to connect clients to support systems they must help their clients explore relationships with family and friends to find persons willing and able to provide rides. In some instances transportation may be available from housing facility staff, volunteers or church groups. Several social workers reported this form of transportation works best for short-term purposes but usually does not endure for long-term needs.

Isolation and the attendant feelings of loneliness arise from lack of meaningful interpersonal interaction and separation from support systems such as friends and families. A common expectation is that moving from living alone in a remote rural home to a group living setting will cure loneliness. However, practitioners observed that moving to a housing project usually does not in of itself resolve feelings of loneliness. While the new living situation may offer opportunities for socialization, formerly isolated residents often find becoming part of the group and forming new relationships to be difficult.

Roles social workers fulfill in serving elders residing in rural settings. The unique challenges of rural social work practice bring opportunities for social workers to employ the full gamut of their social work roles and skills. Informants reported acting as advocates, care managers, service coordinators, system navigators, resource finders, consultants, educators, psychotherapists, and family therapists.

Since resource finding is a common function of serving rural elders, awareness of supportive housing options is an important element in the professional social worker's knowledge base. One practitioner observed that a very frail client residing in an independent senior housing apartment was overwhelmed by the numerous service personnel who were coming and going from her apartment while she was receiving extensive home health nursing, physical rehabilitation, along with homemaker and home delivered meals. The social worker was able to refer the client to a newly opened affordable assisted living project in the next town. The client found that moving to the assisted living program with 24 hour on-site support staff delivering services on a regular schedule gave her an increased sense of control. She also noted that having the continuity of the same staff assisting her helped her to feel more comfortable. She observed to her social worker, "I feel like I've never had it so good."

Another informant worked with a client and his wife who lived in their own home in a rural setting; they both were extremely frail. The worker located an opening in an attractive assisted living facility and encouraged them to consider moving to the facility that could offer them support services and a measure of personal security. After several visits and much discussion, the couple decided that they could not leave their home of many years and felt they could get by with the help of a long-term neighbor. In this situation the worker was able to honor the couple's sense of autonomy and choice to remain in their home where they were comfortable.

Often interventions with residents of assisted living settings thrust social workers in the role of acting as a broker in situations where their clients are in conflict with facility staff. These situations raise a host of protocol questions relating on the one hand to helping the client to find the strength to speak up for his or her own interests, while on the other, to guiding the staff in understanding the clients' needs. In cases where the client does not want his or her grievances shared with on-site staff, conflicts may arise for the social worker and treatment options may be narrowed.

Examples of family therapy interventions occurred numerous times during interviews. This affirms the general pattern that families provide the great majority of care and support for elders. This continues to hold true in most cases even after the elder moves to a supported housing or care facility. Yet therapists often noted that family care taking and family relationships for the very old are not uncomplicated. In some cases there may be estrangement, where the cut off is so deep that family involvement is impossible.

Barriers encountered in their work with elders around rural housing issues. The most common barriers reported by informants were treatment limitations imposed by funding programs, client reluctance to accept help and resistance on the part of facility staff to have external interveners work with their residents.

Practitioners related that Medicaid and Medicare reimbursement systems do not cover the time necessary to do collateral work with family members or facility staff, which restricts their ability to help clients. Workers funded by grants have had the opportunity for more collaborative work, and have been able to take the time to make systems interventions with family members or facility staff who work with the client on a daily basis.

Several social workers reported that they have frequently found clients residing in small housing settings to be self conscious about having visits from an outside person in a group living environment. Many elders feel the stigma of being identified as a mental health patient. One respondent, who works with grant funding, notes that in such situations, she begins the intervention very carefully, first developing relationships with staff and then proceeding with the work of providing them with information and ideas on how to respond to client needs.

In some cases clients are referred without adequately being prepared for the social worker's visit. This often leads to confusion and the potential client's refusal of help when the social worker arrives. Several social workers have found this occurs less frequently where housing projects have a resident services coordinator who maintains ongoing relationships with residents and can facilitate a social work visit.

Some housing settings were open to social work interventions, while others were closed to persons other than their own staff assisting residents. Each facility is very different, and taking time to discover how to approach and intervene in each unique setting is important for initiating the helping process. Several workers have found that some small rural residential care facilities function as family settings where they are used to solving problems or meeting resident needs in their own ways and may be distrustful of outside interveners. This may also be a factor in nursing facilities that provide a high level of health services and have formal clinical protocols.

Impact of rurality on their practice. Beyond the obvious inconvenience of extended travel distances, social workers reported that serving elder residents of rural housing programs can be frustrating due to limited local resources for their clients. One practitioner noted, "the therapeutic process can dead-end with no service options available or located a prohibitively long distance away."

Three respondents reported that they found working with isolated clients to be challenging; it is hard to terminate with clients who have no local support such as nearby family members or helpful friends. For clients who do not have a support network, things can be tough for both the client and the therapist. Illustrative of this is an example of an elder who moved from an urban community where there were no available subsidized apartments to a very rural town that had a project with a vacancy. Once he moved in, the client found that he had no informal support system and that local services were not available. He eventually was forced to move back to an urban city when an apartment opened for him.

Impact of rurality on quality of life for elders. Rural social work practice with elder residents of specialized housing programs calls for special sensitivity with regard to understanding rural culture–a culture in which values of self-reliance and personal independence are strongly held. Many long-term rural elder citizens are conditioned to think that there are no resources that could help them and they must take care of themselves on their own. They may define the prospect of professional mental health treatment as something very unfamiliar and perhaps intimidating.

Informants reported that congregate and supportive housing can provide a sense of security to clients which may allow for deeper clinical work than was possible previously. A common finding among the geriatric caseworkers interviewed was that many older women clients from rural areas have been exposed to years of physical and emotional abuse. Living in a supportive housing facility may give older clients the security to accept help in dealing with deep-seeded issues for which they are seeking closure. One practitioner intervened in a case where adult children were pressuring their mother for money to support their substance abuse. The social worker helped the mother to find an apartment in a subsidized multi-unit senior housing project that gave her a sense of security to say no to her children because the entrance doors were kept locked.

Elders aging in place in a rural apartment building with no on site staff can experience anxiety over declining health. One resident expressed this anxiety with repeated calls to 911 for transport to a medical facility. The social worker was able to work with the elder client by reaching out and involving her son. The son found an adult day center that his mother could attend that provided support during the day including medication administration and social activities.

Potential functions and roles for rural social workers in elder facilities. Social workers can provide valuable consultation services to housing staff in understanding resident needs such as recognizing depression, how to make appropriate referrals, and understanding behaviors.

Common referral sources are administrators of housing programs who are seeking help dealing with resident behaviors. In one such case the social worker was referred to work with a resident who had been found smoking in bed on repeated occasions. The administrator had given a final warning that one more incident would lead to eviction. The worker met with staff and made several visits with the client and then met with the family. Social work intervention led to understanding that this behavior occurred when the client felt ignored by family and that she was seeking a closer relationship with certain family members. Work with the client to identify appropriate ways to have increased family contact and more effective relationships, and with the family to help sensitize them to the client's needs, resulted in behavior changes.

Innovations in their practice related to working with elders and housing in rural areas. The multiplicity of challenges that may present in rural settings calls for social workers to be imaginative in their work.

Often this may mean stepping out of the bounds of normal protocols to establish trust with the client. One practitioner discovered that accepting a client's offer of tea or coffee or even a small meal has helped to establish a partnership relationship that has allowed the client to move forward. Whenever possible, flexibility is the key. Doing favors, such as picking up a prescription at the pharmacy for a resident needing medication and having no other way to obtain it, can help build trust.

One therapist found that he had three clients with a similar mental health diagnosis who each held the idea that his or her problems were unique and that no one else could face the same difficulties. To help the three clients find a sense of mutual support and ultimately a sense of empowerment, he plans to bring them together in a confidential location so that they can share their stories, a strategy that has worked successfully for rural community support professionals from another discipline in the area.

One veteran geriatric social worker has turned from her casework therapy practice to organize a new complementary therapy and life enrichment program. After many years of supervising community support and geriatric services programs, the clinician added to her skill base by becoming a licensed massage therapist. Working from the perspective of practicing both as a social work clinician and massage therapist gave her the insight that healing involves the physical, psychological, and spiritual self. The complementary therapies program will connect clients with services such as massage, healing touch and other modalities. Eventually it will be expanded to make these services available to residents of rural housing settings.

POLICY IMPLICATIONS AND PRACTICE GUIDELINES

Helping rural elders to remain as autonomous as possible while still providing safe and secure housing environments can be challenging when housing options are scarce. Social workers in rural areas are often faced with three less than perfect options to offer their clients: remain at home with inadequate supports and home modifications; move to a nursing facility which may unduly compromise autonomy; or leave the area to find more suitable supportive housing. Increasing the availability of low-income congregate and supportive housing in rural areas, as well as the availability of in-home community based care, would allow rural elders more opportunity to reach a natural equilibrium between autonomy and security.

Empowerment-oriented social work involves mobilizing resources and advocating for clients; this is difficult to do in areas where resources are scarce and transportation services are nearly nonexistent. While innovative practitioners may be able to draw on natural support systems and help to create self-help networks–which conceivably could utilize the telephone and even the Internet for much of their communication–ultimately the problem of transportation will surface. Even rural elders in supportive housing need opportunities to leave their homes in order to see old friends, who also may not drive; to go on recreational outings; to shop for necessities; and to get to health appointments. Augmenting existing programs–such as the Senior Companion Program, a federal program supporting low-income senior volunteers who provide companionship and assistance to frail elders–and creating new ones that increase transportation opportunities for rural elders, are important policy interventions, which will aid in preventing loss of autonomy for elders.

The rural social workers interviewed for this chapter mentioned frequently that they had the most liberty to practice client empowerment and service innovation when they were on grant funded projects. Current Medicaid and Medicare funding for social work services is quite constrained. Similar to funding for social work services with other age groups, the focus tends to be crisis oriented and based on a medical model. Funding for more preventative and holistic work would allow rural geriatric social workers to be more creative and empowering in their work with clients.

Despite the restrictive funding streams and the scarce resources available to their clients, the expert social work informants cited here demonstrated creativity and caring in their work with rural elders in specialized housing. Several practice guidelines can be identified from their narratives:

- Take time to develop trust and to understand the client's definition of the problem. This may involve learning to understand a unique rural culture if the practitioner is "from away."
- Work closely with housing staff so that they understand what social workers can provide and so they can facilitate social work interventions.
- Remember that elders are never too old to change, to examine family issues, and to work at resolving past trauma. When they are comfortable with their housing, elders may be more ready to take other personal issues.

- Group work, whether therapeutic or self-help, is an important tool for reducing the isolation characteristic of rural environments.
- Be vigilant in examining the tension between autonomy and security when clients ask that specific information not be divulged to housing staff. Seek peer support and advice when necessary.

Ultimately, social work practice with rural elders in specialized housing must be client-centered and strengths-based.

There are many gaps in the long-term care and specialized housing systems in this country; these are particularly evident in rural areas. Some would say that we are facing a crisis in long-term care and that change and innovation are inevitable. Kane, Kane, and Ladd (1998) outline a list of principles for change, which can be used as guideposts in determining whether future developments in long-term care and specialized housing are moving in a positive direction. Two of these principles will serve as closing thoughts in our discussion regarding social work practice and specialized housing for elders in rural areas.

> Long-term care programs need to be developed in a way that preserves the dignity and autonomy of those who need long-term care and that allows them to live out their lives in as meaningful a way as possible within their families and communities. . . . The good long-term care system has options. Consumer choice is an empty slogan if there is no menu to choose from. These options should include a wide range of ways to get service in one's own home and a wide range of residential settings where services can be efficiently received. Consumer direction is important regardless of where the consumer lives and whether the consumer is receiving care from an agency or an independently employed worker. (p. 303)

These principles should serve to both guide our policy advocacy for future program development and our current practice with rural elders.

REFERENCES

Bolda, E.J., Salley, S.T., Keith, R.G., Richards, M.F., Turyn, R.M., & Dempsey, P. (2000). *Creating affordable rural housing with services: Options and strategies.* Portland, ME: Maine Rural Health Research Center.

Cox, E.O., & Parsons, R.J. (1994). *Empowerment-oriented social work practice with the elderly.* Pacific Grove, CA: Brooks/Cole Publishing Company.

Cvitkovich, Y., & Wister, A. (2001). A comparison of four person-environment fit models applied to older adults. In L.A. Pastalass, & B. Schwarz (Eds.) *Housing choices and well-being of older adults: Proper fit* (pp. 1-25). New York: The Haworth Press, Inc.

Ginsberg, L.H. (1998). Introduction: An overview of rural social work. In L.H. Ginsberg (Ed.) *Social work in rural communities* (3rd ed., pp. 3-22). Alexandria, VA: Council on Social Work Education.

Golant, S.M., & LaGreca, A.J. (1994). City-suburban, metro-nonmetro, and regional differences in the housing quality of U.S. elderly households. *Research on Aging, 16*(3), 322-346.

Hallman, B.C., & Joseph, A.E. (1997). Housing the rural elderly: A place for Abbeyfield? *Journal of Housing for the Elderly, 12*(1/2), 83-103.

Hooyman, N.R., & Kiyak, H.A. (2002). *Social gerontology: A multidisciplinary perspective* (6th ed.). Boston: Allyn and Bacon.

Kane, R.A., Kane, R.L., & Ladd, R.C. (1988). *The heart of long-term care.* New York: Oxford University Press.

Krout, J.A. (2001). Community services and housing for rural elders. *The Public Policy & Aging Report, 2*(1), 6-8.

Lawton, M.P., & Nahemow, L. (1973). Ecology and the aging process. In C. Eisdorfer, & M.P. Lawton (Eds.) *The psychology of adult development and aging* (pp. 619-674). Washington, DC: American Psychology Association.

Lazere, E.B., Leonard, P.A., & Kravitz, L.L. (19889). *The other housing crisis: Sheltering the poor in rural America.* Washington DC: Center on Budget and Policy Priorities.

Norris-Baker, C., & Scheidt, R.J. (1994). From 'our town' to 'ghost town': The changing context of home for rural elders. *International Journal of Aging and Human Development, 38*(3), 181-202.

Parmelee, P.A., & Lawton, M.P. (1990). The design of special environments for the aged. In J.E. Birren, & K.W. Schaie (Eds.) *Handbook of the psychology of aging* (3rd ed., pp. 464-488). San Diego, CA: Academic Press.

Prosper, V., & Clark, S. (1994). Housing American's rural elderly. In J.A. Krout (Ed.) *Providing community-based services to the rural elderly* (pp. 133-155). Thousands Oaks, CA: Sage.

Pynoos, J., & Golant, S. (1996). Housing and living arrangements for the elderly. In R.H. Binstock, & L.K. George *Handbook of aging and the social sciences* (4th ed., pp. 303-324). San Diego: Academic Press.

Schafer, R. (2000). *Housing America's seniors.* Cambridge, MA: Joint Center for Housing Studies of Harvard University.

Chapter 15

Ethical Practice Issues in Rural Perspective

Tara C. Healy, PhD

SUMMARY. Community context has been viewed for more than two decades as the central organizing frame for rural social work practice. Ethical decision-making is complicated by multiple relationships with colleagues, caregiving family members, and elders that are common in rural areas. In order to address these complex situations, a model for multilevel contextual ethical analysis is proposed. The assumption that moral deliberations are based in social relationships is the foundation for contextual ethical analysis. An expanded unit of analysis that includes considering the influence of multiple persons and institutions at multiple levels is an integral part of contextual ethical analysis that supports social workers' efforts to equalize power. Engagement in consciousness raising concerning ethical dimensions of the links between private troubles and public policies is essential. Ethically responsible practice thus includes identifying the ethical foundation for collective political action that promotes social and economic justice by expanding available options when readily available solutions are unjust. *[Article copies available for a fee from The Haworth Document Delivery Service: 1-800-HAWORTH. E-mail address: <docdelivery@haworthpress.com> Website: <http://www.HaworthPress.com> © 2003 by The Haworth Press, Inc. All rights reserved.]*

[Haworth co-indexing entry note]: "Ethical Practice Issues in Rural Perspective." Healy, Tara C. Co-published simultaneously in *Journal of Gerontological Social Work* (The Haworth Social Work Practice Press, an imprint of The Haworth Press, Inc.) Vol. 41, No. 3/4, 2003, pp. 265-285; and: *Gerontological Social Work in Small Towns and Rural Communities* (ed: Sandra S. Butler, and Lenard W. Kaye) The Haworth Social Work Practice Press, an imprint of The Haworth Press, Inc., 2003, pp. 265-285. Single or multiple copies of this article are available for a fee from The Haworth Document Delivery Service [1-800-HAWORTH, 9:00 a.m. - 5:00 p.m. (EST). E-mail address: docdelivery@haworthpress.com].

http://www.haworthpress.com/web/JGSW
© 2003 by The Haworth Press, Inc. All rights reserved.
Digital Object Identifier: 10.1300/J083v41n03_05

KEYWORDS. Ethical practice, rural practice, elders

INTRODUCTION

Community context has been viewed for more than two decades as the central organizing frame for rural social work practice (Ginsberg, 2000; Martinez-Brawley, 1980a, 1985, 2000; Martinez-Brawley & Carlton, 1982; Sundet & Mermelstein, 1983; Waltman, 1986). In fact, "fitting into" the community has been emphasized in guidance offered to social workers planning to practice in rural communities (Ginsberg, 2000; Schmidt, 2000). Moreover, social workers practicing in rural communities are highly visible members of rural communities and are typically engaged in multiple community roles within multiple systems (Miller, 2000). Given the multiple roles social workers assume within rural communities, they should consider themselves as "moral citizens" of their shared communities (Manning, 1997). The communities themselves may be considered moral units just as families are "moral communities" (Fleck-Henderson, 1998). Thus the ethical dimensions of rural social work with community-dwelling elders are inextricably entwined with community context.

In this chapter, I will propose that rural social workers' ethical deliberations should be based on contextual ethical analysis. The assumption that moral deliberations are based in social relationships (Walker, 1998) is the foundation for contextual ethical analysis. A central feature of this model involves considering the influence of the multiple relationships that are common in rural communities. Furthermore, practitioners' integration of generalist multilevel strategies is a necessary component of ethical deliberation in the proposed model of analysis. The conscious equalizing of power (Allen, 1987) wielded by multiple persons and institutions involved with community-dwelling elders is thus assumed to be a major tenet of ethically responsible practice in the rural context. The conceptual foundation for the model of contextual ethical analysis presented in this chapter is derived from an analysis of the literature, social work practice, and research in three rural states (Healy, 1999b; Healy, in press).

First I will discuss the major ethical concepts and concerns pertinent to social work with community-dwelling elders in rural communities. These include the concepts of autonomy and beneficence and concerns about decisional capacity. I will address characteristics of rural communities that influence ethical decision-making including the prevalence of multiple relationships, poverty, and diversity. Next, the tenets of generalist empowerment practice in rural communities will be presented in relationship to contextual ethical analysis. Then contextual ethical analysis will be described using specific examples. In conclusion, I will propose a set of guidelines that may facilitate the implementation of contextual ethical analysis in every day practice with community-dwelling elders in rural communities.

ETHICAL CONCEPTS AND CONCERNS IN RURAL PRACTICE WITH COMMUNITY-DWELLING ELDERS

The "everyday" ethical dimensions involved in social work practice with community-dwelling elders are not as dramatic as the life and death issues typically addressed in bioethics (Kaufman, 1995). Because "everyday ethics" are subtle and pervasive (Egan & Kadushin, 1999), it is essential that social workers be keenly aware of them or "run the risk of having their ethical ideals gradually eroded without realizing how or when this erosion took place" (Rhodes, 1986, p. xii). Miller (2000) points out that the social work literature has not addressed the subtle everyday ethical tensions faced by social workers practicing in rural contexts. Many of these subtle issues may infringe on frail elders' autonomy but may escape the consciousness of social workers who are responding to seemingly more urgent situations in their practice. Although there is an extensive literature emerging concerning everyday ethical tensions faced in social work practice with community dwelling elders (Clemens, Welte, Feltes, Crabtree, & Dubitzky, 1994; Collopy, Dubler, & Zuckerman, 1990; Healy, 1998; Healy, 1999a; Healy, in press; Kane, Penrod, & Kivnick, 1993), these tensions have not been addressed with regard to a rural context of practice.

Autonomy in Rural Communities

As in much of the literature, autonomy and self-determination will be used interchangeably in this chapter. Autonomy is generally defined as the right of individuals or communities to freedom of choice and action concerning various aspects of life (Collopy, 1988; Lynn, 1990). The rugged individualism noted by social workers practicing in rural communities (Gumpert, Saltman, & Sauer-Jones, 2000) parallels the emphasis on support for autonomy in the gerontological literature (Healy, 1998; Healy, 1999a) and on self-determination in the social work literature (Holland &

Kilpatrick, 1991; NASW, 2000; Spicker, 1990). Martinez-Brawley emphasized that rural communities should be self-determining, especially in relation to state and federal policy mandates (1980b). Lynn (1990) notes that it is imperative that social workers acknowledge, work with and reflect the value and knowledge base of the local people (p.16). Today the strengths perspective that has been infused in generalist practice reflects this right of individuals and communities to define and direct problem solving (Miley, O'Melia, & DuBois, 1998).

The distinction between positive and negative autonomy warrants attention (Collopy, 1988). It is common for social workers to think of support of self-determination in terms of negative autonomy, the right to noninterference, to be left alone. But positive autonomy involves the right to the assistance needed to act autonomously. Thus positive autonomy and social and economic justice can be viewed as related concepts. The prevalence of poverty in rural communities in general and among elders of color in particular raises the issue of justice because elders with financial means have long been able to enhance their own autonomy by purchasing needed services. Furthermore, elders have reported a consciousness that financial means is important to maintaining freedom in old age (Horowitz, Silverstone, & Reinhardt, 1991).

Beneficence in Rural Communities

Beneficence, the duty to take action to benefit others, and autonomy are often competing ethical principles in the experience of practitioners responding to the needs of community-dwelling elders (Healy, 1998). This tension between beneficence and autonomy involves practitioners' concern about the safety of elders in contrast to elders' self-determination, the right to define the acceptable level of safety risk (Healy, in press). Because the ethic of care, which is grounded in beneficence, is a foundational value of the social work profession (Baines, 1991), moral pain often arises when social workers are faced with situations in which their own perception of a client's safety is in conflict with that client's wishes or when scarce resources result in unfair choices for elders.

Safety is most often related to the risk of physical harm that could result in exacerbation of illness, suffering, or death (Healy, 1998). As will be discussed later in this chapter, safety risk is often the result of unmet care needs and unsafe housing in rural areas. Practitioners who work with community-dwelling elders have consistently been found to be strongly influenced by safety issues (Clemens et al., 1994; Healy, in press; Kane et al., 1993). Even when practitioners state that they highly value self-determination, safety often takes precedence in their practice decisions (Clemens et al., 1994; Healy, in press; Kane et al., 1993). Thus there may be a bias towards overriding elders' wishes in support of safety that must be questioned methodically.

Decisional Capacity

Because of the possibility of bias toward ensuring safety, practitioners must also guard against assuming impaired decisional capacity on the part of an elder when there exists disagreement concerning acceptable safety risk. Social workers' evaluation of decisional capacity is inextricably linked to support of autonomy (Healy, 1998). In the literature concerning ethical decision-making, it is accepted that an elder must lack the decisional capacity to make a specific decision in order for the principle of beneficence to take precedence over autonomy (Egan & Kadushin, 1999; NASW, 2000). Because cognitive impairment, which is the basis for evaluating decisional capacity (Willis, 1991), strongly influences an elder's ability to remain in the community, the importance of these evaluations cannot be minimized (Aronson & Shiffman, 1995). Kapp (1995) notes that gerontological social workers usually act independently and lack legal sanction for their assessments concerning the decisional capacities of elders. Furthermore, the ongoing collaborative relationships of rural social workers add to the pressure to perceive impaired decisional capacity when elders and others in the community disagree.

Multiple Relationships in Rural Communities

Multiple or dual relationships are defined in the National Association of Social Workers Code of Ethics (NASW, 2000) as occurring when "social workers relate to clients in more than one relationship, whether professional, social or business. Dual or multiple relationships can occur simultaneously or consecutively" (section 1.06). Rural practitioners' multiple relationships with colleagues pose challenges regarding conflict of interest, maintaining the primacy of clients' wishes, and maintaining privacy and confidentiality. In rural areas, the lack of anonymity for residents and social workers has been noted by social workers from Canada (Delaney, Brownlee, Sellick, & Tranter, 1997) and Australia (Lynn, 1990) as well as the United States (Coward, DeWeaver, Schmidt, & Jackson, 1983; Miller, 2000). This visibility and lack of privacy in rural areas has been cited as a central challenge to social workers with regard to attempts to avoid dual or multiple relationships (Miller, 2000) and in maintaining confidentiality (Delaney et al., 1997; Honour,

1979). Practice with community-dwelling elders involves collaborative relationships with multiple persons, both within and outside the community (Collopy et al., 1990; Kapp, 1995); these collaborative relationships form an integral part of community context for rural social workers. Moreover, these multiple relationships among colleagues are normative in many rural communities.

The gerontological literature has grappled with the competing autonomy needs of the multiple persons typically involved in the lives of community-dwelling frail elders (Collopy et al., 1990; Kapp, 1995). Kapp (1995) notes that for gerontological social workers serving community-dwelling elders, the participation of family caregivers is "pragmatically unavoidable" (p. 38). Generally the competing needs of family caregivers can be compelling (Collopy et al., 1990; Kapp, 1995), often raising questions concerning the primacy of elderly clients (Abramson, 1988; Clemens et al., 1994). Furthermore, collaborative relationships with professionals are central to gerontological social work (Bywaters, 1986). Thus social workers in rural communities often confront different perspectives held by professionals, community members, elders, and their family members concerning how problems are defined and ideas for solving those problems.

Elders, family caregivers, and professionals typically rank values differently (McCullough, Wilson, Teasdale, Kolpakchi, & Skelly, 1993). These differences in values cannot be ignored by social workers who practice with community-dwelling elders because they typically collaborate with many persons (Kapp, 1995). When social workers engage in ongoing collaborative relationships, as they do in rural communities (Miller, 2000), their investment in reaching an agreement may be great (Fisher, Ury, & Patton, 1991). Thus, in rural communities, the desire to please colleagues may influence ethical decision-making (Abelson & Levi, 1998; Miller, 2000). An unconscious tendency to agree with opinions of colleagues over those of elders may indeed lead social workers to compromise their own ethical values. Therefore social workers have an ethical obligation to equalize power when there are disagreements among persons holding vastly different degrees of power (Allen, 1987). Typically elders hold the least power in these situations. Family members wield more power than elders, and professionals typically wield more power than family members.

Poverty in Rural Communities

As social workers prepare to address the ethical challenges involved in practice with an expanding cohort of older adults living in rural communities, they need to consider the unique characteristics of these communities. Although Mermelstein and Sundet (2000) contend that the differences between characteristics of rural and urban communities have diminished over the past twenty years, others hold that lack of access to transportation and key health and social services persist to a great degree in rural areas (Coward & Dwyer, 2000; Gumpert et al., 2000; Stunkel, 1997). Krout (1994) notes that elders living in rural communities tend to "have access to a smaller number of and a narrower range of community-based services" and that "clear gaps exist in the continuum of care in rural communities" (p. 70).

Lack of access to health care and home-based community services may lead to premature institutionalization for frail elders living in rural communities (Shaughnessy, 1994). In addition, this lack of access to services may result in unmet care needs that create physically unsafe situations for frail community-dwelling elders (Healy, 1999a). In some situations, safety risk may be caused by inadequate home repair (Coward, McLaughlin, Duncan, & Bull, 1994). Moreover, some rural elders lack access to water and sewerage (Ohio University, 1993). Rural elders have been found to be reluctant to spend their limited resources to make home modifications that would increase safety or reduce the likelihood of falling in their homes (Isberner, Ritzel, Sarvela, Brown, Hu, & Newbolds, 1998). Thus safety risk related to both unmet care needs caused by limited access to services and to lack of safe housing may raise complex ethical issues for rural social workers (Healy, 1999b; Isberner et al., 1998; Macey & Schneider, 1993).

One ethical pitfall for rural practitioners is that decisions might be made based on a bias towards safety without examining whether or not unjust social policies are the root cause of the tension between supporting safety over elders' self-determination. While social workers helping individual elders and their families must address immediate care needs, they must also meet their ethical obligation to work toward social justice.

Poverty itself raises ethical concerns; indeed, poverty among rural elders is greater than among elderly living in metropolitan areas (Coward et al., 1994). As noted earlier, elders who have financial means have always been able to enhance their own autonomy in contrast to poor elders whose autonomy is systematically constrained due to poverty. The common resistance to spending financial resources for assistance may well be related to the lean personal resources available to rural elders. Moreover, elders of color disproportionately experience insufficient economic resources in rural communities (Beckett & Dungee-Anderson, 2000). Those who have suffered chronic poverty may suffer more cumulative effects of poverty than those who have recently become poor in old age. Thus there are cumulative disparities in health status and functional autonomy related to poverty and ethnicity that may be particularly stark in rural areas.

Diversity in Rural Communities

Diversity within the elderly population continues to grow throughout the United States (Schneider, Kropf, & Kisor, 2000). This trend encompasses rural communities as well (Ginsberg, 2000; Summers, 2000). In addition, gay and lesbian elders living in rural areas continue to remain invisible in response to the powerful force of stigma within these communities. Even today, gays and lesbians lack access to many social programs available to their heterosexual counterparts (Barranti & Cohen, 2000; Smith & Mancoske, 1997). Vulnerable populations are likely to confront unique problems in rural communities because many residents in rural communities are wary of diversity (Waltman, 1986).

Although it is beyond the scope of this chapter to analyze, in depth, the particular challenges faced by diverse populations, key factors that are pertinent to contextual ethical analysis warrant consideration. For example, health beliefs and views about aging and social obligation may vary by cultural background and may dramatically influence interactions with professionals whose ethnic backgrounds differ from clients facing health challenges (Nicholson & Kay, 1999; Smith & Mancoske, 1997; Williams & Ellison, 1996). In contrast to an emphasis on individualism in rural communities, clients, families, and professionals from diverse cultural backgrounds might highly value communal decision-making and shared responsibility (Edwards, Drews, Seaman, & Edwards, 1994; Ewalt & Mokuau, 1995). This preference for communal decision-making might be missed by social workers who expect individuals to make independent decisions.

As discussed earlier, the disproportionate degree of poverty among ethnic minorities has a cumulative effect that contributes to the ethical tension concerning equitable access to health care and social services (Crystal & Shea, 1990; Summers, 2000). An example of this is that African American and Hispanic caregivers of frail elders have been found to contend with significantly greater unmet needs than their Caucasian counterparts (Navaie-Waliser, Feldman, Gould, Levine, Kuerbis, & Donelan, 2001). Generally African Americans living in rural communities have been found to "underuse" social services in Carlton-LaNey

(1991). Nonetheless, there is a great deal of diversity among African-Americans living in rural areas (Spence, 1993).The diversity within special populations must be respected as much as the differences between groups of people.

The increasing diversity within rural communities raises questions about the ethical dimensions of multicultural practice. For purposes of ethical deliberation, multiculturalism should be held as a moral virtue rather than a body of knowledge (Walker & Staton, 2000).

Given the expanding array of diversity in society today, we must begin with self-reflection in order to become "culturally responsive" (Hays, 2001). Considering multiculturalism as a virtue requires that we respect all forms of diversity. We must become aware that there are differences in moral deliberation and in ranking values that must be included in our dialogue with elders, families, and colleagues.

GENERALIST EMPOWERMENT PRACTICE IN RURAL COMMUNITIES

Ginsberg notes that generalist practice, that has now gained broad acceptance in social work, originated in rural practice (Ginsberg, 2000). Besides responding to individual and family suffering, generalist practice requires that we address the contextual conditions that create or contribute to that suffering (Gibbs, Locke, & Lohmann, 1990). Thus generalist practitioners intervene through multiple modalities at multiple levels and are skilled in both micro and macro practice.

Martinez-Brawley not only embraced the goodness-of-fit of generalist practice for social workers in rural communities but also promoted empowerment (Lynn, 1990; Martinez-Brawley, 1980b, 1983). Rural social workers should be aware that there are ethical dimensions to be considered at all levels of generalist empowerment practice. Martinez-Brawley's tenets of empowerment may be familiar to social workers embracing more recent versions of empowerment practice (Cox & Parsons, 1994; Gutierrez, Parsons, & Cox, 1998; Lee, 1994). The three tenets of empowerment practice in rural communities include: (1) Empowerment practice requires an emphasis on autonomy and strengths of individuals and communities and views individuals and communities as capable of defining and identifying the means of resolving problem situations. Social workers have a responsibility to give immediate attention to individual, family, group, and community suffering and unmet needs. (2) The second tenet holds that consciousness-raising should be promoted. Conscious awareness of social and economic injustice should be facilitated through a process of linking political and societal forces to present conditions. (3) Political action is the third tenet that follows consciousness raising. After linking political and societal forces to present conditions, collective political action should be taken in order to influence attitudes and change laws, policies, and procedures that perpetuate social and economic injustice at local, state, federal and global levels. Building on this base, rural practitioners are urged to adopt a contextual approach to practice that integrates the "analysis of power relations embedded in clients' everyday environments" (Kemp, Whittaker, & Tracy, 2002). Furthermore, I propose that ethical deliberation must be intertwined with this power analysis and that social workers practicing in rural communities must consider the ethical ramifications of their action or lack of action at all three levels of empowerment generalist practice.

CONTEXTUAL ETHICAL ANALYSIS

Although social work has always been practiced within a moral context, the manner in which we view this context has changed over time (Baines, 1991). Over a decade ago Goldstein (1987) called on social work to address its "neglected moral link." Recently, Reamer (2000) notes that our profession has moved from a focus on the morality of clients to a concern about our own ethical decision-making to our current efforts to establish standards and respond to liability concerns. In light of the increasing acceptance of generalist practice at both foundation and advanced levels (Gibbs et al., 1990; Miley et al., 1998) and as particularly suitable for rural practice (Ginsberg, 2000), reconsideration of our ethical deliberation as generalist practitioners is warranted.

Contextual ethical analysis is grounded on the assumption that moral deliberations are based in social relationships (Walker, 1998). Pertinent to the ethical deliberations of social workers is Walker's contention that "the resolution of a moral problem may be less like . . . the answer to a question than like the outcome of a negotiation" (p. 70). A key factor to remember is that the meaning and ranking of values among persons involved in these negotiations may differ greatly (Ewalt & Mokuau, 1995; McCullough et al., 1993). Thus to consider multiple perspectives is to consider differences in values and especially the ranking of values. How important is physical safety to all those involved? How important is individual freedom? How important are the obligations to care for one another? Culture, position, and power may greatly influence how one responds to these questions.

As noted at the beginning of this chapter, rural social workers are "moral citizens" (Manning, 1997) of communities they serve. Manning defines moral citizenship as "the responsibility to determine right and good behavior as part of the rights and privileges social workers have as members of a community that includes clients, colleagues, agencies, and society" (p. 224). Although practitioners' ethical deliberations focus on what makes one course of social work action morally superior to another (Rhodes, 1986), the moral perspectives of those involved in multilevel generalist assessments are important to consider. For example, the perspectives of care receivers, formal and informal caregivers, and agency-based professionals are all distinct. The stance of a particular state or community agency is represented by individuals who hold their own points of view concerning agency policies, about the moral obligations of society and family members, and about the importance of self-determination. However, we often neglect the moral pain of the persons we serve (Marin, 1981). Social workers must be able to explore diverse moral perspectives in order to decide on an ethical course of action that respects the moral pain of all persons involved. The intense feelings caregivers and professionals bring to the decision-making process are often related to the unspoken moral dimensions of those decisions.

Just as ethical dimensions of practice cannot be separated from practice choices at the micro level (Dean & Rhodes, 1992), the ethical dimensions of multilevel practice cannot be separated from our analysis and action plans. I propose that the unit of analysis for contextual ethical deliberation be expanded to reflect multilevel generalist empowerment-oriented practice. Thus, families (Fleck-Henderson, 1998) and whole communities are viewed as moral units. This means that social workers must consider the ethical implications of policies and procedures at all levels of government in addition to the ethical implications of actions taken with individuals, families, and groups.

Multiple Relationships

The ongoing nature of multiple relationships with neighbors, family members and professionals may complicate social workers' ethical deliberations. These ongoing personal and professional relationships may be viewed as "extra-ethical" factors that influence ethical decision-making (Kugelman, 1992). Social workers are likely to find agreement with persons with whom they are engaged in multiple relationships rather than advocate for a client's position that may differ greatly (Fisher et al., 1991). Because maintaining strong collaborative relationships with other health and social service providers and with key community leaders is integral to rural social work, practitioners are urged to consider how these relationships may be influencing their judgments and actions. How might these ongoing relationships be related to ethical dimensions of practice decision-making? A key question is whether or not practitioners are being unduly dissuaded from advocating for clients in order to reach agreement with other professionals.

Neighbors. Neighbors may become concerned when an individual appears to have neglected hygiene or an elder's home is not maintained in an acceptable manner. Such circumstances may be complicated when social workers have ongoing relationships with clients' neighbors. In a recent study concerning the ethical tensions experienced by rural social workers, one observed:

> The neighbors and church members have [complained] that [their neighbor] . . . is often unkempt . . . She seems to have plenty of food in the house; she hasn't fallen, and she wants to stay there. Her attitude is that if I'm dead I'm dead . . . She doesn't mind the idea . . . that her body might not be found for several days. But her neighbors mind. (Informant quoted in Healy, 1999b)

If a social worker attends the same church as the neighbors who are complaining, she may experience increased pressure to limit her advocacy for an elder's right to self-determination. When neighbors complain about the upkeep of an elder's home, we must raise questions about poverty and economic justice. Expanding the unit of ethical analysis would bring us to critique the lack of public policies that adequately support home repair for low-income elders.

Family members. As noted earlier, social workers routinely collaborate with family members. Abramson (1988) found that social workers tend to spend more time with family members in care planning than with decisionally capable elders. In rural areas, social workers may also be engaged in social relationships with their age peers who are likely to be family caregivers. The presence of dual or multiple relationships with family caregivers may reinforce workers' identification with caregivers' ideas, making it more difficult for social workers to support elders' perspectives when they disagree. In these ethically complex situations, it is most important that social workers be aware of their biases

(Abramson, 1996) and make every effort to equalize the power among those participating in the decision-making process (Allen, 1987).

Health and social service professionals. Disagreements between elders and health care providers can prompt questions about elders' decisional capacity. In a recent study, one social worker noted: "If . . . they are not going to comply . . . that sets in motion this concern for their decision-making abilities" (Healy, 2000). This observation supports Ryden's (1993) view that questions about decisional capacity are usually raised when clients choose a course of action that differs from what medical providers or family members consider to be in their best interest. Although social workers have a clear ethical obligation to equalize the power imbalance in such situations (Allen, 1987), the ethical tensions they experience may be acute. Contextual ethical analysis would lead social workers to question the relationship between the disagreement and the request for evaluation of decisional capacity as a way of beginning a dialogue and engaging in negotiation (Walker, 1998).

Medical providers may exert pressure on social workers when they perceive that elders are not taking medication as prescribed (Healy, in press). Because of ranking values differently, it is possible in such a situation that the physician and the elder differ concerning both problem definition and preferred solution (McCullough et al., 1993). For example, the physician may consider longevity important and a client may find that unpleasant side effects are not worth the promised increased life expectancy. Furthermore, cultural differences concerning the role of western medicine in healing must be considered when the refusal to follow a medical regime is at the heart of pressure to rank beneficence over self-determination (Applewhite, 1995).

Social and Economic Justice

Ethical sensitivity to context requires the inclusion of an analysis of agency, local, state, and federal policies and procedures within the ethical unit of analysis. For example, an elder described by Miller (2000) can no longer manage the physical labor necessary for her to load her wood stove that she uses to heat her home over the winter. The choice discussed with the social worker was to find a way to pay for a board and care facility for the winter. Because problems with wood burning stoves often present safety problems in rural areas (Healy, 1999b), contextual ethical analysis would pose questions concerning the lack of public support to replace wood or coal burning stoves with propane stoves in rural areas. Safety problems with wood stoves may well be one of the major causes of premature institutionalization in rural areas. Therefore, social workers should press state and local policy makers to be responsive to rural needs on ethical grounds supported by concepts of positive autonomy and social justice. Thus barriers to health and social services in rural areas present ethical as well as practice challenges.

If justice is undermined by local, state and federal policies, collective political action is ethically supported. For example, while I participated in a group of social workers serving community-dwelling elders in one rural state, members noticed that barriers created by the state's system of home-based care limited their clients' self-determination. These social workers felt ethically compelled to take political action because of the unmet care needs of their clients; the ethical concept of positive autonomy requires that intrinsic limitations to autonomy created by physical challenges be balanced by equal access to social services. A similar argument for eliminating physical barriers in public accommodations helped support passage of the Americans with Disabilities Act (ADA) in 1990 (*Americans With Disabilities Act*, 1990). If economically privileged individuals and those living in urban areas have greater access to services supporting positive autonomy than do low income, rural individuals, the system of service delivery is unjust. This contextual ethical analysis prompted us, a group of direct service providers, to view the personal problems of individual clients as public issues. We then organized a statewide coalition to address the lack of access to home-based care services faced by many clients. Consciousness-raising concerning the ethical dimensions of state policies helped to gain the direct participation by elders, their families, and professionals in public discourse, politicizing the ethical issue.

CONCLUSION

I propose that we engage in ethical deliberation that is ongoing, active, and an integral part of every day practice decision-making. As visible moral citizens of the rural communities we serve (Manning, 1997), we have responsibilities to elders, families, communities, agencies, and society that may often conflict. Balancing these obligations can be very challenging. Contextual ethical analysis involves an expanded unit of analysis that includes considering the influence of multiple persons and multiple institutions at multiple levels.

Rural social workers have reported reexamining their practice choices in response to community pressure exerted by colleagues (Healy, in press). When we respond to community pressure in this way, we must consider the ethical ramifications of privileging the views of colleagues when we are engaged in ongoing and multiple relationships. These relationships may contribute to our giving more moral weight to the views of colleagues who wield greater power than the elder involved. Thus we may well augment the power of the most powerful and further silence the voices of frail elders. The possibility of privileging the powerful voices of colleagues is inherent in Ryden's (1993) point that professionals question the decisional capacity of elders when there is a disagreement concerning care planning.

In order to develop skill in contextual ethical analysis, I propose that social workers serving the needs of community-dwelling elders in rural communities begin with self-reflection concerning values, ethical principles, and diversity (Abramson, 1996; Hays, 2001). We must ask how our views are similar and different from norms in our rural communities and from those involved in decision-making with community-dwelling elders. Moreover, we must expand self-reflection to include an analysis of the influence of multiple relationships common in rural practice. As rural practitioners, we are more vulnerable to undue influence on our ethical decision-making if we are unaware of the typical wish to please colleagues with whom we have multiple and ongoing relationships (Fisher et al., 1991).

As suggested by Walker and Staton (2000), I propose that we consider multiculturalism as an ethical virtue. Thus our self-reflection must address discrimination and oppression (Hays, 2001), and our analysis of diversity becomes part of our every day ethical deliberation. Multicultural reflection for rural social workers engaged with community-dwelling elders must address the influence of ageism and ableism. The ageism inherent in weighing safety as more important for elders than for younger risk takers must be analyzed as having ethical ramifications. Self-reflection is the beginning of a process of consciousness raising for ourselves as well as with those involved in ethical dialogue. Consciousness raising should be expanded to include an analysis of multiple levels of influence over our practice choices. This means that we must become aware that the links between private troubles and public policies have ethical dimensions (e.g., lack of funding for home repair and heating system conversion in rural areas may lead to premature institutionalization). This expansive consciousness raising can help us identify the ethical foundation for collective political action that promotes social and economic justice. Clearly we are ethically bound to expand available options when readily available solutions are socially and economically unjust (Cox & Parsons, 1994).

While self-reflection serves as the foundation of ethically responsible practice, social workers must create safe environments for ethical dialogue with all involved in the problem situations confronting community-dwelling frail elders (Walker, 1993). Balancing the autonomy rights of individuals, families, and communities (Collopy et al., 1990) can be very challenging. We must begin by exploring the interests and values that form the basis of diverse perspectives. Active inquiry concerning the importance of values for all involved can set the stage for dialogue. As we do so, we must remember that elders, families, and professionals typically rank values differently (McCullough et al., 1993) and that persons from diverse cultures may also rank values differently (Ewalt & Mokuau, 1995). We must realize that we may privilege the perspectives of persons like ourselves and those with whom we are engaged in multiple and ongoing relationships. Therefore, we must seek disconfirming information when we readily reach agreement with persons with whom we have ongoing relationships. To do this, we must systematically seek information that contradicts our assumptions. It is imperative that we ask if decisional capacity is being questioned because there is a disagreement between a disempowered elder and professionals concerning the definition of a problem or the preferred solution to a problem situation (Ryden, 1993). We must also be aware that we may augment the power of those already powerful in these situations (Abramson, 1988) if we do not actively highlight the views of frail elders even when they differ from our own. Thus we must explore the point-of-view of less powerful persons and augment their voices by reiterating their perspectives in the decision-making dialogue (Allen, 1987). We must extend the dialogue to include others in designing a method for evaluating the effects of our actions; we must be prepared to reevaluate our decisions grounded in this evaluation. Once we have engaged in self-reflection and ethical dialogue, we should be prepared to articulate the ethical basis of our practice decisions regarding all three levels of generalist empowerment practice in a language that makes sense to all involved.

Ethically responsible practice requires ongoing, active ethical deliberation as an integral component of practice decision-making. A key concern for rural practitioners is the possibility that multiple relationships may influence decisions that disempower community-dwelling elders. Thus we should require ourselves to carefully examine our decisions when they differ from the wishes of elders in any way. In addition, we have an ethical obligation not to accept the limits placed on rural communities by policies that make sense in urban areas but constrain the choices of rural elders unfairly. The pursuit of social and economic justice may routinely involve collective political action if we are to effectively support the autonomy of elders living in rural communities.

REFERENCES

Abelson, R. P., & Levi, A. (1998). *Decision making and decision theory.* In G. Lindzey, & E.

Abramson, J. S. (1988). Participation of elderly patients in discharge planning: Is self-determination a reality? *Social Work, 33*(5), 443-448.

Abramson, M. (1996). Reflections on knowing oneself ethically: Toward a working framework for social work practice. *Families in Society: The Journal of Contemporary Human Services, 77*(4), 195-202.

Allen, D. (1987). Critical social theory as a model for analyzing ethical issues in family and community health. *Family Community Health, 10*(1), 63-72.

Americans With Disabilities Act. (1990). *United States Department of Justice.* Retrieved April 15, 2002, 2002, from the World Wide Web: *http://www/usdoj.gov. 80/ada/pubs/ada.txt.*

Applewhite, S. L. (1995). Curanderismo: Demystifying the health beliefs and practices of elderly Mexican Americans. *Health & Social Work, 20*(4), 247-253.

Aronson, E. (Ed.), *Handbook of social psychology theory and method* (Vol. 1, pp. 231-309). New York: Random House.

Aronson, M. K., & Shiffman, J. K. (1995). Clinical assessment in home care. *Journal of Gerontological Social Work, 24*(3/4), 213-219.

Baines, C. T. (1991). The professions and an ethic of care. In S. Neysmith (Ed.), *Women's Caring* (pp. 36-72). Toronto: McClelland & Steward.

Barranti, C. C. R., & Cohen, H. L. (2000). Lesbian and gay elders: An invisible minority. In R. L. Schneider, N. P. Kropf, & A. J. Kisor (Eds.), *Gerontological social work* (2nd ed., pp. 343-367). Belmont, CA: Brooks/Cole.

Beckett, J. O., & Dungee-Anderson, D. (2000). Older persons of color: Asian/Pacific Islander Americans, African Americans, Hispanic Americans, and American Indians. In R. L. Schneider, N. P. Kropf, & A. J. Kisor (Eds.), *Gerontological social work* (2nd ed., pp. 257-301). Belmont, CA: Brooks/Cole.

Bywaters, P. (1986). Social work and the medical profession–Arguments against unconditional collaboration. *British Journal of Social Work, 16*, 661-677.

Carlton-LaNey, I. (1991). Some considerations of rural elderly black's underuse of social services. *Journal of Gerontological Social Work, 16*(1/2), 3-17.

Clemens, E., Welte, T., Feltes, M., Crabtree, B., & Dubitzky, D. (1994). Contradictions in case management: Client-centered theory and directive practice with frail elderly. *The Journal of Aging and Health, 6*(1), 70-88.

Collopy, B., Dubler, N., & Zuckerman, C. (1990). The ethics of home care: Autonomy and accommodation. *The Hastings Report, 20*(2), 1-16.

Collopy, B. J. (1988). Autonomy in long term care: Some crucial distinctions. *The Gerontologist, 28*(Supplement), 10-17.

Coward, R. T., DeWeaver, K. L., Schmidt, F. E., & Jackson, R. W. (1983). Distinctive features of rural environments: A frame of reference for mental health practice. *International Journal of Mental Health, 12*(1-2), 3-24.

Coward, R. T., & Dwyer, J. W. (2000). The health and well-being of rural elders. In L. H. Ginsberg (Ed.), *Social work in rural communities* (3rd ed., pp. 213-232). Alexandria, VA: Council on Social Work Education.

Coward, R. T., McLaughlin, D. K., Duncan, R. P., & Bull, C. N. (1994). An overview of health and aging in rural America. In R. T. Coward, C. N. Bull, G. Kukulka, & J. M. Galliher (Eds.), *Health services for rural elders.* (pp. 1-32). New York: Spring Publishing Company.

Cox, E. O., & Parsons, T. J. (1994). *Empowerment-oriented social work practice with the elderly*. Newbury Park, CA: Sage.

Crystal, S., & Shea, D. (1990). Cumulative advantage, cumulative disadvantage, and inequality among elderly people. *The Gerontologist, 30*(4), 437-443.

Dean, R. G., & Rhodes, M. (1992). Ethical-clinical tensions in clinical practice. *Social Work, 37*(2), 128-132.

Delaney, R., Brownlee, K., Sellick, M., & Tranter, D. (1997). Ethical problems facing northern social workers. *Social Worker, 65*(3), 55-65.

Edwards, E. D., Drews, J., Seaman, J. R., & Edwards, M. E. (1994). Community organizing in support of self-determination with Native American communities. *Journal of Multicultural Social Work, 3*(4), 43-60.

Egan, M., & Kadushin, G. (1999). The social worker in the emerging field of home care: Professional activities and ethical concerns. *Health & Social Work, 24*(1), 43-55.

Ewalt, P. L., & Mokuau, N. (1995). Self-determination from a pacific perspective. *Social Work, 40*(2), 168-175.

Fisher, R., Ury, W., & Patton, B. (1991). *Getting to yes, negotiating agreement without giving in* (2nd ed.). New York: Penguin Books.

Fleck-Henderson, A. (1998). The family as moral community: A social work perspective. *Families in Society: The Journal of Contemporary Human Services, 79*(3), 233-240.

Gibbs, P., Locke, B., & Lohmann, R. (1990). Paradigm for the generalist-advanced generalist continuum. *Journal of Social Work Education, 26*(3), 232-243.

Ginsberg, L. H. (2000). Introduction: Overview of Rural Social Work. In L. H. Ginsberg (Ed.), *Social work in rural communities* (3rd ed., pp. 3-26). Alexandria, VA: Council of Social Work Education.

Goldstein, H. (1987). The neglected moral link in social work practice. *Social Work, 32*(3), 181-186.

Gumpert, J., Saltman, J. E., & Sauer-Jones, D. (2000). Toward identifying the unique characteristics of social work practice in rural areas: From the voices of practitioners. *The Journal of Baccalaureate Social Work, 6*(1), 19-35.

Gutierrez, L. M., Parsons, R. J., & Cox, E. O. (1998). *Empowerment in social work practice: A sourcebook*. Pacific Grove, CA: Brooks/Cole.

Hays, P. A. (2001). *Addressing cultural complexities in practice*. Washington, DC: American Psychological Association.

Healy, T. C. (1998). The complexity of everyday ethics in home health care: An analysis of social workers' decisions regarding frail elders' autonomy. *Social Work in Health Care, 27*(4), 19-37.

Healy, T. C. (1999a). Community-dwelling cognitively impaired frail elders: An analysis of social workers' decisions concerning support of autonomy. *Social Work in Health Care, 30*(2), 27-47.

Healy, T. C. (1999b, March). Factors influencing social workers' support of autonomy for elders experiencing cognitive impairment. Paper presented at the 45th Annual Meeting of the American Society on Aging, Orlando, FL.

Healy, T. C. (2000, March). The challenge of everyday evaluation of decisional capacity in home health care. Paper presented at the 46th Annual Meeting of the American Society on Aging, San Diego, CA.

Healy, T. C. (in press). Ethical decision-making: Pressure and uncertainty as complicating factors. *Health & Social Work.*

Holland, T. P., & Kilpatrick, A. C. (1991). Ethical issues in social work: Toward a grounded theory of professional ethics. *Social Work, 36*(2), 138-144.

Honour, R. (1979). The impact of federal policies on rural social service programs. *Human services in the rural environment, 4*(1), 12-19.

Horowitz, A., Silverstone, M., & Reinhardt, J. P. (1991). A conceptual and empirical exploration of personal autonomy issues within family caregiving relationships. *The Gerontologist, 31*(1), 23-31.

Isberner, F., Ritzel, D., Sarvela, P., Brown, K., Hu, P., & Newbolds, D. (1998). Falls of elderly rural home health clients. *Home Health Care Services Quarterly, 17*(2), 41-51.

Kane, R. A., Penrod, J. D., & Kivnick, H. Q. (1993). Ethics and case management: Preliminary results of an empirical study. In R. A. Kane, & A. L. Caplan (Eds.), *Ethical conflicts in the management of home care, the case manager's dilemma* (pp. 3-25). New York: Springer Publishing Company.

Kapp, M. B. (1995). Legal and ethical issues in home-based care. *Journal of Gerontological Social Work, 24*(3/4), 31-45.

Kaufman, S. R. (1995). Decision making, responsibility, and advocacy in geriatric medicine: Physician dilemmas with elderly in the community. *The Gerontologist, 35*(4), 481-488.

Kemp, S. P., Whittaker, J. K., & Tracy, E. M. (2002). Contextual social work practice. In K. K. Miley (Ed.), *Pathways to power: Readings in contextual social work practice* (pp. 15-34). Boston: Allyn and Bacon.

Kugelman, W. (1992). Social work ethics in the practice arena: A qualitative study. *Social Work in Health Care, 17*(4), 59-79.

Lee, J. A. B. (1994). *The empowerment approach to social work practice.* New York: Columbia University Press.

Lynn, M. (1990). Rural social work: Applying Martinez-Brawley's tenets to Gippsland. *Australian Social Work, 43*(1), 15-21.

Macey, S. M., & Schneider, D. F. (1993). Deaths from excessive heat and excessive cold among the elderly. *The Gerontologist, 33*(4), 497-500.

Manning, S. (1997). The social worker as moral citizen: Ethics in action. *Social Work, 42*(3), 223-230.

Marin, P. (1981, November). Living in moral pain. *Psychology Today*, *15*(11), 68-80.

Martinez-Brawley, E. E. (1980a). Identifying and describing the context of rural in social work. *Arete*, *6*(2), 21-32.

Martinez-Brawley, E. E. (1980b). Rural social work tenets in the United States and Latin America: A cross-cultural comparison. *Community Development Journal*, *15*(3), 167-178.

Martinez-Brawley, E. E. (1983). Rural social work, localism, the rural poor and minorities: Local participation or federal withdrawal? *Social Development Issues*, *7*(1), 20-28.

Martinez-Brawley, E. E. (1985). Rural social work as a contextual specialty: Undergraduate focus of graduate concentration? *Journal of Social Work Education*, *1985*(3), 36-42.

Martinez-Brawley, E. E. (2000). Community-oriented practice in rural social work. In L. H. Ginsberg (Ed.), *Social work in rural communities* (3rd ed., pp. 99-114). Alexandria, VA: Council of Social Work Education.

Martinez-Brawley, E. E., & Carlton, M. (1982). Systemic characteristics of the rural milieu: A review of social work related research. *Arete*, *6*(4), 23-34.

McCullough, L. B., Wilson, N. L., Teasdale, T. A., Kolpakchi, A. L., & Skelly, J. R. (1993). Mapping personal, familial, and professional values in long-term care decisions. *The Gerontologist*, *33*(3), 324-332.

Mermelstein, J., & Sundet, P. A. (2000). Rural social work is an anachronism: The perspective of twenty years of experience and debate. In L. H. Ginsberg (Ed.), *Social work in rural communities* (3rd ed., pp. 63-80). Alexandria, VA: Council on Social Work Education.

Miley, K. K., O'Melia, M., & DuBois, B. L. (1998). *Generalist social work practice, An empowering approach* (2nd ed.). Boston: Allyn and Bacon.

Miller, P. J. (2000). Dual relationships in rural practice: A dilemma of ethics and culture. In L. H. Ginsberg (Ed.), *Social work in rural communities* (3rd ed.). Alexandria, VA: Council on Social Work Education.

National Association of Social Workers (NASW). (2000). *Code of ethics of the National Association of Social Workers*. Washington, DC: Author.

Navaie-Waliser, M., Feldman, P. H., Gould, D. A., Levine, C., Kuerbis, A. N., & Donelan, K. (2001). The experiences and challenges of informal caregivers: Common themes and differences among whites, blacks, and Hispanics. *The Gerontologist*, *41*(6), 733-741.

Nicholson, B. L., & Kay, D. M. (1999). Group treatment of traumatized Cambodian women: A culture-specific approach. *Social Work*, *44*(5), 470-479.

Ohio University. (1993). *Rural communities: Legacy and change: Capacity to care* [video]. S. Burlington: Ohio University and the Rural Clearinghouse at Kansas State University: Author.

Reamer, F. G. (2000). The social work ethics audit: A risk-management strategy. *Social Work*, *45*(4), 355-366.

Rhodes, M. L. (1986). *Ethical dilemmas in social work practice*. Milwaukee, Wisconsin: Family Service of America.

Ryden, M. (1993). Clinical determination of competency and existential advocacy. In A. Caplan (Ed.), *Ethical conflicts in the management of home care* (pp. 68-75). New York: Springer.

Schmidt, G. G. (2000). Remote, northern communities. *International Social Work, 43*(3), 337-349.
Schneider, R. L., Kropf, N. P., & Kisor, A. J. (Eds.). (2000). *Gerontological social work* (2nd. ed.). Belmont, CA: Brooks/Cole.
Shaughnessy, P. W. (1994). Changing institutional long-term care to improve rural health care. In J. M. Galliher (Ed.), *Health services for rural elders* (pp. 144-181). New York: Springer Publishing Company.
Smith, J. D., & Mancoske, R. J. (1997). *Rural gays and lesbians: Building on the strengths of communities.* New York: Harrington Park Press.
Spence, S. A. (1993). Rural elderly African Americans and service delivery: A study of health and social services needs and service accessibility. *Journal of Gerontological Social Work, 20*(3/4), 187-202.
Spicker, P. (1990). Social work and self-determination. *British Journal of Social Work, 20*, 221-236.
Stunkel, E. (1997). Rural public transportation and the mobility of older persons: Paradigms for policy. *Journal of Aging & Social Policy, 9*(3), 67-85.
Summers, G. F. (2000). Minorities in rural society. In L. H. Ginsberg (Ed.), *Social Work in Rural Communities* (3rd ed., pp. 165-175). Alexandria, VA: Council on Social Work Education.
Sundet, P. A., & Mermelstein, J. (1983). The meaning of community in rural mental health. *International Journal of Mental Health, 12*(1-2), 25-44.
Walker, M. U. (1993). Keeping moral space open: New images of ethics consulting. *Hasting Center Report, 23*, 33-40.
Walker, M. U. (1998). *Moral understandings: A feminist study in ethics.* New York: Routledge.
Walker, R., & Staton, M. (2000). Multiculturalism in social work ethics. *Journal of Social Work Education, 36*(3), 449-462.
Waltman, G. H. (1986). Main street revisited: Social work practice in rural areas. *Social Casework: The Journal of Contemporary Social Work, 67* (8), 466-473.
Williams, E. E., & Ellison, F. (1996). Culturally informed social work practice with American Indian clients: Guidelines for non-Indian social workers. *Social Work, 41*(2), 147-151.
Willis, S. L. (Ed.). (1991). *Cognition and everyday competence* (Vol. 11). New York: Springer Publishing Co.

SECTION V
LOOKING AHEAD: TRAINING AND POLICY RECOMMENDATIONS

Chapter 16

Future Training and Education Recommendations for Rural Gerontological Social Workers

Nancy P. Kropf, PhD

SUMMARY. With the increasing number of older adults, social work students need to be prepared to work with this population in a variety of settings. Rural areas may have high concentrations of older adults including those who age-in-place, and those who relocate to retirement areas in small towns and rural communities. Within the curriculum, content on health care, economics, and leadership/decision making need to be included to prepare students for practice in these areas. In addition,

[Haworth co-indexing entry note]: "Future Training and Education Recommendations for Rural Gerontological Social Workers." Kropf, Nancy P. Co-published simultaneously in *Journal of Gerontological Social Work* (The Haworth Social Work Practice Press, an imprint of The Haworth Press, Inc.) Vol. 41, No. 3/4, 2003, pp. 287-299; and: *Gerontological Social Work in Small Towns and Rural Communities* (ed: Sandra S. Butler, and Lenard W. Kaye) The Haworth Social Work Practice Press, an imprint of The Haworth Press, Inc., 2003, pp. 287-299. Single or multiple copies of this article are available for a fee from The Haworth Document Delivery Service [1-800-HAWORTH, 9:00 a.m. - 5:00 p.m. (EST). E-mail address: docdelivery@haworthpress.com].

http://www.haworthpress.com/web/JGSW
© 2003 by The Haworth Press, Inc. All rights reserved.
Digital Object Identifier: 10.1300/J083v41n03_06

programs need to actively seek students who have an interest in working within more rural practice settings. *[Article copies available for a fee from The Haworth Document Delivery Service: 1-800-HAWORTH. E-mail address: <docdelivery@haworthpress.com> Website: <http://www.Haworth Press.com>* *© 2003 by The Haworth Press, Inc. All rights reserved.]*

KEYWORDS. Training, gerontological social work, rural curriculum content

INTRODUCTION

As the number of older adults increases, the diversity within the later life population will also expand. In social work education, students need to be exposed to various issues of diversity and multiculturalism in an effort to sensitize them to similarities and differences among clients. Too frequently, diversity is solely defined by variables of race/ethnicity, gender, sexual orientation, and age. While these are important characteristics, other significant variables are omitted, such as community context. Older adults who live in rural or remote areas, for example, may have different life histories, social support systems, and experiences with formal service networks than similarly aged cohorts who live in more urban locations. Therefore, diversity within the older population needs to be broadly defined within the context of assessment, practice, and policy courses.

Unfortunately, many students graduate from social work programs with limited exposure to issues of aging (Damron-Rodriguez & Lubben, 1997; Kropf, Schneider, & Stahlman, 1993; Scharlach, Damron-Rodriguez, Robinson, & Feldman, 2000; Wendt & Peterson, 1993). Various initiatives are currently underway to increase capacity for practice with older adults such as the John A. Hartford funded projects for curriculum innovation, student education, and faculty development (Rosen & Zlotnik, 2001). Although all social work programs are not part of these formal initiatives, there is a great deal that can be done within social work programs to prepare students to practice with older adults (Kropf, in press). As part of these efforts, students need to be exposed to the issues facing older adults and communities within non-urban locations.

IMPORTANCE OF TEACHING CONTENT ON RURAL OLDER ADULTS

This chapter will focus on issues in preparing social work students to become rural gerontological social workers. An assumption is that many practitioners will find themselves working with increased numbers of older adults, and these clients will become part of diverse social service networks. The National Association of Social Workers has promulgated a position statement on practice with rural populations in an effort to promote practice in underserved communities. Particular issues that are especially relevant in rural areas are understanding dual relationships in areas with high densities of social networks and improving rural communities' infrastructures (NASW, 2002). In order to prepare students for practice roles, content on older adults (including those who reside in rural areas) needs to become more visible within the curriculum. In the remaining sections of this chapter, content on methods to increase knowledge and skills will be presented.

DESCRIPTION OF THE AGING RURAL POPULATION

An important issue in educating students about this older population is to define and describe the aging population that lives in rural areas. Like older adults who live in cities and metropolitan areas, not all of these contexts are the same. Individuals who live in suburban communities have different experiences than those who live in downtown or inner city areas. Likewise, people who live in large urban areas (e.g., New York City, Los Angeles) may have difference lifestyles than those who live in moderate ones (e.g., Richmond, Santa Fe). As all urban areas are not alike, rural areas have different characteristics, populations, structures, and cultural features. Therefore, one aspect of educating students about this population is to define the rural population in different areas and community types.

An important factor in defining the older population is studying various contexts within rural life. For example, there are different reasons why older adults live in rural communities. Some older adults "age-in-place"; that is, the surrounding community changes yet they remain in the same area. The situation of aging-in-place typically involves out migration of younger cohorts from an area, and often is based upon labor force or quality of life issues. Older adults who age in place may find themselves in communities that lack a viable infrastructure as the tax base erodes.

Other communities actively seek older adults to migrate to the area. These "in migrators" typically are in good enough health and have economic resources to relocate to areas that offer a better quality of life. For example, the snowbirds of the North and Mid West may migrate to areas in the South where the weather is more temperate and offers a higher quality of life (van den Hoonaard, 2002). While this population may be attractive to small communities as in-migrators bring economic resources to an area, there are other impacts that must be anticipated. In times of a health crisis, for example if a person becomes ill, in-migrators have limited informal supports available as family and friends live elsewhere. This situation may place a strain on the health and social service network as the need for formal services are great.

ISSUES FOR SOCIAL WORK EDUCATION

The population of older adults who reside in rural areas poses important issues for inclusion in social work education. Some of the most significant issues for social work include health status and care, economics, and availability of social supports. As in other areas of social work, these factors may be different for diverse segments of the older rural population including persons of color and women.

Health status and care. Probably the most pressing problem for older adults in rural areas is access to quality health care. Rural areas are notoriously underserved in relation to health care providers and services, and many communities are without hospitals, community based services (e.g., home health care providers), or long term care options. In a recent international conference on health and rural elders, four themes were elucidated and coalesced into a strategy to promote health in rural areas (Mitka, 2000). These were:

1. Need for greater and better research on local, national, and worldwide consequences of increased aging in rural areas,
2. Need to establish strategies for preventing illness and injury, and establish a base of good health among this population,
3. Need to educate all health care providers about special aspects of aging in rural areas, and
4. Need to abolish inequities in access to health care and other services that are essential to maintaining independence among rural older adults.

Students in social work programs need to face the challenges that older adults experience in living in communities with scarce health resources.

In addition, students need be aware that cultural issues may be related to the lack of participation in formalized health care programs. For example, older African Americans who live in the rural South engage in cultural practices and rituals that are believed to be more effective than established medical practices. The older population in the Sea Islands of South Carolina have a saying that "the doctor can't do me no good" (Ralston, 1993). These older adults tend to remain out of the formal health care system, fearing doctors and hospitals as places where people go to die.

Long term care issues are also challenging for older adults in rural areas. Often, patient care may be compromised when resources are unavailable in the communities after discharge from an acute care setting (Botsford, 1993). In addition to the lack of health care options that are available, the limited economic resources of many older adults in rural areas may be an additional barrier in accessing long term care services (Coburn & Bolda, 2001). Clearly, social workers have a role in advocating for changes to make health care resources more available and affordable for older adults in rural areas.

Challenges in health care are not confined to the physical health domain, as psychiatric conditions are often untreated in rural communities as well. Students also need to explore challenges related to mental health functioning of older adults in rural areas. The most prevalent mental health problem of late life is depression, and this condition often is manifested somatically in the older population. In an attempt to estimate the prevalence of depression and eating disorders in older Midwestern rural women, a study analyzed eating content and patterns of this population (Pollina & McKee, 2000). Within this study, older women with certain nutritional risk factors were found to have higher depression scores. In addition, this study found that this community dwelling population was more at risk for obesity than for being significantly underweight.

Within the older population, a significant health care issue is assessment of cognitive status. Differential diagnosis between depression, delirium, and dementia is complex, and mental health practitioners need valid assessment measures to use with diverse older populations. For example, a study in rural Colorado was undertaken to assess the distribution of cognitive functioning of both Hispanic and non-Hispanic older adults (Mulgrew, Morgenstern, Shetterly, Baxter, Baron, & Hamman, 1999). As the rural population becomes more diverse, rural communities will experience even more complex and challenging issues in terms of assessment and diagnosis of late life mental health conditions. Students in health and mental health courses can explore some of these complex issues within the context of rural health care systems.

Economics. In addition to learning about health care issues and resources, students also need to understand the economics of rural areas. Poverty is a pervasive problem in many rural communities, and poverty rates have been higher among older adults who live in rural areas compared to urban dwelling elders. Coward and Dwyer (1998) report that the combined interaction of age and community residence are significant predictors of poor economic status. That is, older adults who live in rural areas have less income and lower quality of housing than those who live in urban areas (van Nostrand, 1993).

In addition to fewer economic inputs, older adults in rural areas may have additional expenses that erode their household budgets. For example, the price of gasoline has increased, which puts a strain on budgets of families in rural areas. Routine trips in remote areas (e.g., grocery store, pharmacy) have inflated costs due to the amount spent on fuel. In addition, resources that are available in small towns may have less competition which can keep the price of items higher than in urban areas. These types of factors may quickly drain the incomes of older adults (Myers, Kropf, & Robinson, 2002).

Social supports. As people age, there may be a need for additional support to conduct their activities of daily living. In addition, the older adult may also need to have support after an acute health crisis such as hospitalization or recent diagnosis. While a common perception is that older adults in rural areas are surrounded by available kin, the reality is that these older adults may have limited sources of support (Botsford, 1993). In rural areas, older adults may have less access to sources of informal supports, which is partially explained by the increased distance between members of the social network.

In addition to informal sources of support, older adults may require assistance from formal services and programs. Unfortunately, a comprehensive system of care may be unavailable for older adults regardless of community type. For older adults in rural areas, the continuum of formalized services may be especially abbreviated. A major problem with access to services for rural older adults is related to health care financing, as greater numbers are dependent on public programs (Medicare and Medicaid) for services (Coburn & Bolda, 2001). In evaluating service gaps within the older population, some of the most extensive differences between urban and rural services were formal supports such as adult day care centers, homemaker and chore services, hospice and respite services, and home health nursing, which are often lacking in more rural communities (Coward & Dwyer, 1998). These stresses place tremendous pressure on rural areas to seek creative methods of financing to serve older adults in these communities.

TEACHING CONTENT ON RURAL OLDER ADULTS

In order to cover the spectrum of issues within the social work curriculum, courses need to include content on rural older adults from a practice, policy, and research perspective. This section will highlight social work roles and skills that are particularly relevant to gerontological social workers in rural areas. Within the curriculum, students should be sensitized to the importance of both direct and macro practice interventions with older adults. In addition, instructional methods that can be employed to teach this content are presented.

Models of social work practice. Due to the breadth of social work practice in rural areas, social work students need to have an orientation to practice across multi-system levels. Case management is a method of practice that is commonly used within small communities as the target of intervention may be the individual, family system, or surrounding community itself. In addition, social workers need to develop leadership skills in order to exert influence in communities that often may have characteristics of closed systems. Finally, technology provides opportunities in innovative intervention models such as telemedicine or telehealth. Due to geographical distance and the lack of resources, these innovations may be particularly useful for delivering service in rural areas. Social work courses can educate students in understanding and employing intervention approaches that have specific utility with older adults in rural areas.

Case management. In rural communities, a major issue of practice is linking older adults and their families to needed resources. Case management is a practice model that is used extensively in rural areas to help with linkage and provide a method to help older adults secure services that might be unknown or misunderstood. In order to demonstrate the importance of case management in varying contexts, two rural case management programs will be highlighted.

In one model, support to informal caregivers was used as an adjunct to formal case management services within a rural hospital in New York (Botsford, 1993). Due to the demands on a relatively small case management staff, the hospital undertook a training program for families on care coordination. Social work and medical staff provided training to family care providers on psychological aspects of care, physical aspects of aging, identifying and securing community resources, and developing advocacy skills. Based upon self reports of the program, care providers reported reduced stress in their role after completing the support program and were able to obtain assistance from formal agencies to reduce caregiving demands. This type of program provides an example of a creative way to engage families in rural areas to effectively assume some case management tasks for their older family members.

Case management has also been developed for custodial grandparents who are raising grandchildren in rural communities (Myers et al., 2002; Robinson, Kropf, & Myers, 2000). Families who participate within this case management program are assisted in interfacing with the multiple service networks that are typically part of this caregiving situation (e.g., schools, public welfare, mental health). In addition, the service model includes a monthly support group to help link custodial grandparents to each other in an effort to decrease isolation and alienation which accompanies this role.

Administration and leadership skills. In preparing students for practice in rural areas, the curriculum also needs to include content which helps students develop leadership skills. Social workers who practice in small towns need to be aware of the local decision-making factors, processes, and power structures as a way to enact change. This process includes understanding the decision making networks in community structures and sources of influential leadership.

Within administration courses, various issues related to rural practice can be explored and discussed. Often, part of the service agenda in rural areas focuses on change within the current service network or system. Part of the assessment process is understanding the concept of power within small communities, such as the distribution within the population and key community players. For example, influential people within the community may hold multiple roles that exert influence in many areas of community life. Martinez-Brawley (2000) describes one area where powerful community actors held influential roles in several domains of community life such as environmental boards, funding sources (e.g., United Way), and local service providers (e.g., hospital). In preparing students to hold administrative and leadership positions in this type of community, they need to have a clear perspective on the dense decision making networks that may exist and influence factors such as resource allocation and service priorities.

Telemedicine interventions. As technology becomes more advanced, social workers may be involved with telemedicine or telehealth interventions. Most broadly defined, "telemedicine" is the use of telecommunications to provide medical information and services (Perednia & Allen, 1995). However, Kaye (1997) argues that "the term 'telehealth' may well be more accurate in describing telemedicine applications . . . , given the likelihood that professions other than medicine (such as nursing) will be major participants in its implementation" (p. 243). In fact, the US Department of Health and Human Services (DHHS) recently established an Office for the Advancement of Telehealth "to support the agency's push to use telecommunications . . . among grantees, clinicians and other health care professionals" (HRSA focuses agency, 1998).

Telemedicine approaches have several beneficial outcomes for older adults in rural areas. These include access to services for those who live in remote areas, possible cost reduction in providing services, and outreach and support to family caregivers. As Dezendorf and Green (1999) describe, information technology offers various potentials in service delivery including eradicating barriers to service, raising awareness of outcomes and options, and partially offsetting the barrier of poverty as greater improvements are made in technology efficiency and efficacy. Four types of telemedicine programs have been identified for older adults (Kropf & Grigsby, 1999), which seem to have specific utility for social workers in rural community settings:

1. *Health maintenance programs*. These telemedicine services provide quality care that is accessible and affordable for older adults. Example include physical and psychosocial services to older adults with varying health care conditions such as patients with cancer (Allen & Hayes, 1994), psychological or psychiatric conditions (Ball, 1996; Burke, Roccaforte, Wengel, Conly, & Potter, 1995; Montani et al., 1997), patients with pacemakers (Barbaro, Bartolini, & Bernarducci, 1997) and diabetics (Owens, 1997).
2. *Emergency response programs.* These programs provide timely and direct links to health care sources that can provide aid in emergency situations. For example, cardiac patients may wear a device that would link them to an emergency system in cases of arrest or problem (Roth, Carthy, & Benedek, 1997). In another emergency response model, older adults can link to a community resource center via broadband video communication in a situation where they feel unsafe, or in the midst of a dangerous situation (Erkert, 1997).
3. *Psychiatric or psychological.* In addition to programs that target physical health, telemedicine has also been used for psychiatric and psychological purposes. These telemedicine programs can be used for screening (as in mental status) or actually providing intervention, such as reassurance.

4. *Support to caregivers.* Another function of telemedicine is to provide support to care providers of older adults such as reducing isolation, providing support in times of a crisis, providing access to expert knowledge, and linking to other care providers (Ball, 1996).

METHODS TO ATTRACT STUDENTS TO RURAL PRACTICE

Another educational issue in preparing students for rural practice is recruitment. The scarcity of resources within rural locations is related to the inadequate number of professionals who deliver services in these areas. Specifically, social work needs to develop and retain qualified professionals to administer and provide social welfare services in rural communities (Daley & Avant, 1999). In this section, additional methods to attract students to practice in rural communities are explored.

One method of attracting students to this field of practice is providing students with an opportunity to learn more about rural social work through exposure to issues found within these communities. First person accounts, or hearing rural stories, help students develop a sensitivity and appreciation of different ways of living, knowing, and being. Carawan, Bass, and Bunch (1999) provide examples of using narratives within classes to give voice to the inner lives of rural people and provide more contextual understanding of life in a rural area. By inviting various speakers from rural communities into the classroom, students become aware of personal and social narratives that exist. Stories may include various themes such as sense of community and place, subculture issues (e.g., people of color in rural areas, persons who are gay/lesbian who live in these communities), and the dynamics and politics of these places.

Strategies have also been developed to "home grow" professionals from persons who are part of rural areas. The home grown approach may have advantages in retaining a workforce as people are already familiar with life and experiences within these community contexts. However, few programs have been developed that afford the community-university partnership that is needed within this approach (Daley & Avant, 1999; Zlotnik, 1998). Social work program should take the lead in developing courses, curriculum, and internship experiences that focus on particular aspects of social work practice in rural areas. In addition, social work programs need to develop networks to and relationships with key organizations within communities and provide methods for individuals to enroll in social work programs. Distance education resources (e.g., online courses, satellite courses) can increase access to university programs without requiring students to leave their communities in order to complete course work.

In summary, social work needs to examine various methods and strategies to educate students for work in rural areas and small communities. Within the social work curriculum, direct practice methods and administrative/leadership skill courses need to include content on contexts, skills, roles, and knowledge that is necessary for effective practice in rural areas. In addition, innovative programs such as telemedicine can also be included as a way to help students consider creative ways to provide cost effective and efficacious services within these community settings.

As the older population continues to grow, people in rural areas will increasingly be clients of social services. Some of these rural communities face an eroding tax base, with labor force aged adults moving to more prosperous locations. This situation may cause problems for social workers, as few formal services may be available to assist older adults with late life health and social issues. Other communities attract older adults of retirement age who relocate to be in more desirable communities (e.g., Sunbelt areas). In these high retirement areas, the in-migrators arrive in good health with economic resources but may turn to formal services quickly in times of a crisis situation. In both of these scenarios, social workers must be educated and prepared to deal with the psychosocial, resource, and economic issues of providing services to older adults in small towns and rural areas.

REFERENCES

Allen, A., & Hayes, J. (1994). Patient satisfaction with telemedicine in a rural clinic. *American Journal of Public Health, 84*, 1693.

Ball, C. J. (1996). Telepsychiatry: The potential for communications technology in old age psychiatry. *Journal of Telemedicine and Telecare, 2*(Supp. 1), 117-118.

Barbaro, V., Bartolini, P., & Bernarducci, R. (1997). A portable unit for remote monitoring of pacemaker patients. *Journal of Telemedicine and Telecare, 3*(1), 96-102.

Botsford, A. L. (1993). Caregiver support in rural areas: A stepping stone to case management for rural hospitals. *Journal of Gerontological Social Work, 20*(3/4), 147-165.

Burke, W. J., Roccaforte, W. H., Wengel, S. P., Conly, D. M., & Potter, J. F. (1995). The reliability and validity of the Geriatric Depression Rating Scale administered by telephone. *Journal of the American Geriatric Society, 43*, 674-679.

Carawan, L. W., Bass, L. L., & Bunch, S. G. (1999). Using narratives in educating social workers for rural practice. In I. B. Carlton-LaNey, R. L. Edwards, & P. M. Reid (Eds.). *Preserving and strengthening small towns and rural communities.* (pp. 355-366). Washington, DC: NASW Press.

Coburn, A. F., & Bolda, E. J. (2001). Rural elders and long term care. *Western Journal of Medicine, 174,* 209-213.

Coward, R. T., & Dwyer, J. W. (1998). The health and well-being of rural elders. In L. H. Ginsberg (Ed.). *Social work in rural communities.* (213-232). (3rd ed.). Alexandria, VA: Council on Social Work Education.

Daley, J., & Avant, F. (1999). Attracting and retaining professionals for social work practice in rural areas: An example from East Texas. In I. B. Carlton-LaNey, R. L. Edwards, & P. M. Reid (Eds.). *Preserving and strengthening small towns and rural communities.* (pp. 335-345). Washington, DC: NASW Press.

Damron-Rodriguez, J., & Lubben, J. (1997). The 1995 WHCoA: An agenda for social work education and training. In C. Saltz (Ed.). *Social work response to the 1995 White House Conference on Aging: From issues to actions* (pp. 65-77). New York: The Haworth Press, Inc.

Dezendorf, P. K., & Green, R. K. (1999). Using electronic social work to serve the rural elderly population. In I. B. Carlton-LaNey, R. L. Edwards, & P. M. Reid (Eds.). *Preserving and strengthening small towns and rural communities.* (pp. 298-312). Washington, DC: NASW Press.

Erkert, T. (1997). High-quality television links for home-based support for the elderly. *Journal of Telemedicine and Telecare, 3*(Supp. 1), 26-28.

HRSA focuses agency resources on telehealth. (1998, May 22). *HRSA News.* U.S. Department of Health & Human Services Health Resources and Services Administration. Washington, DC. *http://www.hrsa.dhhs.gov/Newsroom/releases/oat.htm.*

Kaye, L. W. (1997). Telemedicine: Extension to home care? *Telemedicine Journal, 3,* 243-246.

Kropf, N. P. (in press). Strategies to increase student interest in aging. *Journal of Gerontological Social Work.*

Kropf, N. P., & Grigsby, R. K. (1999). Telemedicine for older adults. *Home Health Care Services Quarterly, 17*(4), 1-11.

Kropf, N. P., Schneider, R. L., & Stahlman, S. D. (1993). Status of gerontology in baccalaureate social work education. *Educational Gerontology, 19* (7), 623-634.

Martinez-Brawley, E. E. (2000). *Close to home: Human services and the small community.* Washington DC: National Association of Social Workers.

Mitka, M. (2000). International conference considers health needs of the rural elderly. *Journal of the American Medical Association, 4,* 423-424.

Montani, C., Billaud, N., Tyrrell, J., Fluchaire, I., Malterre, C., Lauvernay, N., Couturier, P., & Franco, A. (1997). Psychological impact of a remote psychometric consultation with hospitalized elderly people. *Journal of Telemedicine and Telecare, 3,* 140-145.

Mulgrew, C. L., Morgenstern, N., Shetterly, S. M., Baxter, J., Baron A. E., & Hamman, R. (1999). Cognitive functioning and impairment among rural elderly Hispanics and non-Hispanic whites as assessed by the Mini-Mental State Examination. *Journals of Gerontology, 54B,* P222-P230.

Myers, L., Kropf, N. P., & Robinson, M. M. (2002). Grandparents raising grandchildren: Case management in a rural setting. *Journal of Human Behavior in the Social Environment*, *5*(1), 53-71.

NASW. (2002, March). Rural social work. Proposed Public and Professional Policies. NASW News, p. 5.

Owens, D. R. (1997). Telemedicine in screening and monitoring of diabetic eye disease. *Journal of Telemedicine and Telecare*, *3*(Supp. 1), 89.

Perednia, D. A., & Allen, A. (1995). Telemedicine technology and clinical applications. *Journal of the American Medical Association*, *273*, 483-488.

Pollina, L., & McKee, D. M. (2000). Nutritional risk among elderly rural Midwestern women. *Family and Consumer Sciences Research Journal*, *29*, 3-18.

Ralston, P. (1993). Health promotion for rural black elderly: A comprehensive review. *Journal of Gerontological Social Work*, *20*(1/2), 53-78.

Robinson, M. M., Kropf, N. P., & Myers, L. (2000). Grandparents raising grandchildren in rural communities. *Journal of Aging and Mental Health*, *6*(4), 1-13.

Rosen, A., & Zlotnik, J. L. (2001). Social work's response to the growing older population. *Generations*, *25*(1), 69-72.

Roth, A., Carthy, Z., & Benedek, M. (1997). Telemedicine in emergency home care–the 'Shahal' experience. *Journal of Telemedicine and Telecare*, *3*(Supp. 1), 58-59.

Scharlach, A., Damron-Rodriguez, J., Robinson, B., & Feldman, R. (2000). Educating social workers for an aging society: A vision for the 21st century. *Journal of Social Work Education*, *36*(3), 521-538.

van den Hoonaard, D. K. (2002). Life on the margins of a Florida retirement community: The experience of snowbirds, newcomers, and widowed persons. *Research on Aging*, *24*(1), 50-66.

van Nostrand, J. F. (Ed.). (1993). *Common beliefs about the rural elderly: What do national data tell us?* Washington DC: National Center for Health Statistics.

Wendt, P. F., & Peterson, D. A. (1993). Developing gerontological expertise among higher education faculty. *Educational Gerontology*, *19*, 59-70.

Zlotnik, J. L. (1998). Preparing human service workers for the 21st century: A challenge to professional education. In J. Zlotnik & S. Jones (Eds.), *Preparing helping professionals to meet community needs: Generalizing from the rural experience.* Alexandria, VA: Council on Social Work Education.

Chapter 17

Rural Mental Health: A Discussion of Service Capacity Building for Rural Elders

Eloise Rathbone-McCuan, PhD
Share Bane, PhD

SUMMARY. Mental health services available in many rural communities are too limited in scope and availability to meet the needs of rural citizens. The future of mental health services for the rural poor will be impacted by state government decisions about Medicaid funding priorities. It is important that rural practitioners, especially those that work in the fields of mental health, health, and aging services, engage in advocacy for better coverage of the rural poor and low-income elderly persons. This chapter discusses issues of advocacy related to improving the provision of mental health services to older rural citizens as an important goal in the larger effort to expand and improve rural mental health service delivery throughout the nation. *[Article copies available for a fee from The Haworth Document Delivery Service: 1-800-HAWORTH. E-mail address: <docdelivery@haworthpress.com> Website: <http://www.HaworthPress.com> © 2003 by The Haworth Press, Inc. All rights reserved.]*

KEYWORDS. Medicaid, rural elders, advocacy

[Haworth co-indexing entry note]: "Rural Mental Health: A Discussion of Service Capacity Building for Rural Elders." Rathbone-McCuan, Eloise, and Share Bane. Co-published simultaneously in *Journal of Gerontological Social Work* (The Haworth Social Work Practice Press, an imprint of The Haworth Press, Inc.) Vol. 41, No. 3/4, 2003, pp. 301-312; and: *Gerontological Social Work in Small Towns and Rural Communities* (ed: Sandra S. Butler, and Lenard W. Kaye) The Haworth Social Work Practice Press, an imprint of The Haworth Press, Inc., 2003, pp. 301-312. Single or multiple copies of this article are available for a fee from The Haworth Document Delivery Service [1-800-HAWORTH, 9:00 a.m. - 5:00 p.m. (EST). E-mail address: docdelivery@haworthpress.com].

http://www.haworthpress.com/web/JGSW
© 2003 by The Haworth Press, Inc. All rights reserved.
Digital Object Identifier: 10.1300/J083v41n03_07

INTRODUCTION

The authoritative volume, *Mental Health: A Report of the Surgeon General* (Surgeon General, 1999), devotes extensive discussion to the mental health needs of older Americans. It verifies that there are subgroups in the elderly population that face special psychiatric care and general mental health problems. The rural elderly are continuously identified as among the most under-served and at-risk groups of older Americans. Solutions for providing better mental health services to the rural elderly require changes in the structure of service delivery and significant service provision development (Rathbone-McCuan, 2001). There is agreement among rural advocates, service providers, and policy makers about the steps that can be taken to improve service provision. This chapter discusses the type of capacity-building that will enhance the delivery of needed rural mental health services.

Social workers providing services to low income rural elderly are consistently engaged in client advocacy efforts to obtain a myriad of resources to meet health, social and emotional client needs. In their practice with the rural elderly, advocacy consists of helping actions taken on behalf of individual elderly clients, groups of elderly rural citizens, families and other informal care giving support networks, and community-wide concerns. No matter what the social worker's specific job description–adult protective services case manager, nursing home consultant, mental health counselor, economic and social development specialist, or aging network service administrator–advocacy is a primary service delivery goal and professional ethical obligation.

This chapter proposes that advocacy functions are essential for planning and delivering mental health services to older rural adults. It considers how the configuration of rural mental health services in most areas lacks sufficient resources to serve the elderly population, and discusses how Medicaid resources must be preserved and expanded as a funding vehicle to deliver needed services.

RURAL MENTAL HEALTH DELIVERY CONCERNS

Comprehensive assessment and diagnostic services, psychotherapy treatment, group and family counseling, well monitored medication regimes, adequate and diverse service reimbursement options, and an array of formal and informal community resources need to be in place if rural communities are to have adequate mental health service coverage. Services should be arranged on a continuum to meet acute and long-term care needs as well as offer prevention and mental health education. Mental health services should be well integrated into other community service networks such as schools, social welfare agencies, primary care units, and long-term care facilities to improve care for children, adolescents, and elderly persons. Persons with addictions and those with accompanying mental health issues need treatment access in geographic areas close to their family and community.

Access to mental health care among rural persons has been a long standing concern of practitioners, policy makers, and rural advocates (Lambert & Agger, 1995). Rural communities often face serious problems in obtaining mental health services. Geographic distance, limited mental health resources, fear and stigma of mental health problems (Wagenfeld, Murray, Mohatt, & DeBruyn, 1994), and affordable care are barriers that older people and others in need of service face (Bane & Bull, 2001). A stronger rural mental health delivery system would benefit all those in need of care. Managed behavioral health care arrangements are less well developed in rural areas because of the shortage of licensed mental health care providers, which is less true in metropolitan areas.

Community mental health centers (CMHC) were once the anchor point for providing rural mental health services to rural persons. Capacity to serve the general mental health needs of rural populations has been reduced, however, after several decades of intensive mandated services to those with severe and persistent mental illness (Lambert & Agger, 1995). In addition, serving rural areas is affected by limited state funding, a phenomenon that is growing more critical with state budget crises and cutbacks in many health and human services. Community mental health centers are struggling to maintain key service functions such as comprehensive case management services when they face hiring freezes for staff replacements. Budget reductions limit the purchase of psychiatric service consultations; reduce community outreach efforts; and preclude the development of new programs that more effectively integrate mental health and addiction services, community corrections and outpatient mental health services, mental health consultation in long term care settings, and comprehensive mental health assessment access.

In the absence of geriatric psychiatrists and other aging mental health specialists (Colenda, Mickus, Marcus, Tanielian, & Pincus, 2002) in rural communities, older persons and other rural residents needing specialized mental health care rely on physicians as their first contact when emotional problems are confronted. Sometimes rural physicians are the only source of mental health care available or the single professional with whom older people will share information about emotional and distressful behavioral symptoms (Merwin, Hinton, Dembling, & Stern, 2003). The number of rural physicians in private practice is decreasing, the group-practice arrangements are stretched very thin, allowing only limited physician contact, and the low level of patient reimbursement from Medicare and Medicaid is precluding further inclusion of low-income, rural aged patients into physician practice. Many rural elderly face both medical and mental health care crises (Judd & Malcom, 2002).

FEDERAL AND STATE MENTAL HEALTH LEGISLATION

The fragmented and insufficient mental health service delivery system in the United States is the result of complex federal and state legislation and funding arrangements. The deinstitutionalization movement of the mentally ill from large state funded and private psychiatric hospitals began in the early 1960s, at which time the Community Mental Health Centers Act of 1963 was passed by Congress. This act was subsequently amended in 1976 and then replaced by the Mental Health Systems Act of 1980, which continued to support the operation of CMHCs throughout the country. The Community Mental Health Centers Act was repealed in 1981 and replaced by the Mental Health Block Grant Act of 1981 (Lambert & Agger, 1995). The use of block grant funds by states gave them greater discretion regarding expenditure of capped funds within a more flexible set of federal guidelines. Original block funding was intended to give federal financial support to states for providing community-based mental health services to adults with severe and persistent mental illness and children with serious emotional disturbances, but the elderly were not specifically identified. Only those older individuals with severe and persistent mental illness were specifically impacted by federal provision guidelines.

The 1986 Amendments to the Mental Health Block Grant established the requirement for states to establish a comprehensive mental health plan that emphasized how states would care for people living in rural areas (Stein, 2001). Efforts for extending services into rural areas were at the discretion priority of each state. In 2000 Congress converted the mental health block grant to the Community Mental Health Services Performance Partnership grant (P.L. 106-310). This act now requires states to develop new service delivery performance targets while also maintaining the requirement that each state have a mental health planning council with 51 percent of its membership consisting of service consumers, family members, and non-treating professionals.

According to a recent analysis by the National Alliance for the Mentally Ill (2002), many states face a dilemma in meeting new accountability, standards with evidence-based unduplicated data on mental health provision. Many states lack a good mechanism of accountability, and this precludes those states from being able to report precise data on who is served with what services over what time duration. As the result of limitations of state mental health data systems, it is difficult to undertake mental health utilization research studies that are needed to give an accurate picture of rural mental health delivery and a more accurate estimate of the number of older persons served by community mental health centers.

RECOMMENDATIONS FOR RURAL MENTAL HEALTH DELIVERY

Over the past four decades of evolving mental health legislation, there has been inconsistent attention to and recommendations for improving rural mental health service delivery. An examination of the findings of the National Rural Health Association (1999) and the Rural Mental Health Provider Group convened by the Center for Mental Health Services in the Substance Abuse and Mental Health Services Administration of the U.S. Department of Health and Human Services (1997) indicate two general themes within the recommendations to improve rural mental health services. One theme is the increased service access to mental health resources, and the second is the severe shortage of qualified rural mental health providers. Less consistent, however, is attention to the lack of service reimbursement equity which should be a priority in rural mental health services research and planning.

Access to Mental Health Services

The adoption of urban mental health service delivery models in rural areas has not produced adequate rural mental health service programming. Beeson (1998) explains why rural service delivery models have not evolved separately from urban service patterns, attributing this to policy decisions, planning processes, and professional influences. Health and human service policy is rarely established specifically for rural environments. Providers often face program guidelines that assume a community services infrastructure available in urban areas, but which rural communities lack. Rural providers continuously face making adaptations that often intersperse informal resources in place of meager formal resources.

For example, rural mental health case management for those with severe and enduring mental illness must rely heavily on the mobilization of patient support alternatives different from those in urban areas. Stable living arrangements are difficult to find because rural areas lack specialized housing for mentally ill persons, and there is a severe shortage of public low-income housing. Older persons with a history of mental illness may be excluded from senior housing complexes because federal law may have designated the units as exclusively senior citizen housing (Karaim, 2002).

Family living arrangements may often be the only alternative even though those arrangements are not in the best interest of the patient or the family. The rural tradition of "taking care of your own" is increasingly difficult to sustain as the increased employment of rural women has added new demands on the caregiving functions within all stages of the intergenerational family life cycle. Services noted as helpful to caregivers of older persons such as counseling, family meetings, and support groups (Zarit & Zarit, 1998) are less easily accessed by family members living outside of metropolitan areas even though they carry the same caregiving burdens.

Specialized vocational opportunities that match well with the interests and capacities of patients must be located and accessed from within the community's general employment opportunity field. Rural shelter work situations may be difficult to sustain because of the limited supply of work that can be solicited from a rural area appropriate for production in sheltered settings (Missouri Association of Sheltered Work Shops, 2002). Opportunities for extended and alternative employment for older rural residents are less common in depressed rural economic sectors. Some of the stressors of aging in rural communities relate to finding supplementary work for income enhancement.

Urban models of best mental health practice, especially those that are well suited for older persons and individuals with combined physical and psychiatric disabilities, are not immediately transferable to rural communities. The resources for adapting urban care models to fit non-metropolitan areas could make these services effective. On the other hand, costs of rural area implementation may far exceed personal resources of low-income rural elderly, and reimbursement may be too low to sustain program operations (Beeson, 1998).

Rural Personnel Shortages

Incentives for rural mental health manpower recruitment have been available for many years through federal programs, foundations, and to a lesser extent, state-level initiatives. Financial support for rural specialty practice training programs through scholarships and loan forgiveness incentives have been and continue to be offered. The impact of these, however, has not achieved a sustained widespread solution to rural health provider shortages. Programs have come and gone depending on funding priorities. Short term episodic grants have been awarded to universities and medical centers, but funding has been inadequate. This has been especially true as the shortage of rural mental health professions continues (Merwin et al., 2003).

More effort must be made to identify and recruit young people from rural areas who have an interest in returning to their rural areas or transplanting themselves to alternative rural environments that offer a personally desired quality of life. In addition, more effort should be made to attract rural social work and allied human service personnel who are interested in career advancement through graduate degree training and have every intention to practice in their rural roots area. Both groups should have internships within rural service settings where they could eventually practice or where they have current lower level positions from which they would advance after further training (National Rural Health Association, 1999).

Federal and state rural practitioner employment incentive and training programs should be consolidated in order to better meet the needs of specific rural areas. These programs should be strictly monitored and evaluated by state departments of health and mental health in partnership with academic institutions and future rural agency employment sites. Rural communities should be given greater flexibility in recruiting their own trainee applicants based on a better knowledge of professional long range commitments for rural practice.

Academic training programs with external funding for special rural manpower training programs, often based in urban areas, might build in stronger mechanisms for initial local rural applicant recruitment.

Rural graduate alumni can also be very effective consultants for the design and implementation of rural training programs.

Rural Service Reimbursement Equity

There should be much greater equity in third party reimbursement between urban and rural service provision when services are delivered by equally credentialed providers. For example, Medicaid rates for rural nursing homes serving elderly persons with psychiatric conditions should be much more equal between urban and rural nursing homes. There is often no real cost-effective justification for negotiating lower rural provider rates when the mental health care needs for psychiatric care consultation, medications, and more intensive personal care needs are constant between rural and urban facility patient populations (Beeson, 1998). Rate equity issues between rural and urban long term care centers is also becoming a point of concern, as more individuals with long term care insurance are experiencing nursing home care episodes.

Medicaid is a major source of service reimbursement for many of the rural poor as it covers their health care costs. Medicaid was originally passed in 1965 as part of the Social Security Act and was conceived as a federal-state partnership. In 1996, Medicaid provided health coverage to approximately 12 percent of the population, excluding those in institutions, and close to 45 percent of people with incomes below the poverty line (Stein, 2001). In 1999, over 40 million Americans had Medicaid coverage. During the 1990s, states achieved rapid transfer of Medicaid patients into managed care programs. Managed care covered about 14 percent of Medicaid patients in 1993, and by 2000 it covered 56 percent of patients (Weissert & Goggins, 2002).

As the devolution of federal Medicaid policies are transferred to state level policy decisions (Linhorst, 2002), states will further intensify their scrutiny over Medicaid expenditures. States facing very large budget crises are attributing the spiraling costs of health care assumed by state Medicaid contributions as a significant deficit contributor. Managed-care arrangements will be further applied as a means of cost-containment, and eventually all aspects of eligibility and coverage will be reviewed by states for cost-savings (Blau, 1999; Hartman-Stein, 1999). The politics of Medicaid health entitlement can be expected to involve many of the health and human delivery sectors. Major social policy advocacy at the state level will be necessary if the rights and needs of the rural poor are to be well presented in this era of Medicaid devolution and subsequent transformation (Linhorst, 2002).

Rural Mental Health Research

Rural mental health providers and advocates would be well served to reach consensus about priority research questions that can better guide service delivery. Of importance is to better understand the issue of mental health stigma among older rural persons which is frequently identified as a barrier to the use of rural mental health services. Some of the specific issues of stigma that we need to understand within the older rural population include: (1) Is stigma associated with lingering images of state mental institutions as they existed when the current cohort of elderly were younger? (2) Are social relationships valued most by older people affected by receipt of mental health services? (3) Are younger generations of family members and other care providers contributing to issues of stigma based on their own perceptions of mental health and illness? and (4) What is the relationship between the elder's own spiritual framework and sense of duty to cope with grief, anxiety, and depression? These questions, for example, could be pursued with research samples comparing urban and rural elderly or cross-sectional samples of rural elderly from different sectors of rural America.

ESSENTIAL ELEMENTS OF SOCIAL POLICY ADVOCACY

According to Beeson (1998), social policy is a plan or course of action adopted by government to influence and determine decisions, actions, and strategies. Revisions in a state's Medicaid plan will not automatically safeguard the interests of the rural poor. To give a rural-favorable direction to future state Medicaid expenditure plans, advocacy for the rural poor is of great importance. A report from the Health Resources and Services Administration (2000) indicates that rural communities need to analyze how Medicaid expenditures can be applied more effectively, including merging some rural mental health services into rural health settings. This integration could be a step forward in providing mental health services in the larger context of physical care more readily acceptable to older rural people. Designing care coordination strategies that are more effective and efficient for integrating health and mental health services could offer an important mental health promotion in a more holistic context of well-being and independence so highly valued by older rural persons.

In the process of examining state Medicaid plans, rural advocates may be well positioned to raise the question of urban and rural benefit equity. They need to anticipate how Medicaid policy coverage might be redesigned as an incentive for increasing rather than decreasing the availability of health and mental health service providers. Social policy analysts are anticipating a relatively rapid surge of federal to state Medicaid policy transfer authority. It is necessary to fully analyze the implications for the rural elderly in the larger context of the health care continuum. The time frame for state revisions of Medicaid plans may become one of the most debated domestic social policies issues over the next few years. If a state's agenda is to make large cost-saving decisions about Medicaid service expenditure, a strong rural advocacy voice that encompasses the needs of rural older persons must be in place to make certain that there are enacted policy decisions that work to meet the prevailing needs of poor elders in rural communities.

Rural practitioner involvement in efforts to preserve and enhance rural health and social services will require that social workers apply their expertise of rural community environments for social change using rural agency networks as catalysts for rural political support. Rural state legislators should have a major voice and monitoring function in the restructuring of state health and social service policy. They should take their direction from their political constituency. Front line practitioners and agency administrators are the source of rural expertise necessary to provide direction to rural legislative initiatives in state Medicaid reform. These professionals–including gerontological social workers–are the vital link for helping state policy makers consider all of the major implications for the rural poor, hopefully targeted on the needs of the oldest and youngest generations, in the complex process of Medicaid reform.

CONCLUSION

There is no single model of social advocacy, no one size fits all approach, for small community and nonmetropolitan areas. The diversity of rural areas by geographic, economic production, historical development, cultural and ethnic configuration, and political influence must play a part in planning and implementing rural human service policy advocacy. Social policy reform in the Medicaid context will be a process undertaken without perfect elements of power and influence. Advocacy plans must be flexible and consistently revised to respond to changing political and economic conditions. Because of the policy complexities of Medicaid reform, we need more rural social work and allied health providers to offer effective representation of the needs of all the rural poor. There will be no perfect time frame for advocacy involvement, and no single person or group will have all the needed knowledge and resources for social policy advocacy. Service providers working with the rural elderly need to be in the forefront of advocacy.

Any rural interest Medicaid advocacy group must support the fair distribution of Medicaid funding for the services used by eligible state citizens living in their rural areas. The goals of advocacy would include sufficient policy flexibility to develop service delivery patterns that would be appropriate for rural areas, utilize some component of staff budgets to undertake recruitment of needed personnel, and undertake service performance evaluations that can help answer questions about continuous rural service improvements.

Advocates must work within the state's legislative political structure and gain full support of their rural representatives, asking them to oversee the decisions of policy makers disinclined to give rural citizens and communities priority. Rural advocates must support the involvement of consumers and families to articulate their health and social service needs in a public arena. Local solutions to the general and specific social and health service delivery barriers must be offered by rural advocates within realistic cost effectiveness and efficiency parameters. State Medicaid reforms should be designed and implemented in full recognition of the needs of rural citizens and with an enduring commitment to maintain equity of coverage between rural and urban eligible recipients.

REFERENCES

Bane, S. E. & Bull, C. N. (2001). Innovative rural mental health service delivery for rural elders. *Journal of Applied Gerontology, 20*, 230-240.

Beeson, P.G. (1998). *Policy and rural mental health: Dilemmas and urban bias*. Anniversary publication of the National Association of Rural Mental Health (June, 1998). Retrieved May 8, 2002, from *http://www.narmh.org/pages/refhome.html.*

Blau, D. (1999). Perspectives on managed care. *Journal of Geriatric Psychiatry, 32*, 5-13.

Colenda, C. C., Mickus, M. A., Marcus, S. C., Tanielian, T. L., & Pincus, H. A. (2002). Comparison of adult and geriatric psychiatric practice patterns: Findings from the American Psychiatric Association's Practice Research Network. *American Journal of Geriatric Psychiatry, 10*, 609-617.

Hartman-Stein, P. (1999). Adapting to managed behavioral health care for the elderly: A practitioner's perspective. *Journal of Geriatric Psychiatry, 32*, 48-61.

Health Resources and Services Administration. (2000). *Opportunities to use Medicaid in support of rural health services* (HRSA Publication pp. 1-12). Washington, DC.

Judd, F., & Malcom, H. (2002). Psychiatry and rural general practitioners–Keeping patients and doctors healthy as the key service providers for people with mental health problems in rural communities. *Current Therapeutics, 43*, 7-12.

Karaim, R. (2002). *Housing First, Who Needs Housing? Persons with Mental Illness*. Retrieved 4/21/03 from *http://www.npr.org?new/specials/housingfirst/whoneeds/mentallyill.html.*

Lambert, D., & Agger, M. S. (1995). Access of rural AFDC Medicaid beneficiaries to mental health services. *Health Care Financing Review, 17*, 133-146.

Linhorst, D. M. (2002). Federalism and social justice: Implications for social work. *Social Work, 47*, 201-208.

Merwin, E., Hinton, I., Dembling, B., & Stern, S. (2003). Shortages of rural mental health professionals. *Archives of Psychiatric Nursing, 17*, 42-51.

Missouri Association of Sheltered Workshops. (2002). *Rural shops face unique challenges*. Retrieved April 21, 2003 from *http://www.moworkshops.org/latest folder/Rural Shops.html.*

National Alliance for the Mentally Ill. (2002). *Accountability in the federal mental health block grant*. Retrieved May 8, 2002, from *http://www.ocd.nami.org/update/unitedaccount.html.*

National Rural Health Association. (1999). *The scope of mental health services in rural America*. Retrieved on February 17, 2003, from *http://www.nrharural.org/dc/issuepapers/ipapers.*

Rathbone-McCuan, E. (2001). Mental health care provision for rural elders. *Journal of Applied Gerontology, 20,* 170-183.

Rural Mental Health Provider Group. (1997). *Mental health providers in rural and isolated areas. Center for Mental Health Services, Substance Abuse and Mental Health Administration*, Department of Health and Human Services. Retrieved on February 17, 2003 from *http://www.mentalhealth.org/publications/allpubs/SMA 98-3166.*

Stein, T. J. (2001). *Social policy and policy making by branches of the government and the public at large.* New York: Columbia University Press.

Surgeon General. (1999). *Mental health: A report of the Surgeon General.* (DHHS Publication No. HE 20.402: M). Washington, DC: U.S. Government Printing Office.

Wagenfeld, M., Murray, J., Mohatt, D., & DeBruyn, J. (1994). *Mental health and rural America: 1980-1983*. Washington, DC: Health Resources and Services Administration and National Institutes of Mental Health.

Weissert, C. S., & Goggins, M. L. (2002). Non incremental policy change: Lessons from Michigan's Medicaid managed care initiative. *Public Administration Review, 62*, 206-216.

Zarit, S. H., & Zarit, J. M. (1998). *Mental disorders in older adults: Fundamentals of assessment and treatment*. New York: Guilford Press.

Chapter 18

The Aging Network and the Future of Long-Term Care

The Honorable Josefina Carbonell
Larry Polivka, PhD

SUMMARY. Federal and state governments face a significant challenge in meeting the long-term care needs of an older population that will double in size between 2000 and 2020 and continue to increase through 2050. States have made significant improvements in their long-term care systems for the elderly. However, they are still spending a significant proportion of their long-term care funds on nursing homes. Any effort to improve long-term care for the elderly qualitatively, and not just on the margins, must be focused on developing a more flexible and balanced long-term care system that is responsive to consumer choice.

The Aging Services Network is poised to play a significant role in this transformation process. The strengths of the Network include the ability to develop and manage consumer-driven community-based programs; to assess the needs and resources of individual older persons and provide cost-effective community supports; to operate within fixed, capped budgets; and to identify and maintain roles for informal caregivers. Now is the time for national aging organizations, state units on aging, and area

[Haworth co-indexing entry note]: "The Aging Network and the Future of Long-Term Care." Carbonell, Josefina, and Larry Polivka. Co-published simultaneously in *Journal of Gerontological Social Work* (The Haworth Social Work Practice Press, an imprint of The Haworth Press, Inc.) Vol. 41, No. 3/4, 2003, pp. 313-321; and: *Gerontological Social Work in Small Towns and Rural Communities* (ed: Sandra S. Butler, and Lenard W. Kaye) The Haworth Social Work Practice Press, an imprint of The Haworth Press, Inc., 2003, pp. 313-321. Single or multiple copies of this article are available for a fee from The Haworth Document Delivery Service [1-800-HAWORTH, 9:00 a.m. - 5:00 p.m. (EST). E-mail address: docdelivery@haworthpress.com].

http://www.haworthpress.com/web/JGSW
© 2003 by The Haworth Press, Inc. All rights reserved.
Digital Object Identifier: 10.1300/J083v41n03_08

agencies on aging to use existing opportunities to move towards the establishment of a balanced system of long-term care. *[Article copies available for a fee from The Haworth Document Delivery Service: 1-800-HAWORTH. E-mail address: <docdelivery@haworthpress.com> Website: <http://www.HaworthPress.com> © 2003 by The Haworth Press, Inc. All rights reserved.]*

KEYWORDS. Aging network, long-term care, consumer choice

INTRODUCTION

We have heard a lot of talk about the aging of the baby boomers for the last 10 to 15 years. Much of this talk is about the challenge to federal and state governments and families to meet the long-term care needs of an older population that will double in size between 2000 and 2020 and continue to increase through 2050. Perspectives regarding the progress made thus far by states, local communities and the nation as a whole differ widely. This debate will continue as the aging baby boom increases the demand for long-term care services and specifically for home and community-based service options.

Most states have made significant improvements in their long-term care systems for the elderly. States have used a variety of approaches to increase the amount of home- and community-based service options that they provide to older adults and their family caregivers. One significant mechanism utilized by states is the Medicaid waiver that allows for the funding of home- and community-based services as alternatives to Medicaid-funded nursing home care. However, 75 percent of public funds for long-term care still goes to nursing homes. This proportion has decreased only slightly from the percentage that was spent 10 to 15 years ago.

The U.S. long-term care system for the elderly in both urban and rural communities is largely characterized by a loosely organized and fragmented process of gaining access to care and a bias favoring institutional care for publicly supported long-term care consumers. This bias makes it difficult for states to provide easy and timely access to home and community-based service options. Any effort to improve long-term care for the elderly qualitatively, and not just on the margins, must be focused on developing a more flexible and balanced long-term care system that is responsive to consumer choice.

Our goal should be to make our long-term care system more responsive to the needs and preferences of older people and their families by empowering older people and their families to make informed decisions about their life choices, and creating more flexible service options from which people can choose. Choices that will:

- Help people maintain and improve their health as they age,
- Help families care for their loved ones, and, most importantly,
- Help older people stay at home.

Three factors exist that together provide an impetus for a qualitative transformation of long-term care for the elderly.

(1) *An extensive community-based aging network.* This network includes 56 state units on aging, 655 area agencies on aging, thousands of non-profit, in-home and community-residential service providers and monitoring and advocacy groups like the nursing home ombudsmen. The aging network is over 30 years old and has the capacity in many communities to provide a full range of consumer-oriented home- and community-based long-term care services. A majority of the states have recognized this capacity by giving the aging network, at both the state and service delivery levels, responsibility for administering all or most of the aging-related home- and community-based Medicaid waiver funds.

The aging network in most parts of the country has more experience and expertise in non-medical care management than any other organization. According to one state unit on aging, "this experience has been focused particularly on creating and packaging a wide range of relatively low-cost home and community-based services to minimize frail older persons' use of high-cost institutional resources" (Managed Care Approaches to Long-Term and Integrated Care, New York Office for the Aging, 2002).

(2) *The cost-effectiveness of home- and community-based long-term care services (HCBS).* The cost-effectiveness of HCBS has been demonstrated through research conducted over the last ten years and by the success of a few states in qualitatively shifting the balance of their long-term care system from institutional to community-based care. These efforts have included the implementation of innovative programs such as consumer-directed care and Medicaid waiver-funded assisted living and foster home programs. This research is complemented by the fact that older people vastly prefer community-based alternatives to nursing homes.

In their study of Oregon, Washington and Colorado's successful efforts to contain long-term care costs by expanding home- and community-based services, Alecxih, Lutzky, and Corea (1996) conclude that these states:

> . . . appear to have made home- and community-based care a less expensive alternative to nursing facility care in the following ways:

- . . . targeted home and community-based care to a very impaired population.
- . . . screened all or most people applying for Medicaid-funded nursing facility care to determine if they can remain in the community. Oregon and Washington focus on hospital discharges because a high percentage of nursing home admissions come from hospitals.
- . . . kept per-person spending on home- and community-based care low by using government funds only after tapping all other resources.
- . . . actively developed alternatives to nursing facilities.
- . . . retained state control over the distribution and dispersion of funds, while local agencies have responsibility for the delivery of services. This permits the local agencies or state satellite offices to be more responsive and determine appropriate service providers and payment rates based on their relationships with local providers and their knowledge of each service area.
- . . . instituted comprehensive care management to both assist participants to find the most appropriate care and to monitor spending.
- . . . easily transferred funds from nursing facility to home- and community-based care because they have centralized all aging services at both the state and local level.

(3) *The increasing costs of operating nursing homes*. In Florida, for example, Medicaid nursing home costs grew by $500 million over the last two years and now exceed $2 billion. Much of this increase is due to major increases in staffing standards designed to improve the quality of care. The projected revenue shortfalls facing most states will force them to choose between funding home- and community-based services through expanded waivers or paying increasingly more for their nursing home programs.

IMPROVING ACCESS AND BALANCING LONG-TERM CARE RESOURCES

States may need to make changes in their organizational and administrative structures and the ways they control the use of resources before they can create a more balanced long-term care system that better serves the interests of the long-term care consumer. In many states, the management of long-term care programs is split between departments of aging/senior services (home- and community-based programs) and the departments housing the Medicaid program (nursing homes and some home care). Only a few states have consolidated control over all long-term care programs and funds into one agency. Accountability for long-term care program outcomes would be substantially enhanced by integrating authority and responsibility into a single organizational structure. Accountability for outcomes and administrative efficiency will become an increasingly urgent issue for policymakers at all levels as the need for long-term care services grows over the next several years. As trade-offs become necessary, both efficiency and consumer choice will be better served if decision-making is integrated within an organizational structure with authority over all long-term care resources.

An alternative method of balancing the distribution of long-term care resources is to develop a program at the local or regional level that manages multiple long-term care program funds and operates under a fixed rate. The fixed rate could be constructed through negotiation between representatives of the aging network, under the leadership of the state aging unit, and the state's Medicaid office, and incorporated into a contract. Wisconsin has taken this approach with the Wisconsin Family Care Program, and Arizona has operated this type of a system statewide for several years (Weissert, Lesnick, Musliner, & Foley, 1997).

The Wisconsin Family Care Program has two components–aging and disability resource centers and care management organizations. The resource centers serve as single points of entry into the long-term care system, providing information and counseling on all long-term care, preventive healthcare, and early intervention services. An important feature of the Resource Centers is their long-range goal to serve not only Medicaid-eligible consumers, but also private-pay consumers and their families. Providing information and assistance to the non-Medicaid population is an important element of any strategy to change long-term care systems. About 10% of the elderly are Medicaid-eligible and many of these people become Medicaid-eligible after they "spend-down" their own resources on health care and other costs associated with their chronic conditions, including nursing home care. A program that assists private-pay consumers holds great potential for empowering all older people to make informed decisions about their care choices. In addition to having access to help from the Resource Centers, those on private-pay plans will eventually be able to purchase Family Care home- and community-based services through payments based on a sliding scale fee.

In building aging network-based care systems, area agencies on aging and community-based providers are uniquely prepared to play roles which capitalize on both their understanding of older persons and their experience in delivering home- and community-based services. Their strengths include the ability to develop and manage community-based programs; to assess the needs of individual older persons, identify appropriate services and provide cost-effective community supports; to operate within fixed, capped budgets; and to identify and maintain roles for informal caregivers. Now is the time for national aging organizations, state units on aging, area agencies on aging, and community-based providers to use opportunities such as gradually expanded demonstration projects to move towards the establishment of balanced systems of long-term care.

IMPROVING LONG-TERM CARE IN RURAL COMMUNITIES

The need to balance the distribution of our scarce long-term care resources is especially evident in our rural communities. It is more difficult to provide home- and community-based care in rural environments because of transportation expenses, acute labor market shortages and other "economies of scale" limitations that drive up the costs of serving persons in their own homes or smaller congregate care settings. As a result, rural communities are often more dependent on nursing homes than urban areas.

Aging network-based efforts to coordinate the distribution of long-term care resources across large geographical areas could achieve the "economies of scale" required to provide more community-based services to rural residents. Programs could be redesigned to centralize a number of management functions, including client information systems, financial and personal management, public information services, and administration functions. These efficiency initiatives could generate more resources for services and promote a consumer-centered delivery of care. The additional resources could be used to fund the expansion of consumer-directed care, adult foster homes, and other small congregate providers, including small assisted living facilities (15 beds or fewer), which may be more cost-effective than conventional agency-provided in-home services (personal care, homemaker, respite) in rural environments.

OVERCOMING BARRIERS TO HOME- AND COMMUNITY-BASED CARE

A recent analysis by Wiener, Tilly, and Alecxih (2002) of long-term care systems in seven states identified several major questions that the federal and state governments need to answer as they attempt to balance the distribution of long-term care resources.

1. Can states achieve significant progress in the development of home- and community-based service options in the midst of a significant financial crisis?
2. Can states overcome administrative fragmentation to create a more integrated, uniform method (single entry point) of providing access to services?
3. Will states provide a broader and more flexible set of services in the future? How will states address the increasing frailty and medical complexity of their clients?
4. Will states be able to contain costs while expanding services?
5. Can quality of home- and community-based services be assured?

Government at every level is facing the challenge of providing creative and cost-effective long-term care options for older adults in order to meet existing and future needs. The current economic condition makes it even more important to provide these cost-effective options as alternatives to nursing home care. By doing so, states will also achieve a greater balance in the distribution of long-term care resources.

A potential method for expanding community-based long-term care is to create linkages with the community of faith-based organizations, many of which have long provided a wide range of assistance to the frail elderly. This history, along with the fact that the elderly are a growing percentage of many congregations, could serve as the foundation for a major expansion of long-term care services by faith-based organizations over the next several years. The aging network and faith-based organizations are both driven by a sense of mission defined by an ethic of care. This potential alliance, which has already emerged in some communities across the country, would be supported by efforts of the aging network to balance the use of long-term care resources.

Regardless of the method utilized, the needs, preferences, and capacities of consumers must ultimately determine how long-term care resources are used and to determine the most appropriate use of available services. This is especially true in our attempts to provide home- and community-based services to increasingly frail consumers with complex medical needs. Many states are testing out innovative models to coordinate this care in a consumer-oriented and efficient manner. Such programs include the Program for All-Inclusive Care of the Elderly (PACE), Social Health Maintenance Organizations (SHMO), and the Medicare/Medicaid Integration Projects. Virtually everyone involved in long-term care policy and practice supports the goal of a comprehensive and coordinated continuum of care delivered through a seamless system of acute, chronic and long-term care services. Such a system is some distance in the future, but the aging network can begin to put the building blocks in place now.

IMPLICATIONS FOR SOCIAL WORK

Achieving a balanced long-term care system will depend to a substantial extent on the increased availability of social workers trained to assist the frail elderly to access service options in a way that maintains the consumer's role as central to the process. Social work education should be designed to prepare long-term care case managers to empower consumers through collaborative need and strength assessments and care planning processes that prioritize the preferences of the consumer and maximize the consumer's capacity to direct where, when, and by whom services are provided.

We do not know precisely what percentage of long-term care consumers have the desire and capacity to exercise extensive control over the provision of services, including the power to hire and manage personal care workers. The point, however, is to prepare case managers to help consumers understand all of their options in a community-based system of care, including consumer-direction, and to provide them with the kind of support most consistent with their preferences and capacities. Case managers will still need to monitor the quality of care and to intervene when abuse or fraud occur. But, as advocates for consumer empowerment, they must be willing to accept the risk that comes with greater consumer choice and responsibility and the possibility that their notion of sufficient, high quality care may not be the same as the consumer's.

A key component of the critical role for social workers is to link directly with doctors and nurses in the delivery of care management. An interdisciplinary team approach has been found to be the most effective means to manage the multiple chronic conditions that may be present in an older adult. Care management delivered through such a team ensures that the social support needs–not just the healthcare needs–of the older adult are met. It is equally important for the interdisciplinary team to work closely with an older adult's informal support network in order to help them maintain the highest quality of life and level of independence possible.

CONCLUSION

Changing the direction of long-term care will be very difficult and will require, in most states, a major effort in every year remaining between now and 2020. The task, however, of creating a more consumer-oriented community-based long-term care system will not be as difficult, either politically or fiscally, as trying to maintain the current system for another 20 years. We should marshal the resources of the aging network to modernize long-term care and to take advantage of the opportunities created by the Supreme Court's *Olmstead* decision, the President's New Freedom Initiative, and the CMS Real Choice Systems Change grants program. It is time for the aging network to provide the kind of leadership that can create a coalition of all affected parties by articulating a clear vision for reform based on the needs and preferences of long-term care consumers.

REFERENCES

Alecxih, L., Lutzky, S., & Corea, J. (1996). *Estimated cost savings from the use of home- and community-based alternatives to nursing facility care in three states.* The Lewin Group, Washington, DC: AARP Public Policy Institute.

Wiener, J., Tilly, J., Alecxih, L., & Mario, B. (2002). Home and community-based services in seven states. *Health Care Financing Review, 23* (3).

Weissert, W., Lesnick, T., Musliner, M., & Foley, K. (1997). Cost savings from home and community-based services: Arizona's capitated Medicaid long-term care program. *Journal of Health Politics, Policy and Law, 22* (6), 1329-1357.

Wisconsin Family Care. (2002). Family care options for long-term care can be found at: *http://www.dhfs.state.wi.us/LTCare.*

Appendix

Sources for More Information on Social Work with Rural Older Adults

Elizabeth Johns, MS
Jane Harris-Bartley, MSW

BOOKS, REPORTS, AND WEB PUBLICATIONS

- Administration on Aging. (1996, December). *Home and community-based long-term care in American Indian and Alaska Native communities.* This report, produced by the AoA, Native Elder Health Care Resource Center, University of Colorado, and the National Resource Center on Native American Aging, University of North Dakota, is available online at www.aoa.gov/network/fhcbltc/report.html.
- Administration on Aging and National Institute on Aging. (n.d.) *Resource directory of older people.* Washington, DC: Authors. An interactive version of the directory is available on the website www.nia.hih.gov/health/resource/rd2001.htm. A PDF version is available at www.aoa.dhhs.gov/directory/default.htm.
- Butler, S. S. (2002). Family caregiver experiences with professional home care in a rural state. *Geriatric Care Management Journal, 12*(1), 11-16.

[Haworth co-indexing entry note]: "Appendix. Sources for More Information on Social Work with Rural Older Adults." Johns, Elizabeth, and Jane Harris-Bartley. Co-published simultaneously in *Journal of Gerontological Social Work* (The Haworth Social Work Practice Press, an imprint of The Haworth Press, Inc.) Vol. 41, No. 3/4, 2003, pp. 323-344; and: *Gerontological Social Work in Small Towns and Rural Communities* (ed: Sandra S. Butler, and Lenard W. Kaye) The Haworth Social Work Practice Press, an imprint of The Haworth Press, Inc., 2003, pp. 323-344. Single or multiple copies of this article are available for a fee from The Haworth Document Delivery Service [1-800-HAWORTH, 9:00 a.m. - 5:00 p.m. (EST). E-mail address: docdelivery@haworthpress.com].

http://www.haworthpress.com/web/JGSW
© 2003 by The Haworth Press, Inc. All rights reserved.
Digital Object Identifier: 10.1300/J083v41n03_09

- George, L., & Holden, C. (2001). *Federal programs and local organizations: Meeting the housing needs of rural seniors.* Washington, DC: Housing Assistance Council. Available in HMTL format from www.ruralhome.org/pubs.
- Ginsberg, L. H. (Ed). (1998). *Social work in rural communities* (3rd ed.). Alexandria, VA: Council on Social Work Education.
- Howard, D. M. (1994). *A Handbook on Rural Elderly Transportation Services: A Practical Guide to Operating and Evaluating a Rural Elderly Transportation System.* Kansas City, MO: National Resource Center for Rural Elderly.
- Indian Health Service, Administration on Aging, and National Indian Council on Aging. (2002). *American Indian and Alaska Native roundtable on long-term care: Final report.* The report of an April 2002 conference on American Indian and Alaska Native long-term care. The full text is available online from www.ihs.gov/PublicInfo/PublicAffairs/PressReleases/Press_Release_2002/ Final_LTC_Report_ALL.pdf.
- Kaye, L. W. (Ed.). (2002). Geriatric care management with the rural elderly [Special issue]. *Geriatric Care Management Journal, 12*(1).
- Kaye, L. W., & Sherman, K. (2002). Geriatric practice in rural America: The last frontier. *Social Work Today, 2*, 13-15.
- Kingsley, G. T., Spencer, V., & Simonson, J. (1995). *Assessment of American Indian housing needs and programs: Final report.* Washington, DC: Urban Institute.
- Miles, T. P. (Ed.). (1999). *Full color aging: Facts, goals, and recommendations for America's diverse elders.* Washington, DC: Gerontological Association of America.
- Rogers, C. C. (2000, February). *Changes in the older population and implications for rural areas.* Rural Development and Research Report no. 90. Washington, DC: Economic Research Service, U.S. Department of Agriculture. The full-text version is available from www.ers.usda.gov/publications/rdrr90.
- Turisco, F., & Metzger, J. (2002, December). *Rural health care delivery: Connecting communities through technology.* Oakland: California HealthCare Foundation. This publication is available in PDF format from the publisher's web site, www.chcf.org.

AUDIOVISUAL RESOURCES

Aquarius Health Care Videos
Olde Medfield Square

266 Main Street, Suite 33B
Medfield, MA 02052
888-440-2963
www.aquariusproductions.com

This company distributes videos on a wide range of topics related to aging, including Alzheimer's disease, caregiving, elder abuse, grandparents raising grandchildren, and more.

Films for the Humanities and Sciences
P.O. Box 2053
Princeton, NJ 08543-2053
800-257-5126
www.films.com

This agency offers educational media on a wide range of topics, including many related to aging.

Terra Nova Films
9848 W. Winchester Ave.
Chicago, IL 60643
800-779-8491
www.terranova.org

Terra Nova distributes videos for rental or purchase on many topics related to aging.

AGENCIES AND ORGANIZATIONS

Agencies of the U.S. Government

U.S. Department of Agriculture

Rural Development
Mail Stop 0107
1400 Independence Avenue SW, Room 206-W
Washington, DC 20250-0107
202-720-4581
www.rurdev.usda.gov

This USDA project promotes rural development through various initiatives. One is the Rural Housing Service, which offers home-ownership opportunities to rural Americans, as well as programs for home renovation and repair.

Rural Information Center
National Agricultural Library
10301 Baltimore Ave., Room 304
Beltsville, MD 20705
www.nal.usda.gov/ric/ruralres/aboutric.htm

The Rural Information Center (RIC) provides information and referral services to government officials at all levels, community organizations, rural citizens, and others working to maintain the vitality of America's rural areas.

U.S. Department of Health and Human Services

Administration on Aging
330 Independence Avenue, S.W.
Washington, DC 20201
202-619-0724
www.aoa.gov

The Administration on Aging (AoA) comprises a number of programs relevant to practitioners working with older adults in rural communities. Among these are:

American Indian, Alaskan Native, and Native Hawaiian Program
www.aoa.gov/factsheets/natams.html

Under Title VI of the Old Americans Act, this program advocates for older Native Americans, coordinates activities with other federal departments and agencies, administers grants, and collects and disseminates information related to older Native Americans.

Center for Communication and Consumer Services
www.aoa.gov/naic/about.html

The Center offers extensive public information on research, publications, programs, policies, and services related to aging. A section within the Center's web site (www.aoa.dhhs.gov/naic/Notes/ruralaging.html) offers an extensive list of resources related to rural aging, with links to the corresponding agencies, programs, and publications.

Indian Health Service
Reyes Building
801 Thompson Avenue, Suite 400
Rockville, MD 20852
301-443-3593
www.ihs.gov

The IHS, part of the U.S. Department of Health and Human Services, operates a comprehensive health service program for American Indians and Alaska Natives. Services include hospital and community-based medical care, rehabilitation, and disease prevention. The IHS provides health services to approximately 1.5 million American Indians and Alaska Natives who belong to more than 557 federally recognized tribes in 35 states.

National Advisory Committee on Rural Health and Human Services
http://ruralcommittee.hrsa.gov

This advisory committee provides recommendations to the Secretary of the Department of Health and Human Services on ways to address issues of rural health. Members of the 16-person committee come from the public and private sectors, and bring expertise in medicine, nursing, law, administration, research, and public health. Chartered in 1987, the committee meets three times yearly. Copies of its reports are available on the web site.

National Institute on Aging (NIA)
National Institutes of Health
9000 Rockville Pike
Bethesda, MD 20892
www.nia.nih.gov

One of the agencies within the National Institutes of Health, the NIA conducts and supports research, provides training, and disseminates information on health issues of particular relevance to older people. NIA offers free information on specific health issues for health professionals as well as the general public.

Office of Minority Health
OMH Resource Center
P.O. Box 37337
Washington, DC 20013-7337
www.omhrc.org

The Office of Minority Health Resource Center serves as an information and referral service on minority health issues for professionals, community groups, consumers, and students.

Office of Rural Health Policy
5600 Fishers Lane, 9A-55
Rockville, MD 20857
301-443-0835
www.ruralhealth.hrsa.gov

Located in the Health Resources and Services Administration of the Department of Health and Human Services, the Office of Rural Health Policy maintains a national clearinghouse of information on rural health policy issues, works with minority rural populations, promotes research, and funds innovative programs. It also provides funding to 50 state offices of rural health, listed at ruralhealth.hrsa.gov/funding/50sorh.htm. This site also lists state rural health associations and rural health research centers nationwide.

U.S. Department of Housing and Urban Development (HUD)
www.hud.gov

HUD sponsors a wide range of housing programs of potential interest to older residents of rural areas and the agencies that serve them. Its informative web site includes a section specifically for older adults: www.hud.gov/groups/seniors/cfm.

Office of Native American Programs (ONAP)
www.hud.gov/offices/pih/ih/onap/index.cfm

The mission of ONAP, which is located within HUD's Office of Public and Indian Housing, is to make decent, affordable housing available to Native American families, develop economic opportunities, and promote community development.

Other Organizations and Agencies

Association of Programs for Rural Independent Living (APRIL)
5903 Powerdermill Road
Kent, OH 44240
330-678-7648
www.april-rural.org

APRIL is a national network of rural centers for independent living. Members include other organizations and individuals working to promote rights and benefits for individuals with disabilities living in rural environments.

Center on Ethnic and Minority Aging
5398 Wynnefield Ave.
Philadelphia, PA 19131
215-477-5719
www.cemainfo.net

The center focuses on research, consultation, training, development of practice models, and creation of alternative service delivery-approaches to benefit ethnic and minority individuals, families, and communities. A membership organization, CEMA, also publishes a newsletter and sponsors conferences and other events.

Center on Minority Aging
University of North Carolina
Campus Box 3465
730 Airport Road, Suite 204
Chapel Hill, NC 27599-3465
919-966-6818
www.unc.edu/depts/cmaweb

This is one of six Resource Centers for Minority Aging (RCMARs) funded by the National Institute on Aging (NIA), the National Institute of Nursing Research, and the Office of Research on Minority Health. The goal of the RCMARs is to reduce differences in health outcomes between minority and non-minority elders by focusing research on health promotion and prevention of disease and disability.

Community Action Agencies (CAAs)

These are nonprofit private and public organizations established under the Economic Opportunity Act of 1964 to fight the war on poverty. There are approximately 1,000 Community Action Agencies in the United States, more than half of them in rural areas. With a primary focus on the needs of people living in poverty, CAAs are involved in a broad range of service areas, including family supports, health care, housing, job training, and the like. More information is available through the website of the Community Action Network: www.communityactionpartnership.com.

Community Transportation Association of America (CTAA)
1341 G Street, N.W., 10th floor
Washington, DC 20005
202-628-1480
www.ctaa.org

CTAA is a national professional membership association of organizations and individuals committed to eliminating isolation and improving mobility for all people. CTAA conducts research, provides technical assistance, offers educational programs, and advocates to make coordinated community transportation available, affordable, and accessible. Among the CTAA's areas of interest is rural and senior transportation.

Housing Assistance Council (HAC)
1025 Vermont Avenue, N.W., Suite 606
Washington, DC 20005
www.ruralhome.org

This nonprofit corporation assists local organizations to build and manage affordable housing in rural America. The HAC provides loans, technical assistance, and training, sponsors research and demonstration projects, and maintains an extensive publication program.

National Adult Day Services Association (NADSA)
8201 Greensboro Drive, Suite 300
McLean, VA 22102
866-890-7357
www.nadsa.org

According to its website, the mission of NADSA "is to enhance the success of its members through advocacy, education, technical assistance, research, and communication services." This site offers education and training materials, videotapes, publications, and brochures.

National Alliance for Hispanic Health (NAHH)
1501 16th Street, N.W.
Washington, DC 20036
www.hispanichealth.org

This member organization of some 1300 health and human service providers conducts policy research and develops and distributes bilingual resources. NAHH operates HispanicHealth.org, a website devoted to health-related information, and publishes a newsletter, the *Hispanic Health Reporter,* available online.

National AHEC (Area Health Education Centers) Organization
500 Commonwealth Drive
Warrendale, PA 15086
888-412-7424
www.nationalahec.org

The mission of AHECs, and of their national organization, is to expand access to health care in underserved areas, including rural ones.

National Asian-Pacific Center on Aging
1511 Third Ave., Suite 914
Seattle, WA 98010
206-624-1221
www.napca.org

This advocacy organization for Asian Pacific Americans describes itself as working with "elders, policy makers, program administrators, and community leaders to prepare not only for an aging American society, but also for the increasing diversity of senior populations."

National Association for Hispanic Elderly/Asociación Nacional Pro Personas Mayores
234 E. Colorado Blvd., Suite 300
Pasadena, CA 91101
626-564-1988

The programs of this private, nonprofit organization include a national research center, assistance to organizations seeking to reach Spanish-speaking elders, and dissemination of informational materials in English and Spanish. The Association also administers Project Ayuda, which provides employment counseling and placement services.

National Association of Professional Geriatric Care Managers (GCM)
1604 N. Country Club Road
Tucson, AZ 85716-3102
520-881-8008
www.caremanager.org

The organization's web site offers information about professional care managers and their services as well as tips on finding a qualified geriatric care manager. Its web site describes GCM as "a non-profit, professional organization of practitioners whose goal is the advancement of dignified care for the elderly and their families."

National Association for Rural Mental Health (NARMH)
3700 W. Division Street, Suite 105
St. Cloud, MN 56301
320-202-1820
www.narmh.org

NARMH is a national membership organization of organizations and individuals focused on strengthening rural mental health and substance abuse services and supporting mental health service providers in rural areas. The organization sponsors a website and listserv, an annual conference, and a publications program.

National Association of Social Workers
750 First Street, N.E., Suite 700
Washington, DC 20002-4241
202-336-8258
www.socialworkers.org

National Association of Spanish Speaking Elderly
2025 I Street, N.W., Suite 219
Washington, DC 20006

National Caucus and Center on Black Aged
1220 L Street, N.W., Suite 800
Washington, DC 20005
202-637-8400
www.ncba-aged.org

This organization is dedicated to improving life for African American and other low-income minority elderly persons, with a particular focus on employment and housing.

National Center on Elder Abuse (NCEA)
1225 I Street, N.W., Suite 725
Washington, DC 20005
202-898-2586
www.elderabusecenter.org

The NCEA's helpful website offers extensive resources on elder abuse, including basic fact sheets and other publications, data on elder abuse, guidance on reporting abuse, information about abuse in nursing homes and other institutions, and among particular populations.

National Council on the Aging, Inc. (NCOA)
409 3rd Street, N.W., Suite 200
Washington, DC 20024
202-479-1200
www.ncoa.org

NCOA is a private, nonprofit organization providing information, training, and advocacy in all aspects of aging services and issues. It publishes material on a range of issues related to aging, including senior housing and rural issues. Two of its "constituent units" of particular interest to persons in rural areas are the National Coalition on Rural Aging (NCRA) and the National Institute of Senior Centers. Information about these and others is provided on the NCOA web site.

National Hispanic Council on Aging
2713 Ontario Road, N.W.
Washington, DC 20009
202-265-1288
www.nhcoa.org

According to the organization's web site, the National Hispanic Council on Aging is "dedicated to improving the quality of life for Latino elderly, families, and communities through advocacy, capacity and institution building, development of educational materials, technical assistance, demonstration projects, policy analysis, and research." The website reproduces the newsletter *Noticias,* and offers information about a variety of other topics of interest to Hispanic elders and their families.

National Indian Council on Aging (NICOA)
10501 Montgomery Blvd., N.E., Suite 210
Albuquerque, NM 87111-3846
505-292-2001
www.nicoa.org

The organization's website describes NICOA as "the nation's foremost nonprofit advocate for the nation's (est.) 296,000 American Indian and Alaska Native elders." It continues, "NICOA strives to better the lives of the nation's indigenous seniors through advocacy, employment training, dissemination of information, and data support." NICOA publishes the newsletter *Elder Visions* as well as reports related to aging in "Indian Country."

National Organization of State Offices of Rural Health (NOSORH)
c/o Nebraska Office of Rural Health
301 Centennial Mall
P.O. Box 95044
Lincoln, NE 68509-5044
402-471-2337
www.nrharural.org/nosorh/offices.html

This national organization works to promote a healthy rural America through state and community leadership. The mission of the national organization is to "foster and promote legislation, information exchange, education, and liaison activities with all State Offices of Rural Health, the Federal Office of Rural Health Policy, the National Rural Health Association, and other organizations. In addition the site includes links to state offices of rural health.

National Resource and Policy Center on Rural Long Term Care
University of Kansas Medical Center on Aging
3901 Rainbow Blvd.
Kansas City, KS 66160
www.kumc.edu/instruction/medicine/NRPC

The university-based program works to improve access to in-home and community-based long-term-care services for elderly and disabled persons living in rural areas of the United States.

National Resource Center on Native American Aging
Center for Rural Health, University of North Dakota
P.O. Box 9037
Grand Forks, ND 58202-9037
800-896-7628 or 701-777-3437
www.und.nodak.edu/dept/nrcnaa

According to its web site, the National Resource Center on Native American Aging "is committed to increasing awareness of issues affecting American Indian, Alaskan Native, and Native Hawaiian elders and to be a voice and advocate for their concerns. Through education, training, technical assistance, and research, the center assists in developing community-based solutions to improve the quality of life and deliver of related services to this aging population." Established at the University of North Dakota in 1994, the resource center is a collaboration between the university's Office of Native American Programs and its Center for Rural Health. The Center publishes a newsletter, *Native Aging Visions.*

National Resource Center for Rural Elderly
Center on Aging Studies
University of Missouri-Kansas City
5215 Rockhill Road
Kansas City, MO 64110
816-235-1747
http://iml.umkc.edu/cas/nrc.htm

The Center focuses on three primary areas of interest to rural practitioners working with older adults: mental health and health-care coordination services; housing programs and assistance mechanisms; and access and transportation services. The Center staff represents a mix of field practitioners with practical experience in service provision, as well as experts in the field of academic gerontology. The Center has produced a series of publications of interest to practitioners and publishes a newsletter called *The Rural Networker*.

National Rural Health Association (NRHA)
1 West Armour Blvd., Suite 203
Kansas City, MO 64111
816-756-3140
www.nrharural.org

NRHA is a nonprofit, professional organization targeting health care problems unique to rural areas and serving as a liaison between rural health care providers and older people. It offers information on health-care delivery to rural providers and publishes the quarterly *Journal of Rural Health*. The organization sponsors national rural health conferences and an annual rural health policy institute, and has a particular emphasis on the health status of rural minority populations.

The National Senior Service Corps Program (Senior Corps)
Corporation for National and Community Service
1201 New York Avenue, N.W.
Washington, DC 20525
www.seniorcorps.org

Senior Corps administers three national programs that provide opportunities for older adults through which they can volunteer their experience and skills in local communities: the Foster Grandparent Program, the Retired and Senior Volunteer Program (RSVP), and the Senior Companion Program.

Native Elder Health Resource Center
University of Colorado Health Sciences Center
P.O. Box 6508, Mail Stop F800
Aurora, CO 80045-0508
303-724-1414
www.uchsc.edu/ai/nehcrc

According to its web site, this national resource center for older American Indians, Alaska Natives, and Native Hawaiians places "special emphasis on culturally competent health care." Its priorities include "ascertaining health status and conditions, improving practice standards, increasing access to care, and mobilizing community resources." The organization's web site lists bibliographic material and offers links to exemplary programs and other Native American sites.

Resource Center for Minority Aging Research (RCMAR)
www.rcmar.ucla.edu

The National Institute on Aging established the Resource Centers for Minority Aging Research (RCMAR) initiative in 1997, as part of an effort to reduce health disparities between minority and other older adults. The central coordinating center at UCLA provides logistical support to the six RCMAR centers around the United States. Two with a rural focus are:

The Center on Minority Aging, University of North Carolina, Chapel Hill (CMA)
Campus Box 3465
730 Airport Road, Suite 204
Chapel Hill, NC 27599-3465
919-966-6818
www.unc.edu/depts/cmaweb

The Center on Minority Aging describes its mission as reducing "racial disparities in health by focusing on research in disease prevention, health promotion, and disability prevention for minority elders." The CMA is affiliated with the University of North Carolina's Institute on Aging.

Native Elder Research Center
University of Colorado Health Sciences Center
American Indian and Alaska Native Programs
Nighthorse Campbell Native Health Building
Mail Stop F800
P.O. Box 6508
Aurora, CO 80045-0508
www.uchsc.edu/ai/nerc

The Native Elder Research Center sponsors research, training, continuing education, technical assistance, and information dissemination focused on improving the health and well-being of older American Indians and emphasizing the unique cultural characteristics of Native American populations.

Rural Assistance Center
University of North Dakota
P.O. Box 9037
Grand Forks, ND 58202
800-270-1898
www.raconline.org

Funded by the federal Office of Rural Health Policy, in the U.S. Department of Health and Human Services, the RAC is intended to be a single point of entry to more than two hundred HHS programs serving rural areas. The Center sponsors a listserv and publishes a newsletter, *The Rural Monitor,* available through its web site.

Rural Victimization Project
Institute for Family Violence Studies
Florida State University School of Social Work
C-2500 University Center
Tallahassee, FL 32306-2750
850-644-6303
http://familyvio.ssw.fsu.edu/rural

The Institute conducts workshops and publishes domestic violence training manuals and online tutorials, including "Domestic Abuse in Later Life: A Competency-Based Training Manual for Meals on Wheels Volunteers and Other Elder Services Staff" and "Escaping the Shadows: Identifying and Assisting Victims of Elder Domestic Abuse" (a video). The Institute web site contains many useful references to resources on family violence and elder abuse.

SELECTED WEB SITES

AARP
www.aarp.org

At the time this volume was going to press, AARP was planning to add a new online service, Internet Resources on Aging, to its informative and user-friendly web site.

American Psychological Association (APA)
www.apa.org/pi/aging/publications.html

The APA Office on Aging has developed a section of the association's web site listing publications on psychological aspects of aging (brochures, reports, articles, journals, and books).

Code Talk
www.codetalk.fed.us/About.html

This web site, maintained by the Office of Native American Programs of the U.S. Department of Housing and Urban Development, collects and disseminates information from various government agencies and other organizations of importance for Native American communities.

DiversityRx
www.diversityrx.org

Designed for policy makers, health professionals, and advocates challenged with delivering health services to diverse populations, this web site describes itself as "a clearinghouse of information on how to meet the language and cultural needs of minorities, immigrants, refugees, and other diverse populations seeking health care."

FirstGov for Seniors
www.seniors.gov

Maintained by the Social Security Administration, FirstGov for Seniors is designed to be a "virtual agency," a central source of information accessible via the Internet and meant to help users navigate the complex layers of governmental offices and programs offering information and services to older adults. FirstGov for Seniors features direct Internet links to various federal agencies (e.g., National Institutes of Health, Federal Drug Administration, Centers for Disease Control); state government websites and state offices on aging; and nongovernmental information sites, online publications. It also offers information about issues related to health, retirement, and many other topics.

Rural Social Work Caucus
www.uncp.edu/sw/rural

This website features a moderated online discussion group; information on the annual National Institute on Social Work and Human Services in Rural Areas; and extensive links to other sites, including resources on rural transportation and grant opportunities.

SeniorNet
www.seniornet.org

SeniorNet is a nonprofit organization whose goal is to enhance proficiency in the use of computers and communications technology among older adults. In addition to local centers that offer educational programs, SeniorNet maintains a website with learning opportunities as well as discussion "roundtables" on a wide range of topics.

U.S. Administration on Aging

Aging Internet Information Notes: Rural Aging
www.aoa.dhhs.gov/naic/Notes/ruralaging.html

A useful compendium of links to publications, data, research reports, organizations and agencies, and other resources related to rural aging.

Currently and Recently Supported Resources for Policy-Makers, Planners, Agencies, and Practitioners in the Field of Aging
www.aoa.gov/aoa.pages/resrcen.html

A listing of projects involved in a wide range of issues pertaining to aging, including long-term care, legal assistance, and minority aging organizations, with contact information.

Programs and Resources for Native American Elders
www.aoa.gov/AIN/default.htm

A collection of links to aging-related web sites of interest to Native Americans, with an emphasis on federal programs and grants.

Widownet
www.fortnet.org/WidowNet/index.html

Widownet is an information and self-help resource for, and by, widows and widowers. Topics include grief, bereavement, recovery, and other information helpful to those who have suffered the loss of a spouse or life partner.

STATISTICAL RESOURCES

Federal Interagency Forum on Aging-Related Statistics
6525 Belcrest Road, Room 790
Hyattsville, MD 20782
301-458-4460
www.agingstats.gov

This agency assembles statistical information related to aging from ten different federal agencies.

National Center for Health Statistics/Aging Activities
Centers for Disease Control and Prevention
www.cdc.gov/nchs/about/otheract/aging/about_aging.htm

The Aging Activities office of NCHS carries out research and analysis and publishes information on the health of older Americans. Many other useful health-related statistics are also available from the NCHS web site.

U.S. Administration on Aging
www.aoa.gov/aoa/stats/statpage.html

The Administration on Aging maintains links to a variety of statistical information related to the U.S. older adult population.

SELECTED EDUCATIONAL RESOURCES

Stanford Geriatric Education Center
Stanford University School of Medicine
3801 Miranda Avenue
Palo Alto, CA 94304
650-494-3986
www.stanford.edu/dept/medfm/gec/page1.html

The Stanford Geriatric Education Center sponsors a variety of ethnogeriatric programs and curriculum resource materials to assist health-care professionals in understanding cultural issues associated with aging.

Department of Rural Sociology
Texas A&M University
2125 TAMU
College Station, Texas 77843-2125
http://ruralsoc.tamu.edu

The department emphasizes applied research and extension programs for rural people and communities, including the sociology of rural communities and rural minorities. The Hispanic Research Program is directed by Cruz Torres.

Kansas Rural Interdisciplinary Training Program (KS-RIT)
Center on Aging
University of Kansas Medical Center
Kansas City, KS 66160
http://coa.kumc.edu/rit

This project of the University of Kansas Medical Center is designed to enhance the skills of students and practitioners in the field of rural health care. The center's web site contains links to an extensive index of rural service models, including adult day care, community service development, housing, mental health, and senior employment. There are additional links to a Center on Aging lecture series and health screenings. A "rural links" page refers visitors to links to other rural health related sites around the United States.

Center on Aging
University of Maine
5723 D.P. Corbett Bldg.
Orono, ME 04469-5723
207-581-3444
www.mainecenteronaging.org

The UMaine Center on Aging is a co-sponsor of the annual Bar Harbor Rural Geriatric Conference, offers continuing professional education in rural communities, and publishes an online newsletter.

Center for Excellence in Disability Education, Research, and Services
University of Montana Rural Institute
52 Corbin Hall
Missoula, MT 59812-7056
866-424-3822
http://rtc.ruralinstitute.umt.edu

The Rural Institute houses the Research and Training Center on Disability in Rural Communities, which is concerned with issues related to employment and self-employment, independent living, telecommunications, community inclusion, and many others. Another of the Institute's projects is the American Indian Disability Technical Assistance Center. The Institute web site contains a number of links to other disability-related resources.

"Seniors Can" Curriculum
University of Nevada Cooperative Extension
2345 Red Rock Street
Las Vegas, Nevada 89146
702-257-5531

This intensive educational program is designed to assist older adults to live independently at home through the creation and strengthening of social-support networks.

Andrus Gerontology Center
Leonard Davis School of Gerontology
University of Southern California
Los Angeles, CA 90089-0191
213-740-5156
www.ageworks.com

The USC's School of Gerontology offers an online master's program in gerontology and long-term-care administration, a certificate program in gerontology, and online continuing-education modules and "electronic textbooks" for use at other educational institutions.

Maine Rural Health Research Center (MRHC)
Edmund S. Muskie School of Public Service
University of Southern Maine
P.O. Box 9300

Portland, Maine 04104-9300
207-780-4430
http://muskie.usm.maine.edu/centers/centers_mrhrc.jsp

According to its web site, the Maine Rural Health Research Center has as its mission "to inform health care policymaking and the delivery of rural health services through high quality, policy relevant research, policy analysis and technical assistance on rural health issues of regional and national significance." The Center maintains the Database for Rural Health Research in Progress. Also available on the Center's web site is a series of papers titled "Best Practices in Rural Medicaid Managed Behavioral Health."

U.S. Department of Health and Human Services
Substance Abuse and Mental Health Services Administration
Center for Substance Abuse Prevention (CSAP)
http://pathwayscourses.samhsa.gov/samhsa_pathays/courses/courses.htm

The CSAP website offers several online courses of potential interest to professionals who work with older adults. Topics include substance abuse among older adults and program evaluation.

Index

© 2003 by The Haworth Press, Inc. All rights reserved.

BOOK ORDER FORM!

Order a copy of this book with this form or online at:
http://www.haworthpress.com/store/product.asp?sku=5105

Gerontological Social Work in Small Towns and Rural Communities

___ in softbound at $39.95 (ISBN: 0-7890-1693-1)
___ in hardbound at $59.95 (ISBN: 0-7890-1692-3)

COST OF BOOKS ______

POSTAGE & HANDLING ______
US: $4.00 for first book & $1.50 for each additional book
Outside US: $5.00 for first book & $2.00 for each additional book.

SUBTOTAL ______

In Canada: add 7% GST. ______

STATE TAX ______
CA, IL, IN, MN, NY, OH & SD residents please add appropriate local sales tax.

FINAL TOTAL ______
If paying in Canadian funds, convert using the current exchange rate, UNESCO coupons welcome.

❑ **BILL ME LATER:**
Bill-me option is good on US/Canada/Mexico orders only; not good to jobbers, wholesalers, or subscription agencies.

❑ **Signature** ______

❑ **Payment Enclosed: $** ______

❑ **PLEASE CHARGE TO MY CREDIT CARD:**

❑ Visa ❑ MasterCard ❑ AmEx ❑ Discover
❑ Diner's Club ❑ Eurocard ❑ JCB

Account # ______

Exp Date ______

Signature ______

(Prices in US dollars and subject to change without notice.)

PLEASE PRINT ALL INFORMATION OR ATTACH YOUR BUSINESS CARD

Name

Address

City State/Province Zip/Postal Code

Country

Tel Fax

E-Mail

May we use your e-mail address for confirmations and other types of information? ❑ Yes ❑ No We appreciate receiving your e-mail address. Haworth would like to e-mail special discount offers to you, as a preferred customer. **We will never share, rent, or exchange your e-mail address.** We regard such actions as an invasion of your privacy.

Order From Your **Local Bookstore** or Directly From
The Haworth Press, Inc. 10 Alice Street, Binghamton, New York 13904-1580 • USA
Call Our toll-free number (1-800-429-6784) / Outside US/Canada: (607) 722-5857
Fax: 1-800-895-0582 / Outside US/Canada: (607) 771-0012
E-mail your order to us: orders@haworthpress.com

For orders outside US and Canada, you may wish to order through your local sales representative, distributor, or bookseller.
For information, see http://haworthpress.com/distributors

(Discounts are available for individual orders in US and Canada only, not booksellers/distributors.)

Please photocopy this form for your personal use.
www.HaworthPress.com

BOF04